SPRINGHOUSE

MEDICATION
TEACHING AIDS

SECOND EDITION

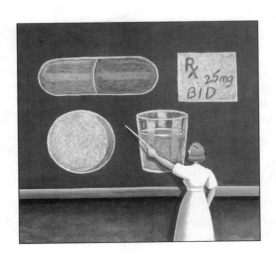

Springhouse Corporation
Springhouse, Pennsylvania

Staff

Senior Vice President, Editorial
Patricia Dwyer Schull, RN, MSN

Publisher
Donna O. Carpenter, ELS

Art Director
John Hubbard

Managing Editor
Andrew T. McPhee, RN, BSN

Clinical Manager
Ann M. Barrow, RN, MSN, CCRN

Drug Information Editor
Lisa Truong, RPh, PharmD

Senior Editor
Naina Chohan

Editor
Mary Lou Ambrose

Clinical Editors
Ann Marie Angelucci, RN, MSN, CCRN; Shirley H. Brownell, RNC, BSN; Lynn Ferchau, RN, MSN, CCRN; Eileen Gallen, RN, BSN; Margaret M. Klein, RN, BSN; Elizabeth D. McNeeley, RN, BSN; Lori Musolf Neri, RN, MSN, CCRN

Associate Acquisitions Editor
Louise E. Quinn

Copy Editors
Cynthia Breuninger (manager), Karen C. Comerford, Brenna H. Mayer, Beth E. Pitcher, Pamela Wingrod

Designers
Arlene Putterman (associate art director), Elaine Kasmer Ezrow, Joseph John Clark, Jackie Facciolo, Don Knauss, Donna S. Morris

Cover Illustration
Terry Widener

Typographers
Diane Paluba (manager), Joyce Rossi Biletz

Manufacturing
Deborah Meiris (director), Patricia K. Dorshaw (manager), Otto Mezei (book production manager)

Editorial Assistants
Carrie R. Cameron, Carol A. Caputo

Indexer
Deborah K. Tourtlotte

The clinical procedures described and recommended in this publication are based on research and consultation with nursing, medical, and legal authorities. To the best of our knowledge, these procedures reflect currently accepted practice; nevertheless, they can't be considered absolute and universal recommendations. For individual application, all recommendations must be considered in light of the patient's clinical condition and, before the administration of new or infrequently used drugs, in light of the latest package-insert information. The authors and publisher disclaim responsibility for adverse effects resulting directly or indirectly from the suggested procedures, from undetected errors, or from a reader's misunderstanding of the text.

℞ A member of the Reed Elsevier plc group

Visit our Web site at http://www.springnet.com

Library of Congress Cataloging-in-Publication Data
Medication teaching aids—2nd ed.
          p. cm.
Includes bibliographical references and index.
1. Drugs—Administration—Handbooks, manuals, etc. 2. Patient education—Handbooks, manuals, etc. I. Springhouse Corporation. [DNLM: 1. Drug Therapy handbooks. 2. Pharmaceutical Preparations—administration & dosage handbooks. 3. Patient Education handbooks. WB 39 M4882 1998]
RM147.M44 1998
615.5'8'071—dc21
DNLM/DLC
for Library of Congress   98-19030
ISBN 0-87434-942-7 (pbk.: alk. paper)   CIP

Contents

Clinical Consultants

Deborah Becker, RN, MSN, CCRN
Lecturer
University of Pennsylvania
School of Nursing
Philadelphia

Rebecca E. Boehne, RN, MSN, PhD
Patient and Family Education
  Coordinator
Portland VA Medical Center
Portland, Ore.

Karna Bramble, BSN, MS, PhD, NP, GNP
Nurse Practitioner Professional
  Leader
Long Beach (Calif.) Veteran Affairs
  Medical Center

Karen T. Bruchak, RN, MSN, MBA
Assistant Administrator, Cancer
  Clinical Programs
University of Pennsylvania Cancer
  Center
Philadelphia

Kathleen C. Byington, RN, MSN, CS
Pediatric Clinical Nurse Specialist,
  Case Manager, Nurse Practitioner
Vanderbilt Children's Hospital
Nashville, Tenn.

James Camamo, PharmD
Clinical Pharmacist for Medication
  Information and Policy
  Development
University Medical Center
Tucson, Ariz.

Lawrence Carey, PharmD
Clinical Pharmacist Coordinator
Jefferson Health System Home
  Infusion Program
Philadelphia

Barbara Ann Costa, RN, MS
Professor Emeritus (retired)
Syracuse University
College of Nursing
Syracuse, N.Y.

Teresa S. Dunsworth, PharmD, BCPS
Associate Professor of Clinical
  Pharmacy
West Virginia University School of
  Pharmacy
Morgantown

Patricia L. Eltz, RN, MSN, CEN
Community Health Educator
Pottstown (Pa.) Memorial Medical
  Center

Belle Erickson, RN,C, MS, PhD
Assistant Professor
Villanova (Pa.) University
College of Nursing

Carmel A. Esposito, RN, MSN, EdD
Coordinator Continuing Education
Nurse Educator
Trinity Health System
School of Nursing
Steubenville, Ohio

Janet Farahmand, CRN, EdD
Associate Professor of Nursing
Neumann College
Division of Nursing
Aston, Pa.

Mary Jo Gerlach, RN, MNEd
Assistant Professor Adult Nursing
Medical College of Georgia
School of Nursing
Athens

Ronald L. Greenberg, PharmD, BCPS
Clinical Pharmacy Coordinator
Fairview Ridges Hospital
Burnsville, Minn.

Margaret K. Hampshire, RN, BSN, OCN
Managing Editor, OncoLink
University of Pennsylvania
Philadelphia

James A. Koestner, PharmD
Clinical Pharmacist—
  Trauma/Surgical Intensive Care
Vanderbilt University Medical Center
Nashville, Tenn.

Nancy L. Gindele Kranzley, RN, MS
Pulmonary Clinical Nurse Specialist
The Christ Hospital
Cincinnati

Catherine Todd Magel, RN,C, EdD
Assistant Professor
Villanova (Pa.) University
College of Nursing

Marie Maloney, PharmD
Clinical Pharmacist
University Medical Center
Tucson, Ariz.

George Melko, RPh, PharmD
Clinical Pharmacist
Jefferson Health System Home
  Infusion Program
Philadelphia

William O'Hara, RPh, PharmD
Clinical Pharmacy Specialist
Thomas Jefferson Hospital
Philadelphia

Theresa Prosser, PharmD, BCPS
Associate Professor
St. Louis College of Pharmacy

Marcia Silkroski, RD, CNSD
President
Nutrition Advantage
West Chester, Pa.

Joseph F. Steiner, RPh, PharmD
Professor and Director of Pharmacy
  Practice
University of Wyoming
School of Pharmacy
Laramie

Margot T. Stock, CNRN, MSN, M.Phil, D.Phil, FNP
Assistant Professor
East Carolina University
School of Nursing
Greenville, N.C.

Foreword

According to a recent study of patients in U.S. hospitals, an average of 106,000 people die each year from adverse drug reactions, and an estimated 2.2 million more are severely injured, ranking adverse drug reactions just behind heart disease, cancer, and stroke as the nation's leading cause of death.

These startling statistics help drive home an important point: The more patients know about the medications they take, the lower their risk of injury or death as a result of adverse drug reactions. For today's nurse, few responsibilities bear as much importance as teaching patients about their drug therapy.

Not all adverse reactions are due to inadequate or incomplete patient teaching, of course. Some patients abuse drugs; others don't comply with their prescribed treatment. But many others land in the hospital because they don't understand how to take their drugs correctly or they fail to recognize the signs and symptoms of a severe drug reaction. Numerous studies indicate that patients who have been informed about their drug therapy comply better with their treatment programs, recover faster, visit the doctor less often, and stay out of the hospital for longer periods than do patients who know little or nothing about the drugs they're taking.

This newest edition of *Medication Teaching Aids* can help prevent or reduce the occurrence of adverse reactions in your patients. In it, you'll find everything you need to teach your patients about their drug therapy.

The book is divided into three sections. The first section contains illustrated teaching aids that explain, step-by-step, how to perform more than 20 drug administration techniques, including how to take tablets; how to use an oral inhaler; how to instill eye, ear, and nose drops; how to give injections; and even how to care for a central venous catheter.

The second section is an A-to-Z compendium of concisely written teaching aids for more than 300 drugs and about 20 drug classes commonly prescribed for home use. More than 45 drugs have been added to this edition, including AIDS drugs, antibiotics, and drugs recently approved by the Food and Drug Administration. For all of these drugs, your patient will learn how to take the drug, how to handle a missed dose, and what other drugs shouldn't be taken at the same time.

The last section contains teaching aids that explain supportive measures augmenting the patient's drug therapy. These aids include measures relating to comfort, diet, health monitoring, and health promotion.

All of the teaching aids in this book have been designed to be photocopied, reviewed with patients, and handed to them when they leave the hospital, doctor's office, pharmacy, extended care facility, or other health care setting. A special binding allows the book to lie flat for easy photocopying. The easy-on-the-eyes large print, the text's uncomplicated language, and the numerous clear and inviting illustrations make the handouts patient-friendly and immediately useful. The in-text logos *Warning* and *Keep in mind* highlight especially critical information, including dangerous drug interactions and cautions for certain patient groups, such as elderly patients or children.

As today's nurse knows only too well, shorter hospital stays, an ever-increasing number of elderly in-patients, and the growing demands of third-party payers make each of us increasingly conscious of the need for exceptional patient teaching. At the same time, we have less and less time to actually do it.

Medication Teaching Aids, Second Edition, helps you efficiently meet that goal of exceptional patient teaching — and in less time that you might imagine. Your patient can refer to a teaching aid to refresh his memory, perfect a technique, or reinforce your teaching. Rest assured that sending your patient home with a handout from *Medication Teaching Aids,* Second Edition, is the next best thing to being there yourself.

Patricia Gonce Morton, RN, PhD
Associate Professor
University of Maryland School of Nursing
Baltimore

Administration techniques

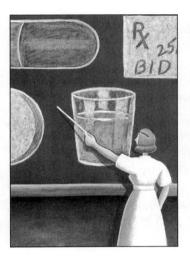

When you measure and administer your patient's medication, you can be sure that he takes it properly. But what about when he goes home? Are you confident that he can continue correct drug administration on his own?

This section of *Medication Teaching Aids,* Second Edition, can help you teach your patient to use proper administration techniques, enabling him to continue effective drug therapy at home. You can photocopy and give him the appropriate teaching aids and review the steps with him. For each administration technique, you'll find step-by-step explanations and illustrations that show your patient exactly how to proceed.

You may want to give the first teaching aid, "Taking your medication correctly," to all patients receiving drug therapy. It provides information to help your patient have a prescription filled, take and store medications, and avoid common problems. The next group of teaching aids covers *oral drugs* and describes how to take tablets, capsules, and liquid medications. Special tips on how to give these medications to a child are also given.

Taking inhaled drugs may seem complicated and confusing to your patient. The teaching aids for *respiratory drugs* can help boost your patient's confidence. They carefully describe each step for using mini-nebulizers, inhalers with holding chambers, AeroVent inhalers, and aerosol equipment. Likewise, the teaching aids for *eye, ear, and nose drugs* provide step-by-step instructions on how to administer eye, ear, and nose drops, apply eye ointment, and use a nasal pump.

The teaching aids for *topical and other drugs* explain how to use medicated bath products, rectal suppositories, and vaginal medications. Administering an enema and giving medications through a gastrostomy tube have also been included.

(continued)

Administration techniques (continued)

The last group, *injections,* can help reinforce your instructions on giving injections. Your patient will gain assurance by studying the appropriate teaching aid on subcutaneous or intramuscular injections, use of an anaphylaxis kit, self-infusion of clotting factors, care of a central venous catheter, or use and care of an implanted port. In addition, instructions for caring for a peripherally inserted central catheter (PICC line) are included.

Other sections on medication safety for children and older adults have been included in this edition, as well as exactly what to do in the event of a suspected drug overdose.

Taking your medication correctly

Dear Patient,

Your primary health care provider has prescribed medication to help treat your condition. This medication will help you only if you take it correctly. Here's how.

Filling your prescription
- Have your prescription filled at the pharmacy you ordinarily use. That way, the pharmacist can keep a complete record of your medications. Tell him if you're allergic to any medications.
- If you need to refill your prescription, don't wait until the last minute. Refill it before you run out of medication.

Taking your medication
- Take your medication in a well-lit room. Double-check the label to make sure you're taking the right medication. If you don't understand the directions, call your pharmacist or primary health care provider.
- If you forget to take a dose or several doses, don't take two or more doses together. Instead, ask your primary health care provider or pharmacist for directions.
- Don't stop taking your medication unless your primary health care provider tells you to. And don't save it for some other time.

Storing your medication
- Keep your medication in its original container. Don't store your medications in a pillbox.
- Store your medication in a cool, dry place or as directed by your pharmacist. Don't keep it in the bathroom medicine cabinet or in the kitchen near the stove. Heat and humidity may cause it to lose its effectiveness.
- If you have children, make sure your medication containers have childproof caps. Always keep the containers out of the reach of children.

Avoiding problems
- Keep the following information about each of your medications on index cards or on a chart: the drug's name, its purpose, its appearance, how to take it, when to take it, how much to take, and special precautions or side effects. Remember, most medications cause some side effects.
- If you have any questions about symptoms you're experiencing while taking your medication, call your primary health care provider right away.

Warning: If you're pregnant or breast-feeding, talk to your primary health care provider before taking any medication or home remedy. Some medications may be harmful to the baby.
- Make sure to remind your primary health care provider and pharmacist about any other medications you take regularly (this includes over-the-counter or prescription medications, herbal medicines, and birth control pills).
- Never take medication that doesn't look right or has passed the expiration date. The medication may not work. Even worse, it may harm you.
- Don't take over-the-counter medications while you're on a prescription medication without first checking with your pharmacist. Another medication can change the way your prescribed medication works.
- Alcoholic beverages and some foods can change the way some medications work. Read the medication label. It may tell you what to avoid. If you are uncertain, ask your pharmacist.
- Your medication has been prescribed just for you. Don't share it with family or friends. They could be hurt by it.

Additional instructions

_____

_____

Giving medication safely to children

Dear Parent or Caregiver,

Here are some safe-administration tips to help you give prescription or over-the-counter medication to children.

Giving the medication

• Always give the medication exactly as prescribed. This includes the amount, the number of doses, and the administration times. Never stop a medication because the child looks better — give the medicine for the entire length of time prescribed.
• Never guess at the amount of medication. Children aren't small adults, and half an adult dose may be too much. Don't pour liquid medication into a teaspoon or tablespoon that you eat with — the measurement won't be accurate. Instead, buy a measured-dose vial at the drugstore or supermarket.
• Don't confuse the abbreviations for teaspoon (tsp.) and tablespoon (Tbs.). If you're giving teaspoons and your vial says ounces, get a measuring device calibrated in teaspoons and tablespoons.
• If you mix medication in food or fluids, use as little food or fluid as possible. Otherwise, the child may not be able to finish it all and won't get the correct dose. Don't mix medication in an infant's formula — he may refuse to take the formula afterwards.
• Don't give chewable tablets to children without teeth. Don't open sustained-release capsules or crush enteric-coated caplets.
• Give infants medication through a medicine dropper. Place the dropper between the gum and cheek and toward the back of the mouth to prevent gagging. Squeeze gently. Don't squirt medication directly into the throat — it may cause choking.

Storing medications

• Follow the storage directions printed on the label.

• Store all medications where children can't see or reach them. Teach your child not to take any medication unless an adult they know and trust gives it to them.

Other precautions

• Make sure you understand what side effects can occur and what constitutes an allergic reaction. Call the primary health care provider if anything new or different happens.
• Don't give one child's medication to another child or to an adult.

! *Warning:* Never describe medication as yummy or candy. This may tempt children to eat it all and overdose.

• Always use the childproof cap and relock the medication after each use. Write down the time of each dose so you'll always know when to give the next one.
• Ask your poison control center to send you poison prevention stickers to apply to all medication containers. Teach children that the sticker means, "Stay away! Only a grownup can give this to me." Post the poison control center's number near your telephone.
• If you're planning to travel, be sure you have enough medicine for the entire trip. Take the pediatrician's telephone number with you.

Additional instructions

_____
_____
_____
_____
_____
_____
_____
_____
_____

Giving medication safely to older adults

Dear Caregiver,

As a person ages, changes in metabolism can increase or decrease a drug's effect. Physical or mental changes can also occur that place older adults at risk for medication-related problems. Here are some tips to help you and other caregivers administer medications to an older adult safely and wisely.

Filling prescriptions
• Have all prescriptions filled at the same pharmacy, so the pharmacist can monitor and keep a record of all medications.
• Don't hesitate to question the primary health care provider or pharmacist about a medication. They're the best sources for drug information.
• Keep track of when medications need refilling so you won't run out of a medication and interrupt the desired effects.
• If the person has poor vision, ask the pharmacist to use large type on the medication containers.
• If the person has trouble opening child-proof containers, ask the pharmacist for easy-to-open containers. Remember to keep them out of reach of children.

Administering medications
• Be sure the person understands why he's taking the medication, when and how he should take it, what side effects may occur and how to handle them, and what special precautions should be taken.
• Try to ensure that the person doesn't stop taking his medication or change the dose without notifying the primary health care provider, even if the person is feeling better.

Storing medications
• Don't store medications in damp places, such as the bathroom or near the kitchen sink. Refrigerate medications if specified.

• Store bulk medications in their original containers to avoid confusion. Then fill pill dispensers from the original containers after double-checking the label.
• If you're caring for a confused older adult, store all medications out of reach in tamper-resistant containers.

Avoiding problems
• Inform the primary health care provider about all the medications being taken (including over-the-counter products), why the person is taking them, and known allergies.
• Keep a list of each medication being taken, the dose, and the name and telephone number of the primary health care provider who prescribed it. Keep a copy handy.
• Inform the primary health care provider immediately of unpleasant or unusual side effects from medication **before** the person stops taking it.
• Ask the person's primary health care provider to review the need for medication at least twice a year or more if necessary.
• Check all medications for expiration dates. Flush old or expired medications down the toilet, and discard the containers.
Warning: Never give the person someone else's medication or give the person's medication to someone else. Medications don't work the same on all people.
• If the patient will be traveling, make sure he brings adequate medications with him and that they are easily accessible. Make sure the person has his prescription cards and his health care provider's telephone number and address with him.
• If you're caring for a older adult, monitor the medication supply and keep the poison control center's telephone number handy.

Additional instructions

_____

_____

Handling and preventing an overdose

Dear Patient or Caregiver,

The information below gives general guidelines on what to do if you think you or someone else has taken extra medication.

Dealing with an overdose

• Call your primary health care provider if you think you've taken an extra dose of medication or have given someone else an extra dose. He will decide if you need further treatment.

• Post the poison control center's number near your telephone. In case of accidental or intended overdosing, remain calm, call poison control, and read the medication label to them so they can identify toxic ingredients. Then do what they instruct. Also, call your primary health care provider for instructions.

• Keep a record of each medication you take or give, the dose, and the name and telephone number of the prescribing primary health care provider. Use this list for reference if you must call poison control or go to the hospital or primary health care provider's office.

• If you find medication or other containers near a person who may have overdosed, take them to the hospital with you. Bring along all pills from the containers, which can provide information about how much medication might have been taken.

• Help the person sit in a comfortable position, and loosen any tight clothing.

! **Warning:** Don't give syrup of ipecac unless instructed to do so by the primary health care provider or poison control center. Never induce vomiting in anyone who has a serious heart condition, has just had a seizure, or is unconscious.

• If the person vomits, help him clear his mouth, if necessary, to prevent choking. Save some vomit for examination if you're going to the hospital or primary health care provider's office. Note whether pill particles are present in the vomitus.

Preventing an overdose

• Keep all medications in their original containers with the labels intact. Read the labels carefully before taking or giving the medications.

• Keep medication out of the reach of children or confused adults. Parents, grandparents, and other caretakers should poison-proof all areas of the home.

• Be sure you understand how to take (or give) the medication, when to take it, how long to take it, and what to do if a problem occurs.

• If you take or give several medications, develop a system to keep track of the times and doses. Tell your family or a friend about your system.

Additional instructions

_____
_____
_____
_____
_____
_____
_____
_____
_____
_____
_____

Taking tablets, capsules, and liquid medications

Dear Patient,

Your primary health care provider has prescribed medication to help treat your condition. Whether your medication comes in a solid form, such as tablets or capsules, or in a liquid form, such as a syrup, elixir, emulsion, or suspension, make sure you take it correctly. Here are some guidelines.

Taking tablets and capsules

First wash your hands. Then gather everything you need, such as the medication, a glass of water or juice and, if you plan to crush a tablet, a commercial pill crusher. If you need to divide a scored tablet, get a knife. Now follow these steps.

1 Look at the medication container to make sure you have the right medication and the right dose.

2 Pour the prescribed number of tablets or capsules into the bottle cap. If too many pour out, drop the extra tablets or capsules back into the container without touching them. Now pour the medication from the cap into your hand.

3 Place the tablets or capsules as far back on your tongue as you can. You may do this with one tablet or capsule at a time or all of them at once.

4 Tip your head slightly *forward,* take a drink of water or juice, and swallow.

Special tips

• Take coated tablets and capsules with plenty of water or juice.
• Avoid touching the extra tablets or capsules you put back into the container. Doing so may contaminate the medication remaining in the bottle.
• If you have trouble swallowing a tablet or capsule, moisten your mouth with some water or juice before you take the tablet. It may also help to crush an uncoated tablet, open a soft capsule, or split a tablet.

❗ *Warning: Never* crush or open tablets or capsules that have a special coating. Doing so may change the medication's effectiveness by changing the way your body absorbs the medication. If you're in doubt, ask your primary health care provider or pharmacist if it's safe for you to crush or open your medication.
• Protect tablets and capsules from light, humidity, and air. If your medication changes color or has an unusual odor, discard it. Also discard all outdated medications.

Taking liquid medication

First wash your hands. Then get the medication bottle and a medicine cup. Look at the container to make sure you have the right medication and to check the prescribed dosage. If the medication is in a suspension, shake it vigorously before proceeding.

1 Uncap the bottle and place the cap upside down on a clean surface.

2 Locate the marking for the prescribed dose on your medicine cup. Keeping your thumbnail on the mark, hold the cup at eye level and pour in the correct amount of medication. Place the cup safely on a flat surface. Check the dose you have measured again. Swallow the medication.

3 Wipe the bottle's lip with a damp paper towel, taking care not to touch the inside of the bottle. Replace the bottle cap.

4 Wash the medicine cup with soap and hot water. Store your medication as directed on the label.

Special tips

• When pouring liquid medication, keep the label next to your palm. This way, if any liquid spills or drips, it won't ruin the label.

(continued)

Taking tablets, capsules, and liquid medications *(continued)*

• If you pour out too much liquid, discard the excess. Don't return it to the bottle.
• If a liquid medication has an unpleasant taste, ask your primary health care provider or pharmacist about diluting the medication with water or juice. Also consider sucking on ice to numb your taste buds before taking your medication. You may also wish to chill an oily liquid before taking it.
• To relieve a bitter taste after swallowing the medication, suck on a piece of sugarless hard candy or chew gum. Gargling or rinsing your mouth with water or mouthwash may also help.

Additional precautions
• Keep all medications out of the reach of children.
• For safety's sake, don't hesitate to ask your primary health care provider or pharmacist about medications and directions you don't understand.
• Never share your medication with anyone else.

Additional instructions

_____

_____

_____

_____

_____

_____

_____

_____

_____

_____

Giving children medication by mouth

Dear Parent or Caregiver,

Giving your child a medication doesn't have to be a problem for you or your child. With patience and care, you can make sure your child gets medication in a calm and careful way.

Take a positive approach

- Make sure you're giving the right medication and dose at the right time to the right child.
- Approach your child in a matter-of-fact but friendly manner to put him at ease. Act as though you expect his cooperation, and praise him when he cooperates.
- Give an older child choices, if possible, to give him a sense of control. For example, offer him a choice of beverage to take with (or after) his medication (unless the primary health care provider tells you not to give the medication with certain beverages or foods).
- Taste a liquid medication (just a drop) before giving it to your child. This gives you an idea of how the medication will taste and whether you'll have to change the taste with flavoring. (Of course, don't taste a medication if you think you may be sensitive to it.)
- Explain the relation between illness and treatment to an older child. He may be more cooperative if he realizes that the medication will help him get better.
- Place a tablet or capsule near the back of your child's tongue, and give him plenty of water or flavored drink to help him swallow it. Then make sure he swallows it.
- Encourage your child to tip his head *forward* when swallowing a tablet or capsule. Throwing his head back increases the risk of inhaling the medication and choking.
- Give medication to an infant in a manner similar to feeding. Giving medication through a bottle's nipple, for example, takes advantage of the infant's natural sucking re-

flex. To make sure the infant gets the full dose, don't mix the medication with formula.
- Closely observe your child to see if the medication has the intended effect or any side effects.

Be honest and careful

- Never try to trick a child into taking medication. Doing so may make him resist you the next time he has to take it and may cause him to distrust you.
- Never tell a child that medication is candy. He may try to take more than the prescribed dose. Or he may not trust you when he learns it isn't candy.
- Don't promise that the medication will taste good if you've never tasted it or if you know that it won't taste good.
- Never threaten, insult, or embarrass your child if he doesn't cooperate. These actions can lead to resistance.
- Keep medication away from a place where your child or others could accidentally take it.
- Don't force your child to swallow his medication or try to hold his nose or mouth shut to promote swallowing. Doing so may cause choking.

Warning: Don't try to give medication to a crying child; he could choke on it.
- If you can't get your child to take his medication, consult your primary health care provider or pharmacist. The medication may come in another form that your child can tolerate.

Additional instructions

_____
_____
_____
_____
_____

Using a mini-nebulizer

Dear Patient,

Your primary health care provider has pre-scribed a medication to help you breathe better. This medication is placed in a nebu-lizer attached to an air compressor that turns the liquid medication into a fine mist that you inhale. Use the nebulizer exactly as your pri-mary health care provider directs at these times:_____. Here's how.

Setting up the treatment

Wash your hands. Remove the nebulizer lid from the cup. Draw up and dilute the amount of medication prescribed by your primary health care provider, following the primary health care provider's instructions.

Add the medication to the cup, and re-place the lid. Attach the tubing to the nebu-lizer and to the outlet on the air compressor (below). Turn on the air compressor and in-crease the flow to 10 to 14 L/minute.

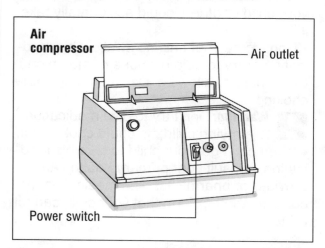

Taking your medication

Place the mouthpiece firmly in your mouth. Breathe slowly and deeply through your mouth until the medication is gone (usually about 10 to 15 minutes).

Turn off the flow when all the medication is gone from the cup.

After each treatment

Remove the tubing from the nebulizer and curl it around the air compressor. Then re-move the lid from the nebulizer cup (below) and rinse the cup with clear water. Place the cup on a clean paper towel until your next treatment.

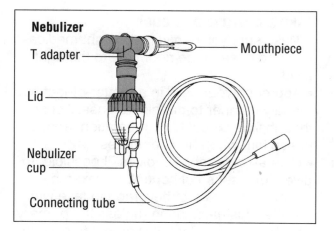

Cleaning the equipment

Clean and disinfect the nebulizer parts every day. First, take apart the pieces of the nebulizer—the lid, cup, T adapter, and mouthpiece. Wash the pieces in warm, soapy water, using a mild, liquid dishwash-ing detergent. Rinse with clear water.

Next soak the pieces in a solution of 1 cup of white vinegar and 1 cup of water for 30 minutes. Rinse well with clear water. Place on a paper towel to dry. You can cover the vinegar-water solution, store it in the re-frigerator, and reuse it for 1 week. If you're using a commercial disinfecting solution, fol-low the manufacturer's directions.

Additional instructions

_____
_____
_____
_____

Using an oral inhaler with a holding chamber

Dear Patient,

Your primary health care provider has prescribed an oral inhaler to help open your breathing passages. In this treatment, you'll inhale a medication through a small device that you put in your mouth. A holding chamber attached to the inhaler helps the medication to reach deeply into your lungs.

Common devices include the InspirEase System and the Aerochamber (some of these have a mask for easier use).

InspirEase System

This system has a holding chamber that collapses when you breathe in and inflates when you breathe out. To operate this inhaler, follow these steps.

1 Insert the inhaler into the mouthpiece, and shake the inhaler. Place the mouthpiece into the opening of the holding chamber, and twist the mouthpiece to lock it.

2 Extend the holding device, breathe out, and place the mouthpiece in your mouth.

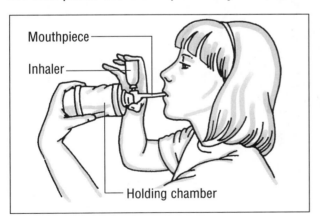

Mouthpiece — Inhaler — Holding chamber

3 Firmly press down once on the inhaler (above). Then breathe in slowly and deeply, collapsing the bag completely. If you breathe too fast, the bag will whistle. Hold your breath for 5 to 10 seconds, then breathe out slowly into the bag. Repeat breathing in and out.

4 Remove the mouthpiece from your mouth. Wait 1 minute. Then shake the inhaler again and repeat the dose, following steps 2 and 3.

Aerochamber systems

These systems use a small cylinder called a valved chamber to trap medication. The device may also include a mask that helps deliver the medication more easily. Follow these steps for use.

1 Remove the cap from the inhaler and from the mouthpiece of the aerochamber. Then insert the inhaler mouthpiece into the wider rubber-sealed end of the aerochamber. Inspect for foreign objects, and check that all parts are secure.

2 Next, shake the device three or four times.

3 Breathe out normally, and close your lips over the mouthpiece (below).
If your device has a mask, place the mask firmly over your nose and mouth.

With either device, aim for a good seal. Leaks will reduce effectiveness.

4 Spray *only one puff* from the inhaler into the holding chamber. Take in one full breath slowly and deeply. If you hear a whistling sound, you're breathing too fast. Now hold your breath for 5 to 10 seconds.

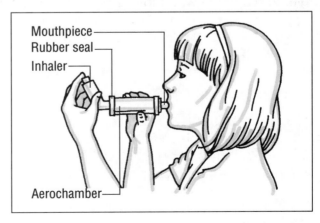

Mouthpiece — Rubber seal — Inhaler — Aerochamber

(continued)

Using an oral inhaler with a holding chamber *(continued)*

If your device has a mask, hold it firmly in place (below), and breathe in at least six times.

❗ *Warning:* Spraying more than one puff at a time into the holding chamber will give you the wrong dose of medication.

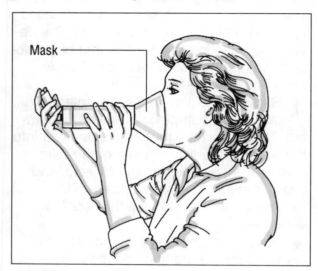

Mask

5 Remove the mouthpiece from your mouth. Wait one minute, and then repeat steps 2 through 4 for each puff prescribed by your primary health care provider.

6 Remove the inhaler. Follow the manufacturer's directions for cleaning and storing it. Rinse any remaining medication from your face. Then rinse your mouth, gargle, and spit the water into a sink or basin.

Additional instructions

_____
_____
_____
_____
_____
_____
_____
_____
_____
_____
_____

Using an AeroVent inhaler

Dear Caregiver,

The primary health care provider has prescribed an AeroVent inhaler to treat the patient's respiratory problem. This device holds medication supplied by a metered-dose inhaler. It delivers the medication through a ventilator breathing circuit. Here are some guidelines for using the device.

Connecting the AeroVent to the circuit

Remove the AeroVent from its box. The device will join the ventilator circuit between the inspiratory tubing and the Y-connector that leads to the patient.

Now gently collapse the AeroVent holding chamber by compressing the device as you would an accordion until the ends come together. Then press the bracketlike clasp down until it clicks into place. Couple one end of the holding chamber to the Y-connector and one end to the ventilator tubing.

! ***Warning:*** Don't use too much force. If you do, you could damage the device or make it difficult to remove.

Be sure that the receptacle port (which holds the inhaler) faces upward and away from the patient.

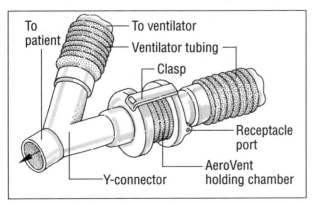

To patient — To ventilator — Ventilator tubing — Clasp — Receptacle port — AeroVent holding chamber — Y-connector

Opening the circuit

Before giving medication, expand the device by unlatching the external clasp (above) and swinging it open.

Grasp the coupled ends of the holding chamber and lightly stretch the device open. Be careful not to bend or rock the AeroVent.

Reposition the receptacle, if needed; it may be displaced when the chamber expands. To give medication, the nozzle of the canister must point directly down. The receptacle port must point up to receive the inhaler.

Giving medication

Shake the inhaler canister and insert its nozzle in the receptacle port. Don't press on the inhaler yet.

When a ventilator exhalation ends, activate the inhaler by pressing on the canister's base once. Have the patient take a deep breath if able; if not, have him take a regular breath or a sigh breath from the ventilator. Wait 1 minute, and then have the patient repeat the process to administer the number of puffs prescribed.

Give only one puff each time, and don't press the inhaler with too much force. This may jam the nozzle and damage the equipment.

After several uses, you may notice cloudiness in the chamber. Don't be alarmed. This results from collected moisture and medication particles.

Finishing your care

Once you've given the medication, remove the inhaler canister and collapse the AeroVent by gently pushing the ends together. Use a slight rotating motion until you compress the device securely. Now relatch the external clasp.

Always replace a damaged AeroVent at once, and attach a new AeroVent when you change the tubing.

Additional instructions

_____

_____

Caring for aerosol equipment

Dear Patient,

Your aerosol equipment includes a compressed air machine and disposable plastic parts: a mouthpiece, a mask, syringes, and medicine cups. All of this equipment must be kept clean. If it isn't, bacteria can enter your lungs along with the mist.

Cleaning the plastic parts

You don't need to clean the parts every time they're used, but you should rinse them in warm or cool water after each use. Allow them to air dry before storing them in a clean plastic bag or another clean container.

Clean the parts *daily,* following the primary health care provider's recommendations or those of the equipment manufacturer. Or use the following procedure:
• Wash the plastic parts in warm water and a mild dishwashing detergent; then rinse. The air compressor doesn't require cleaning. *Never* submerge it in water.
• After rinsing, soak the parts for 30 minutes in a solution of 1 cup white vinegar and 1 cup warm water (above, right). Rinse well in cool water. Or, if you're using a commercially prepared cleaning solution, follow the manufacturer's directions. The vinegar solution may be stored in a covered dish and refrigerated for up to 1 week.
• Let the parts air dry before placing them in a clean storage container.

Maintaining the air compressor

Keeping the compressor in perfect working order promotes better treatments and extends the device's life. How often should you have the compressor serviced? That depends on the type of compressor and the manufacturer's recommendations. Some compressors have a small air filter that should be replaced when it gets dirty.

Troubleshooting problems

If the machine isn't producing enough mist, the problem may be a simple one that you can solve yourself. For example, you might need to:
• change the air filter
• tighten the connections
• try a new aerosol cup.

If these measures fail, take the compressor to your medical equipment supplier to be checked. It may need internal cleaning. However, if the compressor is 8 to 10 years old, it probably needs to be replaced.

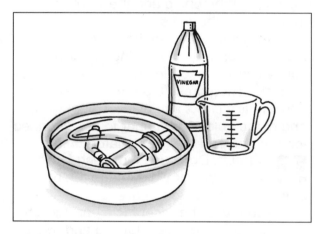

Additional instructions

_____
_____
_____
_____
_____
_____
_____
_____
_____
_____
_____

Giving yourself eyedrops

Dear Patient,

Your primary health care provider has pre-scribed these eyedrops for you.

Medicine #1

Use_____drops_____times a day in your_____eye.

Medicine #2

Use_____drops_____times a day in your_____eye.

Here's how to put drops in your eye.

1 Begin by washing your hands thorough-ly.

2 Check the medication container to make sure you have the right medication and the right dose. Then hold the medication bottle up to the light and examine it. If the medication is discolored or contains sedi-ment, don't use it. Instead, take it back to the pharmacy and have it checked.

If the medication looks okay, warm it to room temperature by holding the bottle be-tween your hands for 2 minutes (below).

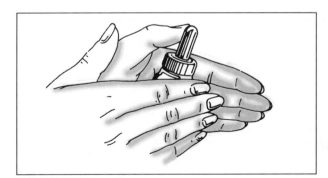

3 Moisten a rayon cosmetic puff or a tis-sue with water, and clean any secre-tions from around your eyes. Use a fresh rayon puff or tissue for each eye. Be sure to wipe outward in one motion, starting from the area nearest your nose (below). Use one tissue or puff per wipe. If you need to wipe again, use a new tissue or puff.

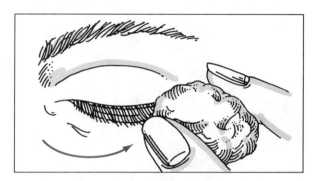

4 Stand or sit before a mirror, or lie on your back, whichever is most comfort-able for you. Squeeze the bulb of the eye-dropper and slowly release it to fill the drop-per with medication.

5 Tilt your head back slightly and toward the eye you're treating. Pull down your lower eyelid (below). This exposes your con-junctival sac (the inside of your lower eyelid).

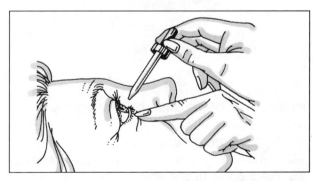

6 Position the dropper over the conjuncti-val sac that you've exposed between your lower lid and the white of your eye. Steady the hand holding the dropper by resting two fingers against your cheek or nose.

7 Look up at the ceiling. Then squeeze the prescribed number of drops into the

(continued)

Giving yourself eyedrops *(continued)*

sac (below). Take care not to touch the dropper to your eye, eyelashes, or fingers. Wipe away excess medication with a clean tissue.

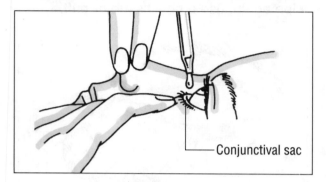
Conjunctival sac

8 Release the lower lid. Try to keep your eye open without blinking for at least 30 seconds. Apply gentle pressure to the corner of your eye at the bridge of your nose (below) for 1 minute. This will prevent the med-

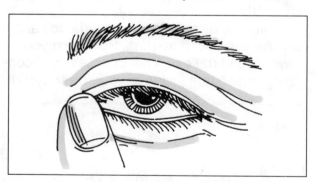

ication from being absorbed through your tear ducts.

9 Repeat the procedure in the other eye, if the primary health care provider orders.

10 Recap the bottle and store it away from light and heat.

If you're using more than one kind of drop, wait 5 minutes before you use the next one.

Important: Call your primary health care provider immediately if you notice any of these side effects:

_____

_____

_____

_____

_____

Remember, never put medication in your eyes unless the label reads "For Ophthalmic Use" or "For Use in Eyes."

Additional instructions

_____

_____

_____

_____

_____

_____

_____

_____

_____

_____

_____

Putting ointment in your eye

Dear Patient,

Your primary health care provider has prescribed this eye ointment for you:

Name of medication: _____

Use this ointment _____ times a day

in your _____ eye.

Here's how to apply the ointment.

1 Wash your hands thoroughly. Make sure you have the right medication and dose. Hold the ointment in your hand for several minutes to warm it before use (unless the label says not to do so).

2 Moisten a rayon cosmetic puff or a tissue with water, and clean secretions from around your eye. Wipe outward in one motion, starting at the side near the nose (below). Use one tissue or puff per wipe. Avoid touching the uninfected eye.

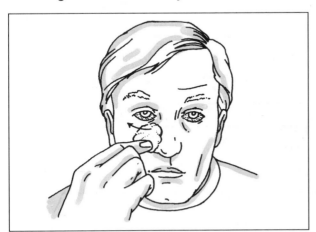

3 Stand or sit comfortably in front of a mirror.

4 Gently pull down your lower eyelid and look up toward the ceiling. Squeeze a small amount of ointment (about ¼ to ½ inch) inside the conjunctival sac — the space between your lower eyelid and the white of your eyeball. Steady the hand that is holding the ointment by resting two fingers against your cheek or nose (below). Hold the tube close to its tip to avoid poking your eye.

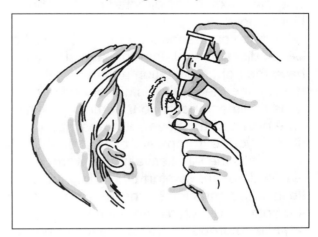

5 Without touching the tube's tip with your eyelashes, close your eye to pinch off the ointment. Roll your eyeball in all directions with your eyes closed (below).

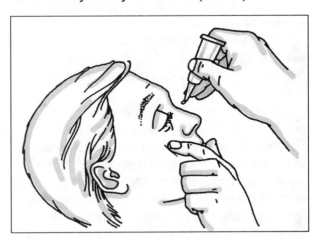

6 Recap the medication. If you're using more than one ointment, wait about 10 minutes before you use the next one. Your vision may be temporarily blurred.

Additional instructions

_____

_____

Giving yourself eardrops

Dear Patient,

Your primary health care provider has prescribed these eardrops:
Use them exactly as directed on the label. Here's how.

1 Wash your hands thoroughly. Check the medication container to make sure you have the right medication and the right dose. If the medication is discolored or contains sediment, notify your primary health care provider and have your prescription refilled. If your eardrops are okay, proceed.

2 Unless the label says not to, warm the eardrops for comfort by holding the bottle in your hands for 2 minutes. Then shake the bottle, if directed, and open it.

3 Fill the dropper; then place the open bottle and dropper within easy reach.

4 Lie on your side to expose the ear you're treating.

5 To straighten your ear canal, gently pull the top of your ear up and back, as shown above, right.

6 Position the dropper above your ear, taking care not to touch it to your ear. Squeeze the dropper's bulb to release 1 drop.

7 Wait until you feel the drop in your ear. Then, if directed, release another drop. Repeat these steps until you have given yourself the prescribed number of drops. To keep the drops from running out of your ear, remain on your side for about 10 minutes.

8 Alternatively, to keep the medication from running out, you may place a cotton ball moistened with the medication *at the very entrance to the ear canal.* However, never place anything in the ear canal. Remove the cotton after 1 hour.

9 As your primary health care provider directs, treat your other ear.

10 Recap the eardrop bottle, and store it away from light and extreme heat, or as directed on the label.

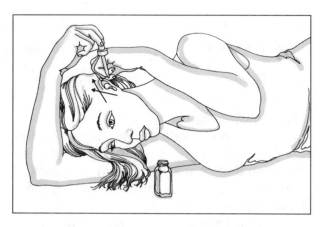

Additional instructions

_____

_____

_____

_____

_____

_____

_____

_____

_____

_____

Giving eardrops to a child

Dear Parent or Caregiver,

To treat your child's ear problem, the primary health care provider has prescribed eardrops. Use them exactly as directed on the label.

Getting ready

1 First wash your hands thoroughly. Then examine the medication container to be sure it's the right medication and the right dose. Does the medication look discolored or contain sediment? If it does, notify the primary health care provider and have the prescription refilled. If it looks normal, you can proceed.

2 Warm the medication (for your child's comfort) by holding the bottle in your hands for about 2 minutes.

3 Then shake the bottle (if directed), open it, and fill the dropper by squeezing the bulb. Place the open bottle and dropper within easy reach.

Giving eardrops

1 Have your child lie on his side to expose the ear you're treating. Now *gently* pull the earlobe down and back (above, right). This will straighten his ear canal.

2 Position the filled dropper above — but not touching — the opening of your child's ear canal. Gently squeeze the dropper's bulb once to release 1 drop.

Watch the drop slide into the ear canal. Or have your child tell you when he feels the drop enter his ear.

Then gently squeeze the dropper's bulb to release the number of drops prescribed.

3 Continue holding your child's ear as the eardrops disappear down the ear canal. Now massage the area in front of the ear. If he is old enough to understand, ask your child to tell you when he no longer feels the drops moving in his ear. Then release his ear.

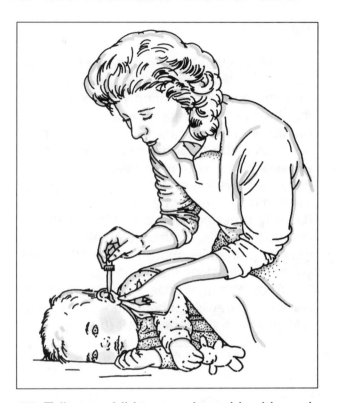

4 Tell your child to remain on his side and to avoid touching his ear for about 10 minutes. If he is too young to do this, hold him in this position and keep his hands away from his ears. You may place a cotton ball moistened with the medication at the *very entrance* to the ear canal, but never place anything *in* the ear canal. Remove the cotton after 1 hour. This will keep the medication from running out. Don't use dry cotton because it may absorb the medication.

If both ears require medication, repeat the procedure in your child's other ear. Finally, return the dropper to the medication bottle (or recap the dropper bottle).

Store the bottle away from light and extreme heat.

Additional instructions

_____

_____

Using a metered-dose nasal pump

Dear Patient,

Your primary health care provider has prescribed medication to be inhaled through a metered-dose nasal pump. Keep in mind that the pump delivers an exact amount of medication. Here's how to use the pump.

1 Look at the medication container to make sure it's the right medication and the right dose. Remove the protective cap, and prime the pump as directed by the manufacturer. (Usually, pressing down about four times primes the pump. If refrigerated, the pump will stay primed for about 1 week. After that, you'll need to prime the pump again.)

2 To get the right dose, tilt the pump bottle so the strawlike tube inside draws medication from the deepest part (below).

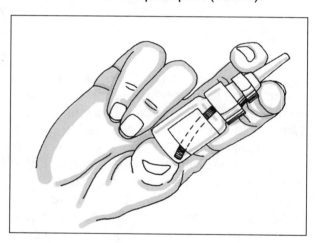

3 Insert the pump's applicator tip about half an inch into your nostril (above, right). Point the tip straight up your nose and toward the inner corner of your eye. (Don't tilt your head, or the medication may run into your throat.)

4 Without inhaling, squeeze the pump once, quickly and firmly. Try to use just enough force to coat the inside of your nostril, but not so much that you inject the medication into your sinuses. (Doing that will

cause a headache.) Spray again if the package directions instruct you to, or repeat the procedure in the other nostril if your primary health care provider directs you to do so.

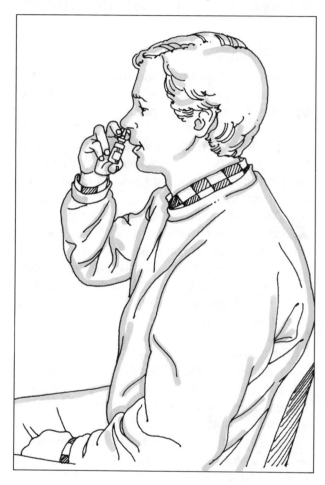

5 Keep your head still for several minutes so the medication has time to work. And don't blow your nose for a while.

6 Store the medication and pump in the refrigerator.

Additional instructions

_____

_____

_____

_____

Giving yourself nose drops

Dear Patient,

Your primary health care provider has prescribed nose drops for you to use at home. Here's what you need to know.

Getting ready

Before you use your nose drops, look at the container to make sure you have the right medication and to check the prescribed dosage. Then follow these steps:

1 Warm the medication container by holding it in your hands for about 2 minutes.

2 With the dropper still in the bottle, squeeze the dropper bulb to load the dropper chamber with medication.

3 The method you use to instill the drops will vary, depending on the problem you're treating.

Treating the nasal passages

If your primary health care provider has prescribed nose drops to treat your nasal passages, position the dropper as shown below. Doing so will help the drops flow down the back of your nose, not your throat. Then proceed.

1 Squeeze the dropper bulb to insert the correct number of drops.

2 Repeat the process in the other nostril, if indicated.

3 Breathe through your mouth so that you don't sniff the drops into your sinuses or your lungs.

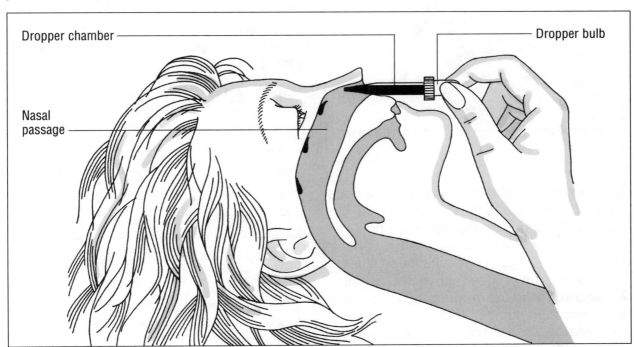

Dropper chamber

Dropper bulb

Nasal passage

(continued)

Giving yourself nose drops *(continued)*

Treating the ethmoid and sphenoid sinuses

To treat a problem in these areas, lie on your back with a pillow under your shoulders and your head tilted *backward,* as shown. Follow these steps:

1 Position the dropper above one nostril (below), and squeeze the dropper bulb to release the prescribed number of drops.

2 Breathe through your nose. This will help the medication move through your sinuses.

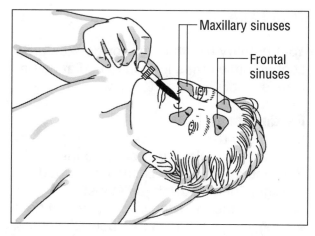

Maxillary sinuses

Frontal sinuses

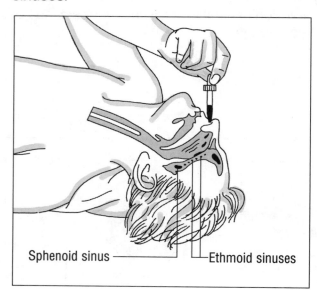

Sphenoid sinus — — Ethmoid sinuses

Treating the frontal and maxillary sinuses

To treat a problem in these areas, lie on your back with a pillow under your shoulders and your head tilted *to one side,* as shown above, right. Then take these steps:

1 Position the dropper above one nostril, and squeeze the dropper bulb to release the prescribed number of drops.

2 Breathe through your nose. This will help the medication move through your sinuses.

Taking precautions

• Follow your primary health care provider's orders exactly. Don't overuse your nose drops.

• Because nose drops are easily contaminated, don't buy more than you'll use in a short time. Discard discolored nose drops and drops that contain sediment.

• Don't share your nose drops with anyone. Doing so may spread germs.

Additional instructions

_____

_____

_____

_____

_____

_____

_____

_____

_____

_____

_____

_____

Using medicated bath products

Dear Patient,

Your primary health care provider has prescribed a medicated bath to help treat your skin problem. A medicated bath:
- relieves itching
- softens scales and crusts (for easier removal).

Preparing the bath

Before beginning, make sure your bathroom is warm and draft-free. Then make sure the bathtub is clean.

Adding the medication

How you'll add medication to your bathwater will vary. Depending on the medication prescribed by your primary health care provider, use one of these methods:
- If you're using a colloidal preparation such as oatmeal, mix 1 measuring cup of oatmeal with a small amount of cool water to form a paste. Then begin filling the tub with warm water. Gradually swirl in the paste as the tub fills.
- If you're using an oil preparation such as mineral oil (with a surfactant), fill the bathtub two-thirds full with warm water. Then add 2 ounces of the oil preparation to the bathwater. Stir the water to distribute the oil.

    Or you may find it more effective to mix ¼ teaspoon of bath oil with ¼ cup of water and then apply it to your skin as you would a lotion.
- If you're using a soda preparation such as baking soda, first fill the bathtub to the correct level with warm water. Then add the powder, stirring until it dissolves.
- If you're using a starch preparation such as cornstarch, first fill the bathtub to the appropriate level with warm water. Meanwhile, slowly dissolve the powder in a small container of water. Then, when the water fills the tub to the prescribed level, add the starch solution.

Taking the bath

Before immersing yourself in the bathwater, be sure the temperature feels warm enough. Then get in the tub carefully, and bathe for about 20 minutes. Don't wash your skin with soap after you finish. This will wash the solution off your skin and defeat the purpose of the medicated bath.

Finishing the bath

After you've finished bathing, be careful not to fall on the slippery tub surfaces as you get out of the tub. Pat yourself dry with a clean, soft towel, removing excess medication in the process. Keep in mind that a skin problem can cause you to lose body heat rapidly, so try not to become chilled. Once you're warm and dry, clean the tub so that it's ready for your next bath.

Additional instructions

_____

_____

_____

_____

_____

_____

_____

_____

_____

_____

_____

Giving medication through a gastrostomy tube

Dear Patient or Caregiver,

The primary health care provider has pre-scribed medication to be given through a gastrostomy tube (G-tube). The following guidelines will help you with this procedure.

Gathering the equipment:
First, assemble the following equipment:
- medication and medication cup
- bulb syringe or small funnel
- warm water
- 4-inch-square gauze pad
- rubber band
- 2-inch-wide surgical tape.

Getting ready
1 Read the instructions on the medication container's label. Then pour the correct amount of medication into the medication cup.

2 Make sure that the patient is in an upright position and not lying flat.

3 Unclamp or uncap the tube. Or, if the patient is receiving continuous feedings, touch the pump's "hold" button to interrupt the feedings, then disconnect the pump tubing from the G-tube.

Note that the absorption of some medications, like Dilantin, is affected by the presence of tube feedings in the stomach. Check with the primary health care provider if the feeding should be stopped for a while before or after giving the medications.

4 Attach the syringe or funnel to the end of the tubing (above, right). If you're using a syringe, remove the bulb first.

Opening a blocked tube
To make sure the tube isn't clogged, pour about 1 ounce of water into it (next page) for adults and about ½ ounce for an infant or child. The water should drain into the stom-

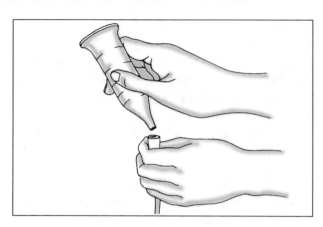

ach by gravity. If it doesn't, try the following actions to unclog the tube:
- Twist the tube gently.
- Change the tube's position. The tube might be pressed against the stomach wall, and changing position will shift it.
- Check each part of the feeding system for kinks, including all connections.
- Flick the tube with your middle finger to remove air bubbles.
- Squeeze the feeding bag to stir up settled formula.
- Flush the tube with water.
- If you're using a pump, turn it off and check for mechanical problems as the manufacturer directs. If a pump feeding still doesn't flow, try letting it flow by gravity.

If none of these actions work, stop the procedure and call the primary health care provider for instructions.

Performing the procedure
1 Pour the medication into the syringe or funnel, letting it flow into the stomach by gravity. Don't force the medication to flow. If medication backs up in the tube or oozes out around the tube, stop giving it and call the primary health care provider for instructions.

2 After you pour all the medication down the tube, pour in about 1 ounce of water

(continued)

Giving medication through a gastrostomy tube *(continued)*

(about ½ ounce for an infant or child). Then remove the syringe or funnel and reclamp or recap the tube or restart the continuous feedings.

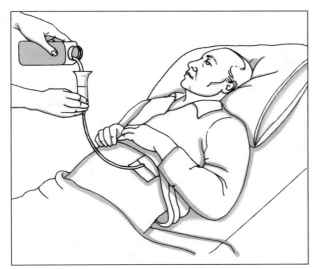

3 If you've recapped or reclamped the tube, wrap a gauze pad around the end of the tube and secure the pad with a rubber band. This keeps the end of the tube clean. Secure the tubing to the abdomen with tape as needed.

Finishing up

1 Check the site where the tube enters the body. If medication has seeped out around the tube, call the primary health care provider for instructions.

2 Rinse all equipment carefully after every use, and store the medication container safely.

3 Notify the primary health care provider if the patient has nausea, vomiting, diarrhea, stomach discomfort, or constipation.

Additional instructions

_____

_____

_____

_____

_____

_____

_____

_____

_____

_____

_____

Inserting a rectal suppository

Dear Patient,

Your primary health care provider has prescribed a rectal suppository. You can learn to insert it quickly and easily in a few steps. Be cautious, though. Unless your primary health care provider orders otherwise, don't use rectal suppositories or other laxatives routinely because you can become dependent on them.

Follow these steps.

1 Wash your hands. Then gather the items you'll need: the suppository, a disposable glove, and a tube of water-soluble lubricating gel.

2 Put the glove on your right hand (or on your left if you're left-handed). Now remove the foil wrapper on the suppository.

If you have trouble doing this, the suppository may be too soft to insert. Hold it under cold running water until it becomes firm, or put it in the freezer for a minute or two before inserting it — just don't let it get too cold and hard. Better yet, store your suppositories in the refrigerator.

3 Once you've removed the foil wrapper, put a generous dab of lubricating gel on the rounded end of the suppository (below). Hold the lubricated suppository in your gloved hand.

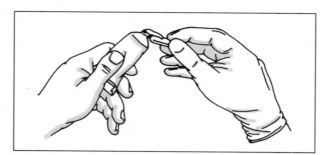

4 Now lie on your side with your knees raised toward your chest. Take a deep breath as you gently insert the suppository —

rounded end first — into the anus with your gloved hand (below). Push the suppository in slowly, just far enough so that it doesn't slip out.

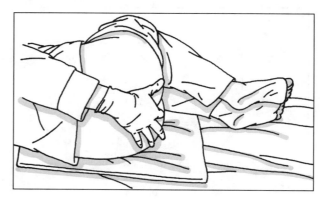

5 Once the suppository is in place, you'll feel an immediate urge to have a bowel movement. Resist the urge by lying still and breathing deeply a few times.

Try to retain the suppository for at least 20 minutes, so your body can absorb it and get the maximum effect from the medication. After you have a bowel movement, discard the glove and wash your hands.

Additional instructions

_____
_____
_____
_____
_____
_____
_____
_____
_____
_____
_____
_____

Giving yourself an enema

Dear Patient,

Your primary health care provider has prescribed an enema for you. Giving yourself an enema is a bit awkward, but it really isn't difficult. Just be sure to give yourself the enema in the morning, so you won't need to use the bathroom during the night. Also be sure you're close to a toilet. Here's what to do.

1 Wash your hands. Open the disposable enema package (the primary health care provider will tell you what brand to buy), and read the instructions carefully.

2 Hold the enema bottle upright, grasping the grooved bottle cap with your fingers. Gently remove the protective shield with your other hand.

3 Lie in bed on your left side with your right knee bent (below). This position helps the enema solution flow into your colon. Place a towel or linen-saver pad under your buttocks to keep the bed dry.

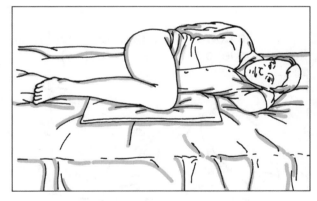

4 Or, you can lie in the knee-chest position, as shown above, right.

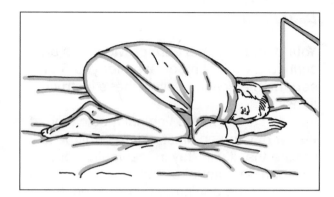

5 Now, gently insert the tip of the enema bottle about 4 inches into your rectum. Take slow, deep breaths as you slowly squeeze the bottle to deposit the solution in your rectum. When the bottle is empty, remove the tip from your rectum.

6 Because your colon is full, you'll feel an immediate urge to have a bowel movement. Try to resist the urge. Hold the solution in for 2 to 5 minutes for a cleansing enema and for as long as you can tolerate for an oil retention enema. Then expel the solution into the toilet.

7 After moving your bowels, clean the rectal area carefully. Then put the used enema bottle in its original box. Discard the box, the linen-saver pad, and other disposable articles.

Additional instructions

_____
_____
_____
_____
_____
_____
_____
_____
_____
_____

Administering a vaginal medication

Dear Patient,

Your primary health care provider has prescribed a vaginal medication for you. To insert the medication, follow these instructions.

1 Plan to insert the vaginal medication after bathing and just before bedtime to ensure that it will stay in the vagina for the appropriate amount of time.

Collect the equipment you'll need: the prescribed medication (suppository, cream, ointment, tablet, or jelly), an applicator, water-soluble lubricating jelly, a towel, a hand mirror, paper towels, and a sanitary pad.

2 Empty your bladder, wash your hands, and place the towel on the bed. Sit on the towel, and open the medication wrapper or container.

3 Using the hand mirror, carefully inspect the area around the insertion site. If you see signs of increased irritation, don't insert the medication. Notify the primary health care provider. He may change your medication.

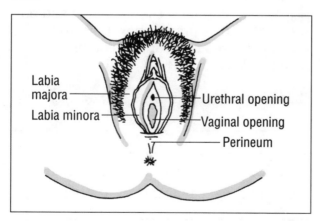

Labia majora
Labia minora
Urethral opening
Vaginal opening
Perineum

4 Place the vaginal suppository or tablet in the applicator (above, right), or fill the applicator with medicated cream, ointment, or jelly.

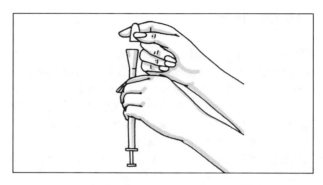

5 To make insertion easier, lubricate the suppository or applicator tip with water or water-soluble lubricating jelly (below).

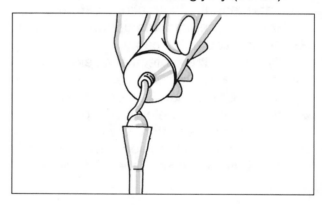

Now lie down on the bed with your knees flexed and legs spread apart (below).

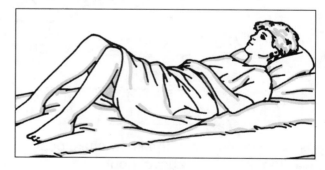

Spread apart your labia with one hand, and insert the applicator tip into the vagina with the other hand (next page, top). Advance the applicator about 2 inches, angling it slightly toward your tailbone.

(continued)

Administering a vaginal medication *(continued)*

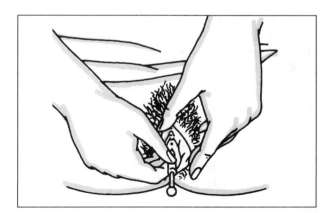

6 Push the plunger to insert the medication (below). Be aware that the medication may feel cold.

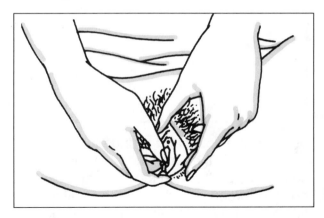

7 Remove the applicator and discard it if it's disposable. If it's reusable, wash it thoroughly with soap and water (below), dry it with a paper towel, and return it to its container.

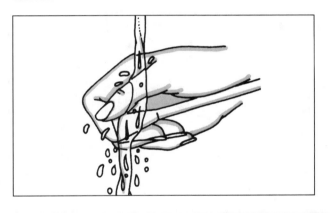

8 If your primary health care provider prescribes it, apply a thin layer of cream, ointment, or jelly to the vulva (the vagina, labia majora, and labia minora).

9 Remain lying down for about 30 minutes so that the medication won't run out of your vagina. If you like, apply a sanitary pad to avoid staining your clothes or bed linens (below).

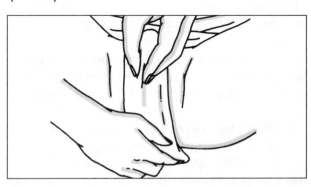

Then check your vagina with a mirror for signs of an allergic reaction. If the area seems unusually red or swollen, contact the primary health care provider.

Additional instructions

_____
_____
_____
_____
_____
_____
_____
_____
_____
_____
_____
_____
_____

Giving yourself a subcutaneous injection

Dear Patient,

Before you can administer your injection, you may need to transfer the correct amount of medication from the bottle to the syringe, unless your medication is premeasured. Follow these guidelines.

1 Wash your hands. Then assemble this equipment in a clean area: a sterile syringe and needle, the medication, and alcohol swabs or wipes (or rubbing alcohol and cotton balls).

2 Check the label on the medication bottle to be sure you have the right medication. For safety, also check the expiration date.

3 Clean the top of the medication bottle with an alcohol swab or wipe.

4 Select an appropriate injection site. Pull the skin taut (below); then, using a circular motion, clean the skin with an alcohol swab or wipe or a cotton ball soaked in alcohol. Leave the alcohol wipe or cotton ball in place (this will help you remember which site you have chosen).

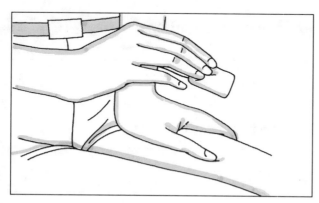

5 Remove the needle cover. *To prevent possible infection, don't touch the needle.* Touch only the barrel and plunger of the syringe. Pull back the plunger slightly to allow air to enter the syringe. The amount of air should equal the amount of medication you're going to take.

Insert the needle into the rubber stopper on the medication bottle, and push in the plunger (below). This pushes the air into the bottle and prevents a vacuum, making it easier to withdraw the medication.

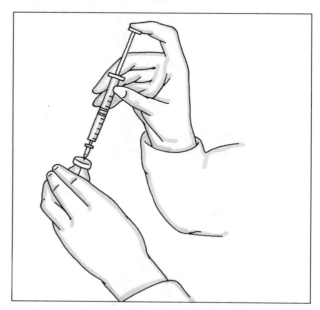

6 Hold the bottle and syringe together in one hand; then turn them upside down so that the bottle is on top. You can hold the bottle between your thumb and forefinger and the syringe between your ring finger and little finger, against your palm. Or you can hold the bottle between your forefinger and middle finger, while holding the syringe between your thumb and little finger (below).

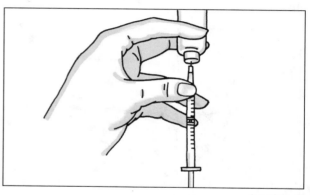

(continued)

Giving yourself a subcutaneous injection *(continued)*

7 Pull back on the plunger until the dose is slightly more than you need. Remove the needle from the vial. Keeping the needle upright, tap the barrel to move air bubbles to the top of the syringe (below). Squirt air bubbles or excess medicine out of the syringe.

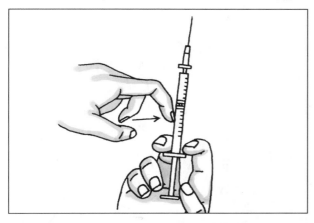

8 Check the dose again to make sure you've withdrawn the correct amount.

9 Remove the swab or cotton ball from your injection site. Using your thumb and forefinger, pinch the skin at the injection site. Then quickly plunge the needle (up to its hub) into the subcutaneous tissue at a 90-degree angle (below). Push the plunger down to inject the medication.

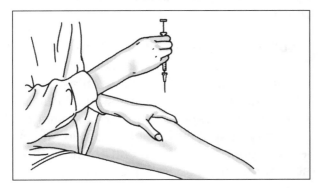

10 Remove the needle at the same angle you used to inject it. Press down on the injection site lightly with a clean alcohol wipe (above, right). Don't rub the injection site when withdrawing the needle.

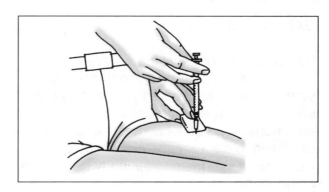

! ***Warning:*** Do not recap the needle. Dispose of the syringe and attached needle in a covered, puncture-resistant container.

Additional instructions

_____
_____
_____
_____
_____
_____
_____
_____
_____
_____
_____
_____

Using an anaphylaxis kit

Dear Patient,

Because you could have a severe reaction to insect stings or certain foods or drugs, your primary health care provider has prescribed an anaphylaxis kit for you to use in an emergency. The kit contains everything you need to treat an allergic reaction:
• a prefilled syringe containing two doses of epinephrine
• alcohol swabs
• a tourniquet
• antihistamine tablets.
    When needed, use the kit as follows. Also, notify the primary health care provider immediately, or ask someone else to call him.

Getting ready
Take the prefilled syringe from the kit and remove the needle cap. Hold the syringe with the needle pointing up. Then push in the plunger until it stops. This will expel any air from the syringe.

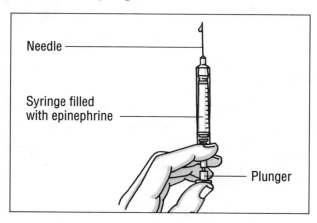

    Next, clean about 4 inches of the skin on your arm or thigh with an alcohol swab. (If you're right-handed, you should clean your left arm or thigh. If you're left-handed, clean your right arm or thigh.)

Injecting the epinephrine
Rotate the plunger one-quarter turn to the right so that it's aligned with the slot. Insert the entire needle—like a dart—into the skin.

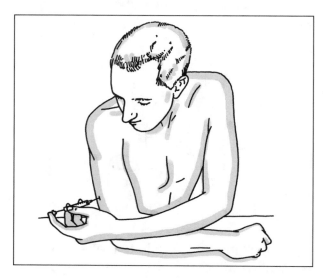

    Push down on the plunger until it stops (above). It will inject 0.3 ml of the drug for an adult or a person over age 12. Withdraw the needle.
    Note: The dose and administration for babies and for children under age 12 must be directed by the primary health care provider.

If you've been stung by an insect
Quickly remove the insect's stinger if you can see it. Use a dull object, such as a fingernail or tweezers, to pull it straight out. Don't pinch, scrape, or squeeze the stinger. This may push it farther into the skin and release more poison. If you can't remove the stinger quickly, stop trying. Go on to the next step.

(continued)

Using an anaphylaxis kit *(continued)*

Applying the tourniquet
If you were stung on your *neck, face,* or *torso,* skip this step and go on to the next one.

If you were stung on an *arm* or a *leg,* apply the tourniquet between the sting site and your heart. Tighten the tourniquet by pulling the string (below).

After 10 minutes, release the tourniquet by pulling on the metal ring.

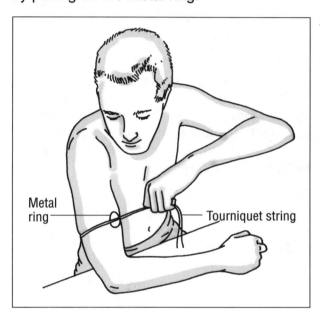

Metal ring

Tourniquet string

Taking the antihistamine tablets
Chew and swallow the antihistamine tablets. (For children age 12 and under, follow the dosage and administration directions supplied by your primary health care provider or provided in the kit.)

What to do next
Next, apply ice packs — if available — to the affected area. Avoid exertion, keep warm, and see a health care provider or go to a hospital immediately.

! ***Warning:*** If you don't notice an improvement within 10 minutes, give yourself a second injection by following the directions in your anaphylaxis kit. If your syringe has a preset second dose, don't depress the plunger until you're ready to give the second injection. Proceed as before, following the instructions to inject the epinephrine.

Special directions
● Keep your kit handy to ensure emergency treatment at all times.
● Ask your pharmacist for storage guidelines. Find out whether the kit can be stored in a car's glove compartment or whether you need to keep it in a cooler place.
● Periodically check the epinephrine in the preloaded syringe. A pinkish brown solution needs to be replaced.
● Make a note of the kit's expiration date. Then renew the kit just before that date.
● Dispose of the used needle and syringe safely and properly.
● Call your primary health care provider to report the incident and obtain another prescription for a fresh kit.

Additional instructions
_____
_____
_____
_____
_____
_____
_____
_____
_____
_____

Learning self-infusion of clotting factors

Dear Patient,

These instructions will help you give your-self clotting factors at home.

Remember, if you're infusing clotting fac-tors for a minor bleeding episode, keep a record of it. Write down when you did the in-fusion, why you needed it, and how much clotting factor you used. Be sure to take this information with you the next time you go to the primary health care provider.

If you give yourself clotting factors for major bleeding, you or someone else must call your primary health care provider right away to tell him about it.

Use these directions to help you do what your nurse or primary health care provider taught you. To avoid infection, be sure to use only new needles and syringes every time you give yourself an infusion.

1 Gather your equipment. Make sure you have your clotting factor concentrate and sterile water, a syringe, a butterfly nee-dle set, a tourniquet, alcohol wipes, gauze pads, and tape.

2 Thoroughly wash your hands with soap and water.

3 Remove the flip-top lids on the clotting factor concentrate bottle and the sterile water bottle. Use the alcohol wipes to clean the stoppers. Add sterile water from the wa-ter bottle to the powder in the concentrate bottle to make a liquid.

4 If you're using *nonvacuum bottles,* inject air into the sterile water bottle and with-draw the water. Inject water into the concen-trate bottle. Direct the water against the bot-tle's side so that you don't make any bub-bles or foam (above, right).

Withdraw air to relieve pressure, and then withdraw the needle. Put a cap on the needle.

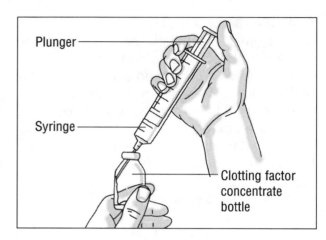

Plunger

Syringe

Clotting factor concentrate bottle

If you're using *vacuum bottles,* the idea is the same. Insert the double-ended needle into the water bottle. Then turn the needle and bottle upside down, and insert the other end of the needle into the bottle that con-tains the concentrate (below).

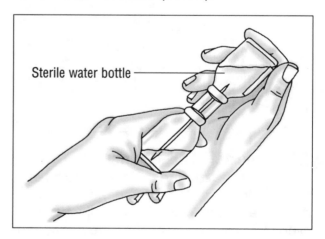

Sterile water bottle

Direct the stream of water against the side of the bottle so that you don't make bubbles or foam.

Lift the water bottle off the needle (to re-lease the vacuum). Pull the needle from the concentrate, and rotate or roll the bottle gently in your hands until the powder dis-solves completely. Clean the stopper of the concentrate bottle with a new alcohol wipe.

(continued)

Learning self-infusion of clotting factors *(continued)*

Next, transfer the dissolved concentrate into your syringe that has a needle and a filter. To do this, use the syringe to inject air into the concentrate bottle. Then pull back on the plunger to draw the reconstituted concentrate into the syringe.

5 Tear a 3" length of tape and set aside. Wrap the tourniquet around your lower arm about 3 inches above the place where you'll insert the needle into your vein. Clean the area with an alcohol wipe and let it dry.

Then loosen the hub at the end of the butterfly needle tubing to break the vacuum. Uncap the needle and insert it at a 30- to 45-degree angle through your skin into the center of the vein (below).

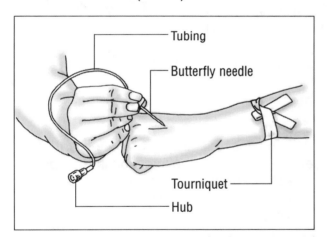

Tubing

Butterfly needle

Tourniquet

Hub

When you see blood return, lower the needle to make it level with your skin. Slide the needle slightly forward so that it won't slip from the vein.

6 Take off the tourniquet and tape the butterfly needle to your skin. Now remove the filter section of your syringe. Attach the syringe part holding the liquid concentrate to the hub of the butterfly needle's tubing. Pull back gently on the plunger of the syringe to fill the tubing with blood. Then infuse the concentrate slowly, as directed by your nurse or primary health care provider.

7 When the infusion is finished, place a gauze pad over the site and remove the needle.

❗ *Warning:* Don't apply pressure to the site as you remove the needle. It can damage the vein.

8 When you've removed the needle, apply firm pressure to the venipuncture site for 3 to 5 minutes. Make sure bleeding has stopped at the site.

9 To prevent the spread of infection, put used equipment into a special box or plastic container. Return it to the hospital or clinic. Wrap other equipment in plastic and return it also.

Additional instructions

_____

_____

_____

_____

_____

_____

_____

_____

_____

_____

_____

Giving an intramuscular injection

Dear Patient or Caregiver,

Use these instructions to review how to give an intramuscular injection.

Selecting the injection site
First choose the injection site. You can use the thigh, hip, buttock, or upper arm. If you're giving yourself the injection, use the front or side of the thigh. If someone else is giving you the injection, he can use the hip, buttock, or upper arm. If possible, though, he should avoid using the upper arm because the muscle there is small and very close to the brachial nerve.

If a series of injections is necessary, rotate the sites. To reduce pain and improve drug absorption, don't use the same site twice in a row.

Thigh
To find the target, place one hand at your knee and your other hand at your groin. As shown below, use the area marked by solid lines for adult injections. Or use the area marked by dotted lines for injections for infants and children.

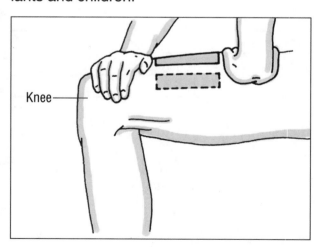

Hip
To find this site, place your right hand on the patient's left hip (or your left hand on the patient's right hip). Then spread your index and middle fingers to form a V. Your middle finger should be on the highest point of the pelvis, known as the iliac crest. The triangular area shown in the illustration below is the injection site.

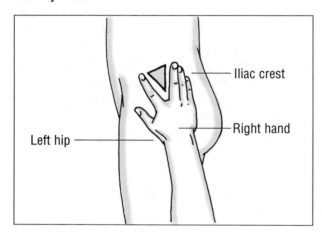

Buttock
Imagine lines dividing each buttock into four equal parts. Give the injection in the upper outermost area near the iliac crest, as shown below. Don't give it in the sciatic nerve area.

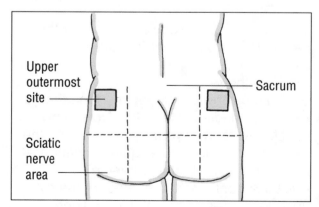

(continued)

Giving an intramuscular injection *(continued)*

Upper arm

Locate the injection site by placing one hand at the top of the patient's shoulder and extending your thumb down the patient's upper arm. Place the other hand at armpit level, as shown below. The triangular space is the injection area.

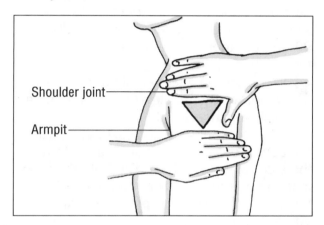

Shoulder joint

Armpit

Giving the injection

1 Wash your hands and gather the medication, alcohol swabs, syringe, and needle. Make sure you have the right medication. For safety, check the expiration date.

2 Remove the top of the medication bottle, and wipe the rubber stopper with an alcohol swab. Unwrap the syringe, and remove the needle cover.

3 Pull back on the plunger of the syringe until you've drawn air into it in an amount equal to the medication you'll be injecting. Insert the needle into the bottle through the rubber stopper. Then inject the air in the syringe into the bottle without withdrawing the needle. This will prevent formation of a vacuum and will make withdrawing the medication easier.

4 Invert the medication bottle. With the needle positioned below the fluid level, draw the medication into the syringe by pulling back on the plunger while you measure the correct amount by checking the markings on the side of the syringe (below). Draw a little extra into the syringe. Then withdraw the needle from the bottle.

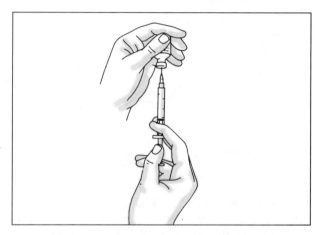

5 Next, check for air bubbles in the syringe. If you see any, hold the syringe with the needle pointing up, and tap the syringe lightly so that the bubbles rise to its top. Then push the plunger to discharge the air. Recheck the dose in the syringe.

Again, hold the syringe with the needle pointing up, and pull back on the plunger just a little bit more. This will cause a tiny air bubble to form inside the syringe; when you inject the medication, this bubble will help clear the needle and keep the medication from seeping out of the injection site. Replace the needle cover.

6 Check the injection site for lumps, depressions, redness, warmth, or bruising on the skin.

(continued)

Giving an intramuscular injection *(continued)*

7 Clean the site with an alcohol swab (below), beginning at the center and wiping outward in a circular pattern to move dirt particles away from the site.

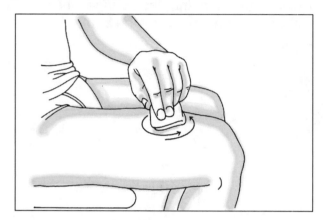

Let the skin dry for 5 to 10 seconds. If it's not dry, the injection might push some of the alcohol into the skin, causing a burning sensation.

8 Remove the needle cover. Now, with one hand, stretch the skin taut around the injection site. This makes inserting the needle easier and helps disperse the medication after the injection.

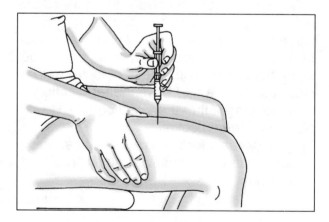

With your other hand, hold the syringe and needle at a 90-degree angle to the injection site (above). Then insert the needle with a quick thrust.

9 Holding the syringe firmly in place, remove the hand stretching your skin and use it to pull back slightly on the plunger. If blood appears in the syringe, you've entered a blood vessel. Take the needle out and press an alcohol swab over the site. Then discard everything and start again. If no blood appears, inject the medication slowly, keeping the syringe and needle at a 90-degree angle. Never push the plunger forcefully.

10 When you've injected all the medication, withdraw the needle at the same angle at which you inserted it.

Using a circular motion (extending from the center outward), massage the site with the alcohol swab to help distribute the medication and promote its absorption (unless the primary health care provider instructs you not to do so).

11 Do not recap the needle. Place the used syringe with the needle attached in a covered, puncture-resistant container reserved only for disposal of needles and syringes. Keep the container in a safe place until you can dispose of it; then dispose of it properly.

Additional instructions

_____

_____

_____

_____

_____

_____

_____

_____

_____

_____

Caring for a central venous catheter

Dear Patient,

To keep your central venous catheter trouble-free, you must flush the catheter and change the dressing regularly.

How to flush the catheter

Flush the catheter at least once a day to prevent blood clots from forming in it.

1 Gather the following equipment: a bottle of heparin flush solution, a disposable syringe with needle, two alcohol or povidone-iodine swabs, several sterile 4-inch-square gauze pads, and tape. Now wash and dry your hands. Open the bottle of heparin flush solution, and wipe the bottle top with an alcohol or povidone-iodine swab. *Don't touch the top after you've cleaned it.*

2 Pick up the syringe, remove the needle cover, and pull back the syringe plunger. Pull back on the plunger until the amount of air in the syringe equals the amount of solution that you'll withdraw from the heparin bottle (below). Then insert the needle into the heparin solution bottle top, and push down on the plunger. Turn the bottle upside down, as shown, and pull back on the syringe plunger to fill the syringe with the correct amount of solution. Remove the needle from the bottle, and put the bottle aside. Replace the needle cover.

3 Remove and discard the gauze pad protecting the end of the catheter. Using a clean povidone-iodine or alcohol swab, wipe the rubber injection cap at the end of the catheter (below). When the cap is dry, open the catheter's clamp. Remove the needle cover, and insert the needle into the rubber injection cap at the end of the catheter.

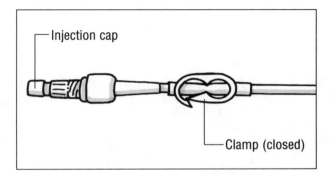

Injection cap

Clamp (closed)

Push down on the syringe plunger to inject the solution into the catheter. Withdraw the needle, and close the clamp. Wrap the catheter end in a sterile gauze pad, and tape it on top of the dressing.

How to change the dressing

Change the dressing over the catheter every other day or whenever it becomes wet or dirty. When you change your dressing, carefully check the skin around the catheter. Call the primary health care provider at once if you see any sign of infection, such as redness, swelling, or pus. Also call him if a fever or pain develops.

1 To change the dressing, obtain a dressing change kit or assemble the supplies recommended by your nurse or primary health care provider. Then wash your hands and remove the soiled dressing. Wash your hands again. (If suggested by your primary

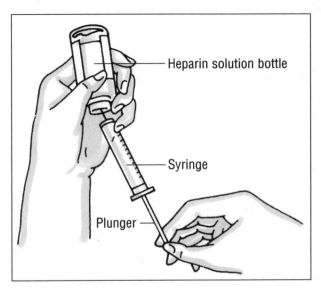

Heparin solution bottle

Syringe

Plunger

(continued)

Caring for a central venous catheter *(continued)*

health care provider, you may want to put on sterile gloves to avoid possible contamination.)

Clean the skin around the catheter with an alcohol swab, beginning near the catheter and working outward in a circular motion (below). Repeat the procedure, using a povidone-iodine swab.

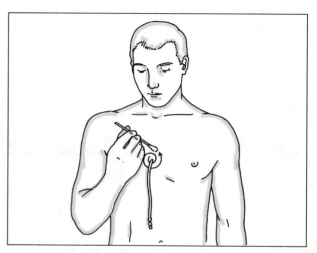

2 Squeeze some povidone-iodine ointment onto a sterile gauze pad (below). Put the pad over the catheter exit site. Cover it with a dry sterile gauze pad. If you're using a transparent dressing, follow the instructions from your nurse or primary health care provider.

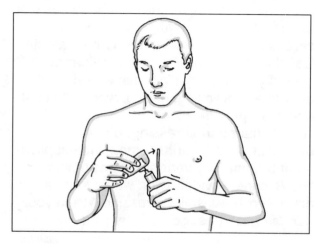

3 Apply adhesive tape over the gauze pads and put an extra layer of tape around the edge (as shown below) to secure the bandage to your skin. Wrap the catheter end in a sterile gauze pad, and tape it on top of the bandage.

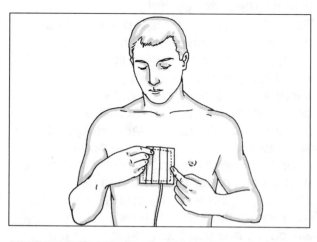

Additional instructions

_____

_____

_____

_____

_____

_____

_____

_____

_____

_____

_____

_____

Caring for an implanted port

Dear Patient,

Here are some guidelines for flushing and injecting medication into your implanted port.

Flushing the port

To keep your implanted port trouble-free, flush the port according to your primary health care provider's instructions (usually monthly). Check with your primary health care provider if you develop a fever or if you observe redness, pain, swelling, or pus at the port site.

1 Gather the following equipment: a 10-ml syringe with needle, a bottle of heparin (if you don't have a prefilled syringe), a special needle (called a Huber needle, which may be bent at a 90-degree angle), one or two alcohol swabs, and one or two povidone-iodine swabs. Wash your hands. Open the bottle of heparin, and wipe the top with an alcohol or povidone-iodine swab. *Don't touch the top after you've cleaned it.*

2 Remove the needle cover from the syringe needle, and pull back the syringe plunger, permitting air to enter the syringe. Pull back on the plunger until the amount of air in the syringe equals the amount of solution that you'll withdraw from the heparin bottle.

   Then insert the needle into the heparin bottle top and push down on the plunger. Turn the bottle upside down, and pull back on the syringe plunger to fill the syringe with solution to the correct amount. Now remove the needle from the bottle and put the bottle aside. Be sure to replace the needle cover until you've prepared the injection site.

   Change the needle on the heparin flush syringe to the Huber needle.

3 Locate your port by feeling for the small bump on your skin. (The site is over a bony area, usually on the upper chest.)

4 Clean the injection site with an alcohol swab (allow the site to air dry) and then a povidone-iodine swab. As shown below, hold the port between two fingers.

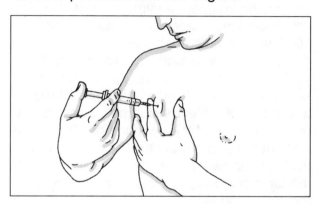

   Push the Huber needle firmly through the skin and port septum until it hits the bottom of the port's chamber. Be sure the needle is inserted at a 90-degree angle (below).

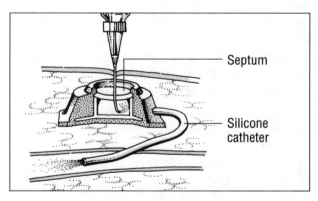

Septum

Silicone catheter

5 Now push down on the syringe plunger, which will inject the heparin solution into the port. You'll normally feel a small amount of resistance. Notify the primary health care provider immediately if the solution will not flow into the port.

6 Remove the needle. To keep the solution from flowing back into the syringe when you remove the needle, continue to push down slowly on the syringe plunger as you withdraw the needle.

(continued)

Caring for an implanted port *(continued)*

Injecting medication into the port

1 Gather the needed equipment: an extension set with a special needle (Huber needle) and a clamp, a 10-ml syringe filled with saline solution, a syringe containing the prescribed medication, a sterile syringe filled with heparin flush solution, a povidone-iodine swab, and two alcohol swabs.

2 Wash and dry your hands. Attach the 10-ml syringe filled with saline solution to the end of the extension set. Gently push on the plunger of the syringe until the extension tubing and needle are filled with solution and all the air is removed. Make sure all the air is removed by flicking the tubing of the extension set.

3 Locate the port by feeling for the small bump on your skin. Hold the port between two fingers. Clean the site with an alcohol swab and then a povidone-iodine swab.

4 Remove the needle cover from the Huber needle. Insert the Huber needle through the skin and port septum until it hits the bottom of the port's chamber. Be sure the needle is inserted at a 90-degree angle.

5 Check for a blood return by pulling back on the syringe that's attached to the extension set.

6 Flush the port with 5 ml of saline solution by pushing down on the plunger of the syringe with the saline solution.

7 Clamp the extension set and remove the saline-filled syringe.

8 Connect the medication-filled syringe to the extension set. Open the clamp and inject the medication, as ordered by your primary health care provider.

9 Check the skin around the needle for swelling and tenderness. If you note these signs, stop the injection and call your primary health care provider.

10 When the injection is complete, clamp the extension set and remove the medication syringe.

11 Attach the saline-filled syringe to the extension set. Then open the clamp and flush the port again with 5 ml of saline solution by pushing down on the plunger of the syringe. Remember to flush the port with saline after each medication injection to minimize medication interactions.

12 Clamp the extension set and remove the syringe. Attach a syringe filled with heparin flush solution to the extension set. Open the clamp and flush the port with heparin, as directed by your nurse or primary health care provider. Clamp the extension set as you finish flushing, and remove the syringe. Put a protective cap on the end of the extension set if you've been directed to leave it in place.

13 Tape the needle in place and apply a dressing, as directed by your nurse or primary health care provider.

Additional instructions

_____
_____
_____
_____
_____
_____
_____
_____
_____
_____
_____
_____

Caring for a PICC at home

Dear Patient,

Your primary health care provider (or a specially trained nurse) has inserted a peripherally inserted central catheter (PICC) into your body to continue intravenous therapy at home. The catheter is typically inserted into a vein in the arm and threaded into a larger blood vessel near the heart, as shown at the right.

Here are some guidelines to help you care for your PICC at home.
• Continue to do your normal daily activities while the catheter is in.
• Flush the PICC line with heparin as instructed by your health care provider. Make sure you understand the I.V. therapy procedure and how to flush the line. Don't be afraid to ask questions until you fully understand all procedures.
• Check the insertion site for fluid, drainage, redness, bleeding, or swelling every 24 hours. Look through the transparent dressing—don't remove the dressing yourself. If you notice any of the above symptoms, call your primary health care provider or home health agency nurse immediately.
• Call your primary health care provider or nurse immediately if you notice an increase in the length of the catheter extending out of your skin.
• Never use scissors near the PICC line.
• If your catheter tears, promptly tape the end to your arm and notify your primary health care provider or nurse.
• Keep a record of the type, brand name, and size of your catheter as well as the insertion site, date, and time. Your primary health care provider or nurse will need this information if complications occur and when it's time to remove the catheter.
• Before showering, wrap the PICC insertion site in plastic wrap and tape both the top and bottom. Don't get the dressing wet.

• Don't have your blood pressure taken in the arm with the PICC. This may damage the catheter.

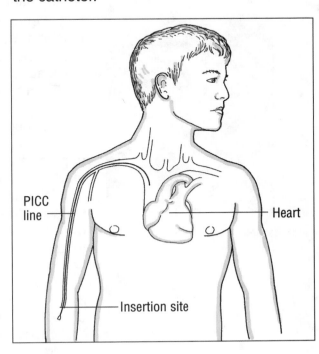

Additional instructions

_____
_____
_____
_____
_____
_____
_____
_____
_____
_____
_____

Medications and drug classes

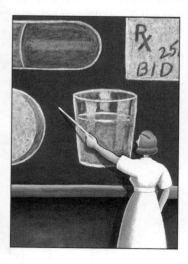

The teaching aids in this section reflect the most commonly prescribed drugs and drug classes taken by patients at home. Designed for easy use, these teaching aids explain in simple terms what the patient can expect during drug therapy. For your quick access, they're arranged in alphabetical order.

Each teaching aid follows the same format. An introduction identifies the conditions the medication treats, such as allergy symptoms or high blood pressure. It then lists a few common trade names. When appropriate, the introduction also mentions how the medication works.

Following the introduction, *How to take this drug* specifies the administration directions. This section may also give special instructions on how and when to take the medication, especially if the medication has more than one form.

If your patient sometimes forgets to take his medication, he can refer to *What to do if you miss a dose*. This section lists what steps to take to get back on schedule — such as skipping a dose or adjusting the timing of the next dose — and usually emphasizes not to take double doses.

The following section, *What to do about side effects*, identifies the medication's common and life-threatening reactions — and tells when to call the primary health care provider right away. Next, the section *What you must know about other drugs* will alert your patient to possible interactions with other drugs or alcohol. He may not think, for instance, that he needs to be concerned about a nonprescription cold medication he's taking. As necessary, the teaching aid will caution him about potentially hazardous nonprescription and prescription drugs.

(continued)

Medications and drug classes (continued)

Special directions covers such topics as other medical conditions the patient should report and tips on how to combat side effects. The *Warning* logo may appear in any of these sections and provides critical information about the drug, including dangerous drug interactions, essential preparation and storage information, and key administration cautions.

In the final section, *Keep in mind*, pregnant or breast-feeding patients, elderly patients, athletes, and others will find specific information about their use of the medication.

Taking acebutolol

Dear Patient,

Acebutolol will help control your high blood pressure or correct your irregular heartbeat. The label may read Sectral.

How to take acebutolol

Acebutolol comes in long-acting capsules. Carefully read the medication label, and follow the directions exactly. Don't break, chew, or crush the capsule. Swallow it whole.

Always check your pulse rate before taking acebutolol. If it's under 50 beats a minute, call your primary health care provider and don't take the dose.

What to do if you miss a dose

If you forget to take your medication, take it as soon as you remember. But if it's within 4 hours of your next dose, skip the dose you missed and take your next dose at the regular time. Don't take two doses together.

What to do about side effects

Call the primary health care provider *right away* if you have trouble breathing or swallowing. Also notify your primary health care provider if you feel very tired or light-headed (a symptom of low blood pressure).

What you must know about other drugs

Tell the primary health care provider what other medications you're taking because they can affect how acebutolol works. For example, taking acebutolol with digoxin (Lanoxin) can slow your heart too much, whereas taking it with indomethacin (Indocin) can reduce acebutolol's effect.

Warning: If you take medication for diabetes, check your blood glucose levels carefully. That's because acebutolol can hide signs of low blood glucose levels.

Special directions

• Be sure you know how you react to this medication before driving or performing activities requiring alertness.
• If you feel tired after taking this medication, plan frequent rest periods.
• Don't abruptly stop taking acebutolol. Doing so may lead to heart problems.
• Before you have surgery, dental work, or emergency treatment, tell the primary health care provider that you're taking acebutolol.
• Check with your primary health care provider or pharmacist before taking nonprescription drugs.

✔ Keep in mind

• Notify your health care provider if you become pregnant while taking acebutolol.
• Tell your primary health care provider about medical conditions you have, such as chronic lung disease, diabetes, heart or blood vessel disease, kidney or liver disease, depression, thyroid problems, or an unusually slow heartbeat.
• If you have diabetes, keep a fast-acting carbohydrate such as a box of raisins nearby in case your blood glucose level drops.
• Tell your primary health care provider and pharmacist if you're allergic to acebutolol or other medications, foods, preservatives, or dyes. Acebutolol may make allergic reactions worse and harder to treat.
• If you're an athlete, you should know that the National Collegiate Athletic Association and the U.S. Olympic Committee have banned acebutolol's use.

Additional instructions

_____
_____
_____
_____

Taking acetaminophen

Dear Patient,

Known by many names (Anacin-3, Panadol, Tylenol, and others), acetaminophen relieves mild pain and fever.

How to take acetaminophen

Acetaminophen comes in many forms: capsule, oral liquid, tablet, chewable tablet, and suppository.

Carefully read and follow precautions listed on the package label. If you're an adult, you can take a dose of acetaminophen every 4 hours as needed, but don't exceed eight tablets a day. You may repeat a child's dose every 4 hours (but don't exceed five doses a day).

If you're using a *suppository* and it's too soft to insert, chill it in the refrigerator for 30 minutes or run cold water over it before you remove the foil wrapper. Then you can insert the medication.

What to do if you miss a dose

If you forget to take your medication, take it as soon as you remember. If it's almost time for your next dose, skip the missed dose and resume your regular schedule. Don't take two doses together.

What to do about side effects

Call the primary health care provider if a rash or hives develop or if your skin turns yellowish.

What you must know about alcohol and other drugs

Don't drink alcoholic beverages when taking acetaminophen because this combination may cause liver damage, especially if you take acetaminophen regularly for a long time.

Check with the primary health care provider or pharmacist before taking any nonprescription drugs. Many contain aceta-

minophen and count toward your total dosage.

Tell your primary health care provider if you're taking diflunisal (Dolobid), which may increase acetaminophen's effects, or warfarin (Coumadin), which may cause bleeding with long-term acetaminophen use.

Special directions

• If acetaminophen doesn't relieve pain after 10 days (adults) or 5 days (children), notify the primary health care provider. If you have new symptoms, if the pain gets worse, or if the pain site appears red and swollen, also contact the primary health care provider.
• If acetaminophen doesn't make a fever go away within 3 days, call the primary health care provider. Also call him if the fever returns or rises or if new symptoms, redness, or swelling occurs.

Warning: Large doses of acetaminophen may cause liver damage. Call the primary health care provider if your skin turns yellowish.

✔ Keep in mind

• Give this medication to a child under age 2 only as prescribed by a primary health care provider.
• Tell the primary health care provider if you have medical problems, particularly if you have diabetes, kidney or liver disease, or blood disorders.
• If you have diabetes, check your blood glucose level carefully. Acetaminophen can affect test results, so contact your primary health care provider about unusual changes.

Additional instructions

_____

_____

_____

Taking acetaminophen with butalbital and caffeine

Dear Patient,

This medication is usually prescribed to treat moderately severe tension headaches. The medication label may read Esgic or Fioricet.

How to take this drug

This medication comes in tablet and capsule forms. Carefully read the medication label and follow the directions exactly. Don't take more than six tablets or capsules in a day. If you don't feel better, call your primary health care provider. Don't increase the dose on your own.

To minimize stomach upset, you may take this medication with milk or meals.

What to do if you miss a dose

If you forget to take your medication, take it as soon as you remember. But if it's almost time for your next dose, skip the missed dose and take the next regular dose. Don't take double doses.

What to do about side effects

If you get allergy symptoms (itching, a rash, difficulty breathing or swallowing), stop taking this medication and notify the primary health care provider *immediately*.

The medication may also cause confusion, dizziness, drowsiness, light-headedness, nausea, stomach pain, and vomiting. If these symptoms persist or increase, contact your primary health care provider.

What you must know about alcohol and other drugs

Don't take this medication with alcoholic beverages, drugs that relax you or make you feel sleepy, antihistamines, or other drugs that may decrease your activity level.

Check with your primary health care provider or pharmacist before taking any nonprescription medications. Many contain acetaminophen and should be counted as part of your total daily dosage. In normal amounts, acetaminophen safely and effectively relieves pain. But in high doses, it can damage the liver.

Tell your primary health care provider if you're taking diflunisal (Dolobid) because it may increase the effects of acetaminophen.

Special directions

● Be aware of your response to this medication before driving or performing other activities requiring alertness.

● *Warning:* Don't stop taking this medication suddenly. Your primary health care provider may recommend reducing the dosage before stopping completely. Don't take more than the prescribed amount, and don't take the medication longer than your primary health care provider directs.

✔ Keep in mind

● If you're pregnant or breast-feeding, check with your primary health care provider before taking this medication.
● Inform the primary health care provider about your medical history, particularly if you have diabetes, kidney or liver disease, or blood disorders.
● If you're an athlete, you should know that the National Collegiate Athletic Association and the U.S. Olympic Committee ban the use of this drug.

Additional instructions

_____

_____

_____

_____

_____

Taking acetaminophen with codeine

Dear Patient,

This medication relieves moderately severe pain. The medication label may read Fiorinal with codeine or Tylenol with codeine.

How to take this drug

You may take this medication as a tablet, capsule, or liquid (usually every 4 to 6 hours). To minimize stomach upset, you may take it with milk or meals.

Carefully read the medication label and follow the directions exactly. If you don't feel better, call the primary health care provider. Don't increase the dose on your own.

What to do if you miss a dose

If you forget to take your medication, take it as soon as you remember. But if it's almost time for your next dose, skip the missed dose and take the next regular dose. Don't take double doses.

What to do about side effects

If you have difficulty breathing or swallowing, a rash, or other signs of an allergic reaction, stop taking this medication and get medical help.

The medication may cause confusion, dizziness, drowsiness, light-headedness, stomach pain, nausea, vomiting, and constipation. If any of these symptoms persist, call the primary health care provider.

What you must know about alcohol and other drugs

Don't take this medication with alcoholic beverages, sedatives, antihistamines, or other drugs that decrease your activity.

Check with the primary health care provider or pharmacist before taking non-prescription medications. Many contain acetaminophen and should be counted toward your daily dosage. In normal amounts, acetaminophen is safe; in high doses, it can damage the liver.

Tell your primary health care provider if you're taking diflunisal (Dolobid) because it may increase acetaminophen's effects.

Special directions

• Avoid driving and other activities that require mental alertness until you know how this medication affects you.
• To avoid possible constipation, include plenty of fluids and fiber in your diet.
• This medication can be habit-forming. Take just the prescribed amount for only as long as directed.
• Sharing this medication is against federal law.

✓ Keep in mind

• If you're breast-feeding or pregnant, talk to your primary health care provider before taking this medication.
• Tell the primary health care provider about your medical history, particularly head injury, severe headaches, diabetes, kidney or liver disease, or blood disorders.
• Don't take this medication if you're allergic to acetaminophen or to codeine, morphine, or other opiates.
• If you're an athlete, you should know that the National Collegiate Athletic Association and the U.S. Olympic Committee ban the use of this medication.

Additional instructions

_____

_____

_____

_____

_____

_____

Taking acetaminophen with hydrocodone/oxycodone

Dear Patient,

This medication helps relieve moderately severe pain. The medication label may read Lortab, Vicodin, Dolacet, or Hydrocet (acetaminophen with hydrocodone), or Percocet (acetaminophen with oxycodone).

How to take this drug

Available in tablets, capsules, and oral liquids, this medication can usually be taken every 4 to 6 hours as needed.

Carefully read the medication label and follow directions exactly. If you don't feel better, call your primary health care provider. Don't increase the dose on your own.

What to do if you miss a dose

If you forget to take your medication, take it as soon as you remember. But if it's almost time for the next dose, skip the missed dose and resume your regular schedule. Don't take double doses.

What to do about side effects

If you have a rash, difficulty breathing, or other signs of an allergic reaction, stop taking the medication and notify your primary health care provider *immediately*.

Other possible side effects include confusion, dizziness, drowsiness, light-headedness, itching, stomach pain, nausea, vomiting, and constipation. If these symptoms continue or become severe, call your health care provider.

What you must know about alcohol and other drugs

Avoid taking this medication with alcoholic beverages, medications that relax or sedate you, antihistamines, and other drugs that decrease your activity level.

Check with the primary health care provider or pharmacist before taking any nonprescription medications. Many contain acetaminophen and should be counted toward your daily dosage. In normal doses, acetaminophen is safe and effective; in high doses, it can damage the liver.

Tell your primary health care provider if you're taking diflunisal (Dolobid) because it may increase acetaminophen's effect.

Special directions

• Avoid driving and other activities that require mental alertness until you know how this medication affects you.
• To combat possible constipation, consume plenty of fluids and fiber.
• This medication may be habit-forming. Take just the amount prescribed only as long as directed.
• Sharing this medication is against federal law.

✓ Keep in mind

• If you're pregnant or breast-feeding, talk to your primary health care provider before taking this medication.
• Inform the primary health care provider about your medical history, especially head injury, severe headaches, diabetes, kidney or liver disease, or blood disorders.
• Don't take this medication if you're allergic to acetaminophen or to codeine, morphine, or other opiates.
• If you're an athlete, you should know that the National Collegiate Athletic Association and the U.S. Olympic Committee ban this medication's use.

Additional instructions

_____

_____

_____

_____

Taking acetazolamide

Dear Patient,

This medication helps control glaucoma, certain types of seizures, and heart failure. The medication label may read Dazamide or Diamox.

How to take acetazolamide

This medication comes in tablet, long-acting capsule, and injectable forms.

Carefully check the label, and follow the directions exactly. This medication increases urination, so if you take it once a day, take it in the morning with breakfast. If you take it more than once a day, take the last dose no later than 6 p.m., unless the primary health care provider tells you otherwise.

Take acetazolamide with food or milk to minimize the chance of an upset stomach. If you have difficulty swallowing tablets, you can mix a tablet in 2 teaspoons of hot water and 2 teaspoons of honey or syrup. If you have trouble swallowing capsules, call the primary health care provider.

What to do if you miss a dose

Take it as soon as you remember. But if it's almost time for your next dose, skip the missed dose and take the next dose at the regular time. Don't take double doses.

What to do about side effects

Notify your health care provider as soon as possible if you start to bruise or bleed easily or if you develop a fever or sore throat.

Special directions

• Take only the amount of medication the primary health care provider ordered. If you think you need more, consult your primary health care provider.
• Until you know how this medication affects you, avoid driving or any activity that requires alertness and coordination.

• If this medication causes your body to lose potassium, your primary health care provider may advise consuming potassium-rich foods and fluids, including bananas, potatoes, unsalted peanuts, and orange juice. Or the primary health care provider may order a potassium supplement for you. Don't change your diet, however, without first consulting your primary health care provider.

✓ Keep in mind

• Inform your primary health care provider about your medical history, especially if you have Addison's disease, diabetes, gout, or kidney, liver, or lung disease.
• If you have diabetes, carefully monitor glucose levels in your blood and urine. This medication may increase glucose levels.
• If you're taking acetazolamide to control seizures, don't suddenly stop taking it.
• If you become pregnant while taking this medication, notify your primary health care provider.
• If you're an athlete, you should know that the National Collegiate Athletic Association and the U.S. Olympic Committee ban acetazolamide's use.

Additional instructions

_____
_____
_____
_____
_____
_____
_____
_____
_____
_____

Taking acyclovir

Dear Patient,

This medication, which is also called Zovirax, treats infections caused by the herpes virus, such as genital herpes and shingles. It's also given for chickenpox. Although this medication won't cure you, it will make you feel more comfortable and shorten your illness.

How to take acyclovir

Carefully read the label on your medication, which may be in capsule, tablet, liquid (oral suspension), or ointment form. Follow the directions exactly.

Take acyclovir until your prescription is finished, even if your symptoms subside and you begin to feel better. Try not to miss any doses, but don't take the medication more often or longer than directed.

Take the *capsule, tablet,* or *liquid* form of acyclovir with meals to minimize possible stomach upset. If you're taking *liquid* acyclovir, measure each dose accurately by using a measuring spoon. Don't use a household teaspoon.

If you're using *ointment,* wear a disposable glove to apply the medication. Doing this helps prevent spreading the infection to other body areas. Apply enough ointment to cover each herpes blister. A ½-inch strip of ointment will cover about 2 square inches.

What to do if you miss a dose

Take the dose as soon as you remember. But if it's almost time for your next dose, skip the missed one and take the next one at your regularly scheduled time. Don't take two doses together.

What to do about side effects

The medication may cause nausea and vomiting. If these symptoms persist or become worse, contact your primary health care provider.

What you must know about other drugs

Be sure to tell the primary health care provider what other medications you're taking — especially probenecid (Benemid), which may make acyclovir's effects stronger. Also tell the primary health care provider if you're taking zidovudine (also called AZT or Retrovir) because this combination may cause drowsiness.

Special directions

• Avoid sexual activity if either you or your partner has herpes symptoms. Acyclovir will not prevent the spread of herpes between partners. Using a latex condom may help prevent the spread of herpes, but using a spermicidal jelly or a diaphragm probably won't.
• Keep the areas affected by herpes clean and dry. Also, wear loose-fitting clothing to avoid irritating the sores.
• Never apply the ointment form of acyclovir to your eyes.

✓ Keep in mind

• If you're a woman and have genital herpes, be sure to have a Pap test at least once a year.
• Tell your primary health care provider if you have kidney disease, as this may increase the amount of acyclovir in your blood.

Additional instructions

_____
_____
_____
_____
_____
_____

Taking albuterol

Dear Patient,

Albuterol is prescribed for bronchial asthma, chronic bronchitis, emphysema, and other lung disorders. It relieves coughing, wheezing, shortness of breath, and breathing difficulties by improving the flow of air in the lungs. Albuterol is also known as Proventil and Ventolin.

How to take albuterol

You may take albuterol in syrup, tablet, extended-release tablet, or aerosol form. Or you may use an albuterol solution with a nebulizer.

Carefully read the medication label. Follow the directions exactly. Don't increase the amount or frequency of your dose without consulting your primary health care provider.

Don't break or chew an *extended-release tablet;* swallow it whole.

Use your nebulizer or other breathing device exactly as you were taught. Don't take more than two inhalations at a time, unless directed. Wait 1 to 2 minutes after the first inhalation to be sure you need another. If you need another breathing device in less than 2 weeks, you may be taking too much medication. As needed, check with your primary health care provider or pharmacist.

What to do if you miss a dose

Take a missed dose as soon as possible. Take any remaining doses for that day at regularly spaced intervals. Don't take double doses.

What to do about side effects

You may experience tremors, nervousness, dizziness, difficulty sleeping, headaches, or an unusual taste in your mouth. If these symptoms persist, call your primary health care provider.

What you must know about other drugs

Tell your primary health care provider what other medications you're taking because they may affect the way albuterol works. For example, some medications for depression may affect the heart and blood vessels. And some heart medications may keep albuterol from working properly.

Special directions

• If you still have trouble breathing after using albuterol or if your condition is worse, contact your primary health care provider.
• If you're taking two aerosol medications — such as albuterol and an adrenocorticoid medication or ipratropium (Atrovent) — inhale the albuterol first. Wait about 5 minutes and then use the adrenocorticoid or the ipratropium. Taking albuterol first opens your air passages and helps the next medication work better.

✓ Keep in mind

• Tell your primary health care provider if you become pregnant while taking this medication.
• *Warning:* If you have diabetes, albuterol may increase your glucose level. Contact your primary health care provider if you notice a change in your blood or urine test results.
• If you're an athlete, you should know that the U.S. Olympic Committee permits the use of inhalation aerosol and inhalation solution forms of albuterol.

Additional instructions

_____

_____

_____

_____

Taking alendronate

Dear Patient,

Your primary health care provider has prescribed alendronate because you have osteoporosis or Paget's disease. This medication will improve your condition by helping to maximize bone formation. The brand name of this medication is Fosamax.

How to take alendronate

This medication is available as a tablet. Take it with 6 to 8 ounces of plain water, first thing in the morning. Wait at least 30 minutes before you eat, drink, or take any other medication.

What to do if you miss a dose

Do not take the missed medication later in the day. Continue your usual dosing schedule the next day.

What to do about side effects

You may experience flatulence (gas), indigestion-like symptoms, headache, and muscle or bone pain. Contact your primary health care provider or pharmacist if these symptoms persist or become severe.

What you must know about other drugs

If you regularly take antacids or calcium supplements, don't take them until 30 minutes after you take alendronate. Taking both medications together will decrease the benefit of alendronate.

Tell your primary health care provider if you take aspirin or aspirin-like pain relievers, such as a group of drugs called nonsteroidal anti-inflammatory drugs (NSAIDs). Taking these drugs with alendronate may increase your chance of stomach upset.

Inform your primary health care provider if you're on hormone replacement therapy — you shouldn't be taking alendronate.

Special directions

• Don't take this medication with any liquid other than plain water. Other liquids, such as coffee, orange juice, or mineral water, may decrease the medication's effectiveness.

! *Warning:* Don't lie down for 30 minutes after taking alendronate because stomach upset may occur.

• Tell the primary health care provider if you don't eat enough foods rich in vitamin D or calcium. He may prescribe vitamin supplements.

• Increasing the amount you exercise and cutting down on smoking and alcohol may help your condition. Ask your primary health care provider about this.

✔ Keep in mind

• If you're pregnant or breast-feeding, be sure to tell your primary health care provider before taking this medication.

• Older adults are more likely to experience side effects with alendronate.

Additional instructions

_____
_____
_____
_____
_____
_____
_____
_____
_____
_____
_____

Taking allopurinol

Dear Patient,

Allopurinol treats chronic gout (gouty arthritis) by decreasing the amount of uric acid produced by the body. The name on your medication may be Lopurin or Zyloprim.

How to take allopurinol
This medication is available as a tablet. Carefully read the label, and follow the directions exactly. To work effectively, allopurinol must be taken regularly as directed by your primary health care provider.

Take allopurinol after a meal if you find that it upsets your stomach. Drink ten to twelve 8-ounce glasses of liquid each day unless your primary health care provider directs otherwise. And continue to take allopurinol even if you take another medication for gout attacks.

What to do if you miss a dose
Take the dose as soon as you remember. But if it's almost time for your next dose, skip the missed dose and take the next dose at the regular time. Don't take double doses.

What to do about side effects
Contact your primary health care provider *immediately* if you have a rash, skin ulcers, hives, itching, blood in your urine, trouble breathing, chest tightness, or unusual bruising, bleeding, or weakness.

Common side effects include drowsiness, diarrhea, nausea, and vomiting. If any of these symptoms persist or become worse, call your primary health care provider.

What you must know about alcohol and other drugs
Avoid alcoholic beverages or limit the amount you drink. Too much alcohol may increase the uric acid in your blood and decrease the benefit of allopurinol.

Inform your primary health care provider about other medications that you're taking. Combining oral anticoagulants (blood thinners) and allopurinol may increase your risk for abnormal bleeding. Taken with allopurinol, medications such as azathioprine (Imuran) or mercaptopurine (Purinethol) may increase the chance of serious side effects.

Also consult your primary health care provider before taking nonprescription preparations. Taking too much vitamin C, for instance, may increase your risk for kidney stones.

Special directions
- Until you know how allopurinol affects you, avoid driving and other activities that require alertness.
- Have regular checkups so your primary health care provider can monitor your progress and the effects of allopurinol.

✔ Keep in mind
- Tell the primary health care provider about any other medical problems you have, especially diabetes, high blood pressure, or kidney disease. Your allopurinol dosage may need to be adjusted.
- *Warning:* If you have diabetes, albuterol may increase your glucose level. Contact your primary health care provider if you notice a change in your blood or urine test results.
- Allopurinol is used to prevent gout attacks and will not relieve an attack that has already started.

Additional instructions
_____
_____
_____

Taking alprazolam

Dear Patient,

This medication relieves anxiety or tension caused by unusual stress. Alprazolam is also known as Xanax.

How to take alprazolam
This medication is available as a tablet. Carefully read the label, and follow the directions exactly.

What to do if you miss a dose
If you're using this medication regularly and you miss a dose, take it right way if it's within an hour or so of the scheduled time. Later than that, skip the missed dose and take the next dose at the regular time. Don't take double doses.

What to do about side effects
Alprazolam may make you feel drowsy, dizzy, light-headed, clumsy, unsteady, or less alert than usual. Even if you take this medication at bedtime, you may feel drowsy or sluggish when you wake up. If these feelings persist or become severe, contact your primary health care provider.

What you must know about alcohol and other drugs
Avoid alcoholic beverages and other central nervous system depressants (including hay fever, allergy, or cold remedies), which may cause excessive drowsiness. When taken with alprazolam, cimetidine (Tagamet) may also increase drowsiness.

Tell your primary health care provider about other medications you're taking. Their dosages may need to be adjusted because of combined effects with alprazolam.

Special directions
• See your primary health care provider at least every 4 months to evaluate whether you need to continue this medication.
• Let all your primary health care providers know that you're taking alprazolam because it may change certain medical test results.
• If you're having dental work that will require an anesthetic, tell your dentist that you're taking alprazolam.

! *Warning:* Don't abruptly stop taking this medication without consulting your primary health care provider. To prevent withdrawal effects, he may reduce your dosage gradually.

• If you think you may have taken an overdose, get emergency help. Overdose signs include continuing slurred speech or confusion, severe drowsiness, and staggering.
• Be sure you know how this medication affects you before you drive or perform other activities requiring alertness.

✔ **Keep in mind**
• If you're breast-feeding or pregnant, be sure to tell your primary health care provider before taking this medication.
• Children and older adults are more likely to experience side effects with alprazolam.
• If you're an athlete, you should know that alprazolam use is banned in most athletic events sponsored by the National Collegiate Athletic Association and the U.S. Olympic Committee.

Additional instructions
_____
_____
_____
_____
_____
_____

Taking aluminum and magnesium hydroxides

Dear Patient,

Called by the brand names Di-Gel, Gelusil, and Maalox, this medication relieves heartburn, acid indigestion, and symptoms of an ulcer. Some of these products contain simethicone, an ingredient that relieves the symptoms of excess gas.

How to take this drug

This medication is available in tablets, capsules, and liquid. Follow the instructions on the package exactly.

If your primary health care provider gave you special instructions on how to use it and how much to take, follow those instructions.

What to do if you miss a dose

If you're taking this medication on a regular schedule, take the missed dose as soon as you remember. However, if it's almost time for your next regular dose, skip the missed dose and resume your regular schedule. Never take two doses together.

What to do about side effects

Constipation or diarrhea may occur. If these problems persist or are bothersome, call your primary health care provider. Stools may also become whitish or speckled, but this is normal with this medication.

What you must know about other drugs

Check with your primary health care provider or pharmacist before taking any other medication because this medication may change the way other medications work or vice versa.

Warning: As a general rule, don't take this medication within 2 hours of taking any other medication by mouth. However, if you're taking tetracycline, ketoconazole (Nizoral), ciprofloxacin (Cipro), or methenamine (Hiprex), you should wait 3 hours after a dose before taking this medication.

Special directions

- Be sure your primary health care provider knows about your medical history, particularly a bone fracture, appendicitis, colitis, severe constipation, hemorrhoids, an inflamed bowel, intestinal blockage or bleeding, rectal bleeding, a colostomy or an ileostomy, diarrhea, edema, or heart, kidney, or liver disease. This medication may make these conditions worse or cause serious problems.
- If your stomach condition doesn't improve or recurs, consult your primary health care provider.
- Have regular checkups so your primary health care provider can check your progress, especially if you're taking this medication for a long time.

✓ Keep in mind

- If you're using this medication to relieve heartburn or acid indigestion, don't take it for more than 2 weeks unless your primary health care provider tells you to.
- If you're using this medication to relieve symptoms of an ulcer, take it exactly as directed and for the full time of treatment ordered by the primary health care provider. For best results, take it 1 and 3 hours after meals and at bedtime (unless the primary health care provider puts you on a different schedule). If you're an older adult and have bone problems, check with your primary health care provider before taking this medication.

Additional instructions

_____

_____

Taking amantadine

Dear Patient,

Amantadine is used to prevent or treat type A influenza (flu) infections. It's also used to treat Parkinson's disease and stiffness and shaking caused by other medications you may take for some nervous or emotional conditions. Other names for amantadine are Symadine and Symmetrel.

How to take amantadine

Amantadine comes as capsules or a syrup. Carefully read your medication label, and follow the directions exactly.

If you're taking amantadine to prevent or treat influenza, finish all of your medication. If you stop taking it too soon, your symptoms may recur. Take the doses at regular intervals — both day and night. Pour the syrup into a measuring spoon for an accurate dose.

What to do if you miss a dose

Take the dose as soon as possible. However, if you're within 4 hours of the next dose, skip the missed dose and go back to your regular dosing schedule. Don't take double doses.

What to do about side effects

Contact the primary health care provider *immediately* if you faint, have blurred vision, feel confused, have difficulty urinating, or experience seizures or hallucinations (see, hear, or feel things that others tell you aren't there).

Common side effects include dizziness, distractibility, irritability, difficulty sleeping, and purplish red, lacy spots on your skin. If any of these side effects persist or become severe, contact your primary health care provider.

What you must know about alcohol and other drugs

Avoid alcoholic beverages because they can increase the side effects of amantadine.

Special directions

- Until you know how this medication affects you, avoid driving or other activities that require alertness and clear vision.
- You may feel dizzy, light-headed, or faint if you get up suddenly from a lying or sitting position. Getting up slowly may help.
- Amantadine may cause mouth, nose, and throat dryness. Try using sugarless hard candy or gum, ice chips, or a saliva substitute. If dryness persists after 2 weeks, check with your primary health care provider.
- If you think amantadine is losing its effectiveness for you, call your primary health care provider. Don't adjust your dosage on your own. And don't stop taking your medication suddenly. If you do, your Parkinson's disease or other symptoms may become worse. Your primary health care provider may reduce your dose gradually.

✔ Keep in mind

- If you're pregnant or breast-feeding, notify your primary health care provider.
- Older adults may be especially sensitive to the medication's side effects.
- If you're taking this medication to prevent or treat flu infections and your symptoms continue or worsen within a few days, contact your primary health care provider
- Tell your primary health care provider if you have kidney disease. Your dose may need to be decreased.

Additional instructions

_____

_____

_____

_____

_____

Taking amiloride

Dear Patient,

This medication helps reduce the amount of water in your body without reducing potassium levels. Amiloride may be used to control high blood pressure. A brand name for this medication is Midamor.

How to take amiloride
Amiloride is available in tablet form. Carefully read the medication label, and follow the directions exactly.

Because amiloride increases urination, take it in the morning if you take a single dose daily. If you take more than one dose daily, take the last dose no later than 6 p.m. If this medication upsets your stomach, take it with meals or milk.

What to do if you miss a dose
Take it as soon as possible. But if it's almost time for your next dose, skip the missed dose and go back to your regular schedule. Don't take double doses.

What to do about side effects
This medication may cause headaches, nausea, vomiting, diarrhea, and loss of appetite. If these effects persist or become severe, contact your primary health care provider.

What you must know about other drugs
Tell your primary health care provider if you're taking another medication for high blood pressure, potassium supplements, or another potassium-sparing water pill. If these medications are taken with amiloride, your potassium level could become dangerously high.

Tell your primary health care provider if you're taking lithium (Lithane) because this combination may increase lithium's side effects.

Check with your primary health care provider before using nonprescription pain relievers because they can interfere with amiloride's effectiveness.

Special directions
• Don't change your diet without checking with your primary health care provider. Increasing your potassium intake by taking a potassium supplement or eating a high-potassium diet is unnecessary and could be dangerous. Symptoms of too much potassium include confusion, nervousness, fatigue, irregular heartbeat, weakness, shortness of breath, and numbness or tingling in your hands, feet, or lips.

Warning: Before surgery (including dental surgery), emergency treatment, or medical tests, tell the primary health care provider or dentist that you're taking amiloride.

• Because amiloride may cause sun sensitivity, avoid direct sunlight when possible, wear protective clothing, and use a sun block with a skin protection factor (SPF) of 15 or higher. If you develop a severe sun reaction, contact your primary health care provider.

✔ Keep in mind
• If you become pregnant while taking this medication, notify your primary health care provider.
• Symptoms of too much potassium are especially likely in older adults because of possible increased sensitivity to amiloride.
• If you're an athlete, you should know that amiloride use is banned by the National Collegiate Athletic Association and the U.S. Olympic Committee.

Additional instructions
_____
_____

Taking amiodarone

Dear Patient,

Your primary health care provider has prescribed amiodarone to correct your irregular heartbeats. The label may read Cordarone.

How to take amiodarone
Amiodarone is available as a tablet. Carefully read the label on your prescription bottle because it tells you how much medication to take. Follow the directions exactly.

What to do if you miss a dose
If you miss a dose of amiodarone, skip the dose completely and go back to your regular dosing schedule. Don't take double doses. If you miss two or more doses in a row, check with your primary health care provider.

What to do about side effects
Check with your primary health care provider *immediately* if you develop a cough, irregular heartbeat, shortness of breath, or painful breathing. Also check with him if you experience malaise, unusual fatigue, nausea, vomiting, increased sensitivity to sunlight, or visual disturbances.

What you must know about other drugs
Tell your primary health care provider if you're taking an anticoagulant (blood thinner), other heart medication, or phenytoin (Dilantin). The effects of these medications may increase if taken with amiodarone.

Special directions
• Visit your primary health care provider regularly to make sure the medication is working properly.
• Carry medical identification that states that you're taking this medication.
• Before surgery (including dental surgery) or emergency treatment, tell the primary

health care provider or dentist that you're taking amiodarone.
• Amiodarone increases your skin's sensitivity to sunlight. Avoid direct sunlight, wear protective clothing including a hat and sunglasses, and use a sun block that contains zinc or titanium dioxide. Contact your primary health care provider if you have a severe sun reaction. Keep in mind that your skin may continue to be sensitive to sunlight for several months after you stop taking this medication.
• After you've taken this medication for a long time, your skin may turn blue-gray where it's been exposed to sunlight. This color usually fades (it may take several months) after amiodarone treatment ends.

✔ Keep in mind
• Tell the primary health care provider if you're breast-feeding or you become pregnant while taking amiodarone.
• Older adults may be especially sensitive to side effects and more likely than younger adults to develop thyroid problems when taking amiodarone.

Additional instructions
_____
_____
_____
_____
_____
_____
_____
_____
_____
_____
_____

Taking amitriptyline

Dear Patient,

Your primary health care provider has prescribed amitriptyline to relieve your depression. The label may read Elavil.

How to take amitriptyline

Amitriptyline comes as a syrup or tablet. Carefully follow the directions on the prescription bottle. They tell you how much and when to take your medication.

Take amitriptyline with food, even for a daily bedtime dose, unless your primary health care provider has told you otherwise.

What to do if you miss a dose

If you miss a dose and you take one dose daily at bedtime, don't take the missed dose in the morning because it may cause disturbing side effects during waking hours. Call your primary health care provider for directions.

If you take more than one dose daily, take the missed dose as soon as possible. But if it's almost time for your next dose, skip the missed dose and go back to your regular schedule. Don't take double doses.

What to do about side effects

Amitriptyline may make you feel dizzy, lightheaded or faint, especially if you get up suddenly from a lying or sitting position. Getting up slowly may help.

You may also experience an irregular or fast pulse, blurred vision, drowsiness, dry mouth, constipation, problems with urinating, or sweating. Notify your primary health care provider if any of these effects persist or become severe.

What you must know about alcohol and other drugs

Check with your primary health care provider before combining amitriptyline with alcoholic beverages or nonprescription medications, such as allergy, cold, or other medications that make you sleepy.

Tell your primary health care provider if you're taking other medications. Barbiturates (antianxiety medication) may decrease amitriptyline's effectiveness.

Cimetidine (Tagamet) and methylphenidate (Ritalin) may increase amitriptyline's effect beyond a safe level.

When taken with amitriptyline, epinephrine (Adrenalin) and norepinephrine (Levophed) may increase your blood pressure, and monoamine oxidase (MAO) inhibitors may cause severe excitation, high fever, or seizures.

Special directions

● Be sure to tell your primary health care provider if you have other medical problems. They may affect the use of amitriptyline.
● You may need to take this medication for several weeks before you begin to feel better. See your primary health care provider at regular intervals so he can check your progress and make dosage adjustments.
● Until you know how amitriptyline affects you, don't drive, use machinery, or do anything else that requires alertness. The drowsiness and dizziness usually go away after a few weeks of taking this medication.
● Increase your fluid and fiber intake to help combat constipation. If these steps don't help, your primary health care provider may prescribe a stool softener.
● If this medication causes mouth dryness, use sugarless gum or hard candy, ice chips, or a saliva substitute. However, if your mouth continues to feel dry for more than 2 weeks, check with your primary health care provider or dentist. Continuing mouth dryness may increase the chance of dental disease, including tooth decay, gum disease, and fungus infections.

(continued)

Taking amitriptyline *(continued)*

• Amitriptyline may make your skin more sensitive to sunlight. Sun exposure may cause a rash, itching, redness, other discoloration, or a severe sunburn. Avoid direct sunlight, wear protective clothing including a hat and sunglasses, and use a sun block with a skin protection factor (SPF) of 15 or higher on your skin and lips. If you have a severe sun reaction, check with your primary health care provider.

• Amitriptyline may affect some medical test results, so tell your primary health care provider that you're taking this medication.

• Also tell the primary health care provider you're taking this medication before you have surgery, dental work, or emergency treatment.

• Don't stop taking this medication without checking with your primary health care provider. He may reduce the dosage gradually to prevent your condition from becoming worse and to lessen the possibility of withdrawal symptoms, such as headache, nausea, and an overall feeling of discomfort.

• Keep in mind that the effects of this medication may last for 3 to 7 days after you stop taking it.

✔ Keep in mind

• If you have diabetes and you notice a change in your blood or urine glucose test results, contact your primary health care provider. This medication may affect your glucose level.

• Notify your primary health care provider if you're pregnant or breast-feeding while taking this medication.

• Children and older adults may be especially sensitive to the medication's effects.

Additional instructions

_____
_____
_____
_____
_____
_____
_____
_____
_____
_____
_____

Taking amitriptyline with perphenazine

Dear Patient,

Amitriptyline with perphenazine is used to treat certain mental and emotional disorders. The label may read Etrafon or Triavil.

How to take this drug

Take this medication with food or right after meals, unless otherwise directed. Don't increase the dose or take it more often than prescribed.

What to do if you miss a dose

Take the dose as soon as you remember. However, if you remember within 2 hours of your next dose, skip the missed dose and go back to your regular schedule. Don't take double doses.

What to do about side effects

Call the primary health care provider *immediately* if you develop a fever, bleeding gums, or mouth sores or if you feel extremely tired.

You may also experience dizziness, drowsiness, uncontrolled movements of the arms or legs, light-headedness when changing position, increased pulse rate, constipation, dry mouth, blurred vision, sensitivity to sunlight, and sweating. Contact the primary health care provider if these effects persist or become severe.

What you must know about alcohol and other drugs

Avoid alcoholic beverages or other medications that make you sleepy or relaxed, such as allergy, hay fever, and cold medications. Use prescription pain products, seizure medications, or anesthetics with this drug only under the advice of your primary health care provider.

Don't take this drug within 2 hours of taking antacids or medication to treat diarrhea. Taking these medications too close together may lessen the effectiveness of amitriptyline with perphenazine.

Special directions

• Be sure to tell your primary health care provider if you have other medical problems. They may affect the use of this medication.
• Before you have surgery, dental work, or emergency treatment, tell the primary health care provider that you're taking this medication.
• This medication can cause drowsiness, so be sure you know how it affects you before you drive a car or perform other activities that require alertness.
• Get up slowly from a lying or sitting position to prevent dizziness.
• Avoid direct sunlight as much as possible. Wear protective clothing, including sunglasses and a hat, and use a sun block with a skin protection factor (SPF) of 15 or higher.

✓ Keep in mind

• If you're breast-feeding or you become pregnant while taking this medication, notify your primary health care provider as soon as possible.
• Teenagers and older adults may be especially sensitive to the effects of this medication.
• Tell your primary health care provider about previous allergic or unusual reactions to perphenazine or other antipsychotics or to amitriptyline (Elavil) or other antidepressants.
• If you're an athlete, you should know that perphenazine use is banned by the National Collegiate Athletic Association and the U.S. Olympic Committee.

Additional instructions

_____

_____

Taking amlodipine

Dear Patient,

Your primary health care provider has prescribed amlodipine because you have angina (chest pain) or high blood pressure. This medication will help improve your condition by relaxing your blood vessels and increasing the amount of oxygen and the blood supply going to your heart. The brand name of this drug is Norvasc.

How to take amlodipine

This medication is available as a tablet. It may be taken with or without food.

What to do if you miss a dose

Take the dose as soon as possible. However, if it is almost time for your next dose, skip the missed dose and take the next scheduled dose. Do not take two doses together.

What to do about side effects

You may be dizzy or feel as if your heart is beating faster than usual. To combat dizziness, rise slowly from a lying to a sitting position; then wait a few minutes before standing.

You may also have swelling of your ankles and feet, flushing, headache, nausea, or fatigue. Your gums may swell and bleed at the beginning of treatment. Contact your primary health care provider or pharmacist if these symptoms persist or become severe.

Because this medication may affect how your liver functions, the primary health care provider will order tests to monitor this.

What you must know about alcohol and other drugs

Tell your primary health care provider or pharmacist if you take any other prescription or nonprescription medications.

Special directions

• Tell your primary health care provider if you have any swelling in your feet and hands or shortness of breath.
• Don't stop taking this medication suddenly. Take all doses as scheduled.
• *Warning:* Don't use this drug for sudden episodes of chest pain. If chest pain becomes severe, call your primary health care provider immediately.
• Brushing and flossing your teeth regularly may help prevent gum bleeding.

✔ Keep in mind

• Older adults may be especially sensitive to this medication.
• If you become pregnant or are breast-feeding, notify your primary health care provider.
• Notify your primary health care provider if you have liver disease.

Additional instructions

_____
_____
_____
_____
_____
_____
_____
_____
_____
_____
_____

Taking amoxicillin

Dear Patient,

Your primary health care provider has prescribed amoxicillin to treat your bacterial infection. Common brand names are Amoxil, Polymox, Trimox, and Wymox.

How to take amoxicillin
Finish all your medication even if you feel better. If you stop it too soon, your symptoms may return.

Take amoxicillin either on a full or an empty stomach at evenly spaced times during the day and night. This medication works best when you have a constant amount in your blood.

Take the *liquid form* straight or mixed with other liquids. To get the full dose, take it immediately after mixing and drink all the liquid.

Don't break, chew, or crush the *capsule form* of the drug. Swallow it whole. The *chewable tablet form* should be chewed or crushed before swallowing.

What to do if you miss a dose
Take the dose as soon as possible. If you take two doses daily and it's almost time for your next dose, space the missed dose and your next dose 5 to 6 hours apart. If you're taking three or more doses a day, space the missed dose and the next dose 2 to 4 hours apart. Then go back to your regular schedule.

What to do about side effects
Contact your primary health care provider *immediately* and stop taking this medication if you develop difficulty breathing, a rash, hives, itching, or wheezing. Such symptoms may mean an allergic reaction.

Common side effects include nausea and diarrhea. If they persist or become severe, notify your primary health care provider.

What you must know about other drugs
Tell your primary health care provider about other medications you're taking. Allopurinol (Zyloprim) taken with amoxicillin may make you more likely to develop a rash. Probenecid (Benemid) increases blood levels of amoxicillin — a beneficial side effect.

Special directions
• If your symptoms don't improve within a few days or if they become worse, check with your primary health care provider.

Warning: If you develop severe diarrhea, don't take diarrhea medication without checking with your primary health care provider. It may make your diarrhea worse or last longer.

Keep in mind
• Inform your primary health care provider if you have kidney, stomach, or intestinal disease or infectious mononucleosis. These conditions may increase the risk of side effects.
• Tell your primary health care provider if you're allergic to other penicillins or cephalosporins, griseofulvin (Fulvicin), or penicillamine (Cuprimine). If you're allergic to amoxicillin, carry medical identification that describes your allergy.
• If you have diabetes, amoxicillin may cause false test results with some urine glucose tests. Call your primary health care provider before changing your diet or the dosage of your diabetes medication.
• If you're breast-feeding, discuss with your primary health care provider whether you should continue while taking amoxicillin.

Additional instructions

_____

_____

Taking amoxicillin with clavulanate potassium

Dear Patient,

The combination of amoxicillin with clavulanate potassium helps treat some bacterial infections. The medication label may read Augmentin.

How to take this drug

Take this medication either on a full or an empty stomach at evenly spaced times during the day and night. This medication works best when you have a constant amount in your blood. Finish all of the medication prescribed.

If you're taking the *chewable tablets,* crush or chew them well before swallowing.

If you're taking the *oral suspension,* use the dropper that comes with the bottle to measure the correct amount. If your medication doesn't have a dropper, use a specially marked measuring spoon.

What to do if you miss a dose

Take the dose as soon as possible. But if it's almost time for your next dose and you usually take two doses daily, space the missed dose and the next one 5 to 6 hours apart. If you take three or more doses daily, space the missed dose and the next one 2 to 4 hours apart. Then go back to your regular schedule.

What to do about side effects

Contact your primary health care provider *immediately* and stop taking this medication if you experience difficulty breathing, itching, a rash, hives, or wheezing. These effects may indicate that you're allergic to this medication.

You may also have nausea and, more commonly, diarrhea. Contact the primary health care provider if these symptoms persist or become severe.

What you must know about other drugs

Tell your primary health care provider about other medications you're taking. Allopurinol (Zyloprim) taken with this medication may increase your chances of developing a rash. Probenecid (Benemid) increases blood levels of amoxicillin — a beneficial side effect.

Special directions

Warning: If you develop severe diarrhea, don't take diarrhea medication without checking with your primary health care provider. Diarrhea medications may make your diarrhea worse or last longer.

Keep in mind

• Inform your primary health care provider if you have kidney, stomach, or intestinal disease or infectious mononucleosis. They may increase the risk of side effects.
• Tell your primary health care provider if you're allergic to other penicillins or cephalosporins, griseofulvin (Fulvicin), or penicillamine (Cuprimine). If you're allergic to this medication, carry medical identification that describes your allergy.
• If you have diabetes, this medication may cause false test results with some urine glucose tests. Call your primary health care provider before changing your diet or the dosage of your diabetes medication.
• If you're breast-feeding, discuss with your primary health care provider whether you should continue taking this medication.

Additional instructions

_____
_____
_____
_____
_____

Taking ampicillin

Dear Patient,

Ampicillin is used to treat bacterial infections. The label may read Omnipen, Polycillin, or Totacillin.

How to take ampicillin

Take all the prescribed medication, even if you feel better. If you stop it too soon, your symptoms may return. Take it at evenly spaced times day and night. Try not to miss a dose because ampicillin works best when you have a constant amount in your blood.

Take ampicillin with a full glass (8 ounces) of water on an empty stomach either 1 hour before or 2 hours after a meal unless otherwise directed.

If you're taking the *liquid form,* use a specially marked measuring spoon to measure the correct dose.

If you're taking the *capsule form,* don't break, chew, or crush the capsules. Swallow them whole.

Don't use ampicillin after the expiration date on the label. It may not work properly.

What to do if you miss a dose

Take the dose as soon as possible. If it's almost time for your next dose and you take two doses daily, space the missed dose and the next dose 5 to 6 hours apart. If you take three or more doses a day, space the missed dose and the next dose 2 to 4 hours apart. Then follow your regular schedule.

What to do about side effects

Contact your primary health care provider *immediately* and stop taking this medication if you have difficulty breathing, a rash, hives, itching, or wheezing. These effects may mean that you're allergic to ampicillin.

You may also have nausea and diarrhea. If these symptoms persist or become severe, notify your primary health care provider.

What you must know about other drugs

Tell your primary health care provider about other medications you're taking. Allopurinol (Zyloprim) taken with this medication may increase your chances of developing a rash. Probenecid (Benemid) increases blood levels of ampicillin — a beneficial side effect.

Special directions

• If your symptoms don't improve within a few days or if they become worse, check with your primary health care provider.

Warning: Ampicillin may interfere with the effectiveness of oral contraceptives (birth control pills) containing estrogen. Use a different or additional birth control while you're taking ampicillin.

• If you develop severe diarrhea, don't take any diarrhea medication without checking with your primary health care provider. Diarrhea medications may make your diarrhea worse or last longer.

✔ Keep in mind

• If you have diabetes, ampicillin may cause false test results with some urine glucose tests. Check with your primary health care provider before changing your diet or the dosage of your diabetes medication.

• Tell your primary health care provider if you're allergic to other penicillins or cephalosporins, griseofulvin (Fulvicin), or penicillamine (Cuprimine). If you're allergic to this medication, carry medical identification that describes your allergy.

• If you're breast-feeding, tell your health care provider before taking this medication.

Additional instructions

_____

_____

_____

Taking antianxiety medications

Dear Patient,

Your primary health care provider has pre-scribed an antianxiety medication for you. These medications are used to relieve ner-vousness or tension and are sometimes used to help patients sleep better. They may be given orally (by mouth) or by injection. In general, antianxiety medications work by slowing down the nervous system and help-ing you relax.

How to take antianxiety medications

These medications are available as tablets, capsules, oral liquids, injections, and sup-positories. Take your medication exactly as your primary health care provider directs — if you take it more often than prescribed, it may become habit-forming. You may have to wait up to 2 weeks for the medication to reach its full effect.

What to do if you miss a dose

If you miss a dose, take it as soon as you remember — but only if it's within an hour of your scheduled dose. If you're more than an hour late, or if it's close to your next sched-uled dose, skip the missed dose and go back to your regular schedule. Don't take double doses.

What to do about side effects

Call your primary health care provider *im-mediately* if you have behavioral changes, difficulty concentrating, hallucinations, con-fusion, shakiness, shortness of breath, or staggering. These may be signs of a drug overdose.

This drug may also cause clumsiness or unsteadiness, dizziness, light-headedness, drowsiness, slurred speech, blurred vision, headache, stomach cramps, or nausea and vomiting.

What you must know about alcohol and other drugs

Don't take this medication with alcohol or other medications that depress your central nervous system. Doing so can cause severe drowsiness. If excessive drowsiness occurs, call your primary health care provider imme-diately. Also, don't take any nonprescription drugs that contain alcohol, antihistamines, or decongestants without first talking to your primary health care provider or pharmacist.

Special directions

• Antianxiety medications can cause ex-treme drowsiness. So know how your body responds to your medication before you drive, operate machinery, or do anything that requires full alertness.

✓ Keep in mind

• Tell your primary health care provider if you're breast-feeding or become pregnant.
• Older adults are especially sensitive to the effects of this medication, so the primary health care provider may adjust the dose.
• Tell your primary health care provider if you have a history of alcohol abuse, drug abuse or dependence, brain disease, chron-ic lung disease, glaucoma, hyperactivity, mental depression, severe mental illness, porphyria, myasthenia gravis, or sleep ap-nea.

Additional instructions

_____
_____
_____
_____
_____
_____
_____

Taking antidepressants

Dear Patient,

Your primary health care provider has prescribed a medication to relieve your depression. Antidepressants usually work by affecting the body's own chemical system.

How to take antidepressants

Antidepressants are available as tablets, capsules, and liquids. Read the medication label carefully, and take the medication exactly as directed by your primary health care provider.

Most antidepressants can be taken either with or without food. However, some work better when taken with food, so ask your primary health care provider or pharmacist for specific instructions.

What to do if you miss a dose

Take the missed dose as soon as you remember unless it's close to your next scheduled dose. If so, skip the missed dose. Don't take double doses. If you usually take this medication at bedtime and miss the dose, don't take it in the morning, because increased side effects may occur during the day.

What to do about side effects

If you have behavioral changes, difficulty concentrating, hallucinations, confusion, shakiness, shortness of breath, or staggering, call your primary health care provider *immediately.* These may be signs of an overdose.

This medication may also cause clumsiness, unsteadiness, dizziness, light-headedness, drowsiness, slurred speech, stomach cramps, constipation, rapid heartbeat, low blood pressure (especially when arising), blurred vision, decreased sexual function (in men), increased sun sensitivity, headache, and nausea and vomiting.

What you must know about alcohol and other drugs

Don't take this medication with alcohol, medications that contain alcohol, or with medications that depress the central nervous system. Doing so can cause severe drowsiness. Don't take antihistamines or decongestants without first talking to your primary health care provider or pharmacist.

Some medications, such as cimetidine and clonidine, as well as tobacco, can increase the levels of antidepressant in your system or cause severe side effects. Avoid these while on an antidepressant, and ask your health care provider for alternatives.

Special directions

• This medication can cause extreme drowsiness, so know how your body responds to it before you drive, operate machinery, or do anything that requires full alertness.
• Be aware that some antidepressants take up to 30 days to reach their full effect.
• Use sunscreen and protective clothing to avoid overexposure to the sun.

🛑 *Warning:* Don't stop this medication abruptly; gradually taper off, following your health care provider's instructions.

✅ Keep in mind

• Tell your primary health care provider if you're breast-feeding or become pregnant.
• Older adults are especially sensitive to the effects of antidepressants, so doses may need to be adjusted.
• Tell your primary health care provider if you have a history of cardiac disease, glaucoma, or urine retention.

Additional instructions

_____

_____

Taking antihistamines

Dear Patient,

Your primary health care provider has prescribed an antihistamine because you have hay fever or other allergies. In general, this medication will improve your condition by preventing the effects of a substance called histamine.

How to take antihistamines

Antihistamines are available as tablets, capsules, liquids, creams, or injections. Most may be taken either with or without food; however, some should be taken on an empty stomach, 1 hour before or 2 hours after a meal. Taking the medication with food may help prevent stomach upset.

What to do if you miss a dose

Take the dose as soon as you remember unless it's close to your next scheduled dose. If it is, skip the missed dose. Don't take double doses.

What to do about side effects

Antihistamines may cause drowsiness, nervousness, increased appetite, and dryness of the mouth, nose and throat. For mouth and throat dryness, try sugarless candy, gum, or ice chips. Contact your primary health care provider if these effects become severe.

What you must know about alcohol and other drugs

Don't drink alcohol while taking antihistamines because this intensifies drowsiness. Tell your primary health care provider or pharmacist if you're taking other medications, especially sedatives, tranquilizers, or medications that cause drowsiness because combining these with antihistamines may also cause severe drowsiness.

Inform the primary health care provider if you take aspirin regularly, because the signs of taking too much aspirin (such as ringing in the ears) will be covered up by antihistamines.

Special directions

• Make sure you know how you react to this medication before you drive, operate machinery, or participate in any activity that requires full alertness.
• Avoid prolonged sun exposure because this medication may make you more sensitive.
• Don't break or crush sustained release forms of antihistamines.

✔ Keep in mind

• Don't breast-feed or become pregnant while on this medication.
• Before starting antihistamines, tell your primary health care provider if you have glaucoma, peptic ulcer disease, or difficulty urinating.
• Tell your primary health care provider if you're having skin testing for allergies because this medication will affect test results.
• Children and older adults are more sensitive to the effects of these drugs.

Additional instructions

_____
_____
_____
_____
_____
_____
_____
_____
_____
_____

Taking antiulcer agents

Dear Patient,

Your primary health care provider has prescribed an antiulcer agent to help keep your ulcer from worsening. In general, this medication can work three ways: by blocking the amount of acid produced by your stomach, by killing bacteria that may cause your ulcer, or by acting as a barrier over the ulcer, protecting it from stomach acid.

How to take antiulcer agents
These medications are available as tablets, capsules, oral liquids, or injections. Some should be taken before meals and at bedtime, and others can be taken any time of the day without regard to food. Check with your primary health care provider or pharmacist to determine which time is right for you.

What to do if you miss a dose
Take the dose as soon as you remember unless it's close to your next scheduled dose. If it is, skip the missed dose. Don't take double doses.

What to do about side effects
This drug may cause abdominal cramping, constipation, diarrhea, drowsiness, headache, nausea, and unusual tiredness or weakness. Contact your primary health care provider if any of these problems become severe.

Some antiulcer agents may cause temporary blackening or whitening of your stools. Patients who also take antacids containing bismuth may have temporary blackening of the tongue and mouth as well.

What you must know about alcohol and other drugs
Antiulcer agents may increase the level of alcohol in your blood, so check with your primary health care provider before drinking.

Tell your primary health care provider if you currently take any other medication, because antiulcer agents change the effectiveness of many medications. Some medications that may be affected include antibiotics known as quinolones, anticoagulants, antidepressants, and blood pressure, asthma, seizure, and antifungal medications.

Antiulcer agents also alter the effects of sucralfate and H_2-receptor antagonists like cimetidine. So don't take these agents 60 minutes before or after taking sucralfate. If you're taking bismuth, don't take aspirin.

Special directions
● Stay away from medications or foods that may irritate your stomach and worsen your condition. These may include aspirin, citrus products, and carbonated drinks.

❗ *Warning:* Cigarette smoking may decrease the effectiveness of antiulcer agents. If you can't stop smoking completely, at least don't smoke after the last dose of the day.

✔ Keep in mind
● Tell your primary health care provider if you're breast-feeding or become pregnant.
● Older adults are especially sensitive to the effects of these drugs, so doses may need to be adjusted.

Additional instructions
_____
_____
_____
_____
_____
_____

Taking aspirin

Dear Patient,

Aspirin is used to relieve pain and reduce fever. It may also be used to relieve some symptoms caused by arthritis (rheumatism).

Aspirin may be used to lessen the chance of heart attack, stroke, or other problems that may occur when blood clots block a blood vessel. However, don't take aspirin for these purposes unless ordered by your primary health care provider because doing so may increase your chance of serious bleeding.

Aspirin has many brand names, including Aspergum, Empirin, and Ecotrin.

How to take aspirin

Aspirin is available in capsules, tablets, chewable tablets, chewing gum tablets, delayed-release (enteric-coated) tablets, extended-release tablets, and suppositories.

Take aspirin after meals or with food (except for enteric-coated tablets and suppositories) to lessen stomach irritation. Take the *tablets* and *capsules* with a full glass (8 ounces) of water. Don't lie down for 15 to 30 minutes after taking the medication to prevent irritation that may lead to trouble swallowing.

Chewable tablets may be chewed, dissolved in liquid, crushed, or swallowed whole. *Enteric-coated tablets* must be swallowed whole. Check with your pharmacist about how *extended-release tablets* should be taken. Some may be broken into pieces (not crushed) before swallowing — others must be swallowed whole.

If you're using a *suppository* and it's too soft to insert, chill it in the refrigerator for 30 minutes or run cold water over it before you remove the foil wrapper. To insert it, first wash your hands; then remove the foil wrapper. Lie on your side and draw your knees up toward your chest. With your index finger,

push the suppository — rounded end first — into your rectum as far as you can.

What to do if you miss a dose

If you're taking this medication regularly and you miss a dose, take it as soon as you remember. However, if it's almost time for your next dose, skip the missed dose and go back to your regular schedule. Don't take double doses.

What to do about side effects

Call your primary health care provider *immediately* and stop taking this medication if you experience difficulty breathing; wheezing; flushing, redness, or other changes in skin color; hives; itching; or swelling of eyelids, face, or lips. These effects may mean that you're allergic to aspirin.

Also, call your primary health care provider *immediately* and stop taking this medication if you have ringing in your ears or hearing loss because you may have too much aspirin in your system (aspirin toxicity).

You may also experience nausea, stomach problems, or easy bruising. If these symptoms persist or become severe, notify your primary health care provider.

What you must know about alcohol and other drugs

Check with your primary health care provider about drinking alcoholic beverages while taking aspirin because this combination may cause stomach problems.

If you're taking other medications, check with your primary health care provider before taking aspirin. Ammonium chloride increases blood levels of aspirin products, which may lead to aspirin toxicity. Antacids in high doses make aspirin less effective. Corticosteroids (for example, prednisone) cause aspirin to be eliminated from the body more rapidly, making aspirin less effective.

(continued)

Taking aspirin (continued)

Anticoagulants (blood thinners) shouldn't be used with aspirin because they may increase your risk of bleeding. Aspirin may increase the effect of oral antidiabetic medication, causing low blood glucose reactions.

Special directions

! ***Warning:*** Tell your primary health care provider if you have other medical problems. They may affect the use of aspirin. Don't give aspirin to children or teenagers who have fever or other symptoms of a viral infection because of the risk of developing Reye's syndrome. Check with the primary health care provider.

• Don't use aspirin if it has a strong, vinegarlike odor. This odor means the medication is breaking down and is no longer effective.

• Don't use the chewable forms of aspirin for 7 days after having your tonsils removed, a tooth pulled, or other dental or mouth surgery.

• Don't place aspirin directly on a tooth or gum surface because it may cause a burn and erode the tooth enamel.

• Check the labels of all nonprescription and prescription medications and skin products, such as shampoo, for aspirin, other salicylates, or salicylic acid. Count these products as part of your total aspirin dosage for the day. Pepto-Bismol (bismuth subsalicylate) is an example of a commonly used nonprescription medication that contains salicylates. Using salicylate-containing products while taking aspirin may lead to an overdose.

• See your primary health care provider at regular intervals if you're taking aspirin for more than 10 days (5 days for children, for pain relief only) or if you're taking large amounts.

• *If you're taking aspirin to relieve pain* and the pain lasts for more than 10 days (5 days for children) or gets worse, new symptoms occur, or redness or swelling occurs, call your primary health care provider.

• *If you're taking aspirin to reduce a fever* and the fever lasts for more than 3 days, returns, or gets worse; new symptoms occur; or redness or swelling occurs, call your primary health care provider.

• *If you're taking aspirin for a sore throat* and your throat is very painful or the pain lasts for more than 2 days or occurs with or is followed by fever, headache, rash, nausea, or vomiting, call your primary health care provider.

• *If you're taking aspirin to lessen the chance of heart attack, stroke, or other problems caused by blood clots,* take only the amount ordered by your primary health care provider. Talk to your primary health care provider if you need medication to relieve pain, fever, or the symptoms of arthritis because he may not want you to take extra aspirin.

• Don't take aspirin to prevent a heart attack or blood clots unless your primary health care provider orders it.

• Don't take aspirin for 5 days before surgery (including dental surgery) unless otherwise directed by your primary health care provider or dentist. Taking aspirin during this time may cause bleeding problems.

• If you have rectal irritation from using suppositories, contact your primary health care provider.

✓ Keep in mind

• Don't take aspirin when you're pregnant, especially in the last three months of pregnancy.

Additional instructions

_____

_____

Taking aspirin with butalbital and caffeine

Dear Patient,

This combination medication helps to relieve the pain of tension headaches and to slow down the nervous system. It's known by several brand names, including Fiorinal.

How to take this drug

This medication is available as tablets and capsules. Take it exactly as ordered. Don't increase your dose or take more of it, and don't take it longer than ordered by the primary health care provider. If you take too much of this medication, it may cause stomach problems, become habit-forming, or lead to medical problems due to an overdose.

To reduce stomach irritation, take this medication with meals or an 8-ounce glass of milk or water.

What to do if you miss a dose

If you take this medication regularly and you miss a dose, take it as soon as you remember. However, if it's almost time for your next dose, skip the missed dose and resume your regular schedule. Never take double doses.

What to do about side effects

If you have breathing difficulties, itching, a rash, or other signs of an allergic reaction, stop taking this medication and notify the primary health care provider *immediately.*

Side effects may include stomach and intestinal symptoms, such as abdominal pain caused by gas, heartburn, indigestion, and nausea. If these side effects persist or become severe, contact the primary health care provider.

What you must know about alcohol and other drugs

Don't drink alcoholic beverages while taking this medication because the mixture may irritate your stomach. Also, the mixture of alcohol and butalbital increases nervous system effects.

Check with the primary health care provider before taking other medications that slow the nervous system. These include medications for colds or hay fever and other allergies; prescription pain and seizure medications; muscle relaxants; and other medications that make you feel relaxed or sleepy. These medications can increase the effect of butalbital.

Special directions

• Don't take this medication if it has a strong, vinegar-like odor. This means the medication is breaking down and is no longer effective.
• Before surgery (including dental surgery) or emergency treatment, tell your primary health care provider or dentist that you're taking this medication. Your primary health care provider may tell you to stop taking it for 5 days before surgery to prevent bleeding problems.
• Because this medication may make you dizzy, drowsy, or light-headed, don't drive, operate machinery, or perform other activities that require alertness until you know how this medication affects you.
• If you think you or anyone else may have taken an overdose, get emergency help immediately. Symptoms of overdose include hearing loss, confusion, ringing or buzzing in the ears, severe excitement or dizziness, seizures, and difficulty breathing.

❗ *Warning:* If you're taking this medication regularly or in large amounts, don't stop it before checking with your primary health care provider. Abruptly stopping this medication may cause withdrawal symptoms.

(continued)

Taking aspirin with butalbital and caffeine *(continued)*

✔ Keep in mind

• Tell your primary health care provider if you have anemia, gout, peptic ulcer or other stomach problems, or heart, kidney, or liver disease because using this medication may make these conditions worse. Also tell him if you have vitamin K deficiency.

• If you have diabetes and take this medication regularly, it may cause false urine glucose test results. Check with your primary health care provider if you notice any unusual changes in the test results.

❗ *Warning:* Children are especially sensitive to the effects of aspirin-containing medications, especially if they have a fever or have lost large amounts of body fluids from vomiting, diarrhea, or sweating. Don't give children or teenagers this medication if they have a fever or other signs of viral infection, such as flu or chickenpox. It may cause a serious illness called Reye's syndrome.

• Older adults are also especially sensitive to the medication's effects and may develop more side effects than younger adults. They may show signs of confusion, depression, or overexcitement.

• Don't use this medication during pregnancy, especially in the third trimester. If you become pregnant or you're breast-feeding while taking this medication, notify your primary health care provider.

• If you're an athlete, you should know that the National Collegiate Athletic Association and the U.S. Olympic Committee limit the amount of caffeine that can be present in the urine of athletes.

Additional instructions

_____
_____
_____
_____
_____
_____
_____
_____
_____
_____
_____

Taking aspirin with codeine

Dear Patient,

This medication is used to treat moderate to severe pain. Brand names include Empirin with Codeine.

How to take aspirin with codeine

To reduce stomach irritation, take this medication with food or an 8-ounce glass of milk or water.

What to do if you miss a dose

If you take this medication regularly and you miss a dose, take it as soon as you remember. But if it's almost time for your next dose, skip the missed dose and go back to your regular schedule. Don't take double doses.

What to do about side effects

If you have breathing difficulty, itching, a rash, or other signs of an allergic reaction, stop taking this medication and notify the primary health care provider *immediately.*

Side effects may include intestinal symptoms, including abdominal pain caused by gas, heartburn, indigestion, and nausea. If these symptoms persist or become severe, contact your primary health care provider.

What you must know about alcohol and other drugs

Don't take this medication with alcoholic beverages because the codeine in it can slow down your nervous system, which could make you extremely drowsy. Also, the mixture of alcohol and aspirin may irritate your stomach.

Tell your primary health care provider about other medications you're taking because some may interact with aspirin with codeine. Medications that make your urine less acidic, such as antacids, also increase urination, which leaves aspirin with codeine less time to work.

Check with your primary health care provider before taking other medications that slow the nervous system, such as medications for colds or hay fever and other allergies, prescription pain and seizure medications, muscle relaxants, and other medications that make you feel relaxed or sleepy.

Taking this medication with anticoagulants (blood thinners) may increase your risk of bleeding.

If you have diabetes, keep in mind that aspirin taken regularly may increase the effects of oral antidiabetic medications. Check with your primary health care provider to see whether your antidiabetic medication dosage needs adjustment.

Taking this medication with acetaminophen (Tylenol) may put you at risk for unwanted side effects.

Special directions

● Tell your primary health care provider if you've ever had an unusual or allergic reaction to aspirin or codeine.
● Check the labels of all nonprescription and prescription medications for aspirin, other salicylates, or salicylic acid. Pepto-Bismol (bismuth subsalicylate) is an example of a commonly used nonprescription medication that contains salicylates. Contact your primary health care provider if you're taking a product that contains a narcotic, aspirin, or other salicylates because combining these medications can lead to overdose.
● Don't take this medication if it smells like vinegar. This means that the aspirin is breaking down and losing its effectiveness.
● Some people become drowsy when taking this medication. Be sure you know how you respond to this medication before you perform activities that require alertness, such as driving or operating machinery.

(continued)

Taking aspirin with codeine *(continued)*

• This medication may cause dizziness and light-headedness. Move slowly when you change from a lying or sitting position.

• Tell your primary health care provider or dentist that you're taking this medication before surgery (including dental surgery) or emergency treatment. Because this medication may cause bleeding problems, your primary health care provider may instruct you to stop taking it 5 days before surgery.

• Don't suddenly stop taking this medication if you've been taking it regularly. Your primary health care provider may want to reduce your dosage gradually to avoid withdrawal effects.

✔ Keep in mind

• Inform the primary health care provider if you have other medical problems, such as gout, because aspirin products can worsen this disorder and reduce the effects of medications used to treat gout. If you have gallbladder disease, the codeine in this medication may cause serious side effects.

• If you're breast-feeding, tell the primary health care provider before taking this medication. If you become pregnant while taking this medication, notify the primary health care provider as soon as possible. Don't take aspirin in the last 3 months of pregnancy unless directed by your primary health care provider.

• Older adults are especially susceptible to the side effects of this medication, particularly breathing problems.

! *Warning:* Children are especially sensitive to the effects of this medication, especially if they have a fever or have lost large amounts of body fluids from vomiting, diarrhea, or sweating. Don't give children or teenagers medication containing aspirin if they have a fever or other signs of a viral infection, such as chickenpox or flu. Aspirin may cause a serious illness called Reye's syndrome. Also, the codeine in this medication may make children unusually excited or restless.

• If you're an athlete, you should know that the National Collegiate Athletic Association and the U.S. Olympic Committee ban the use of codeine.

Additional instructions

_____

_____

_____

_____

_____

_____

_____

_____

_____

_____

Taking astemizole

Dear Patient,

Astemizole is used to relieve or prevent the symptoms of hay fever and other allergies. The brand name for this medication is Hismanal.

How to take astemizole

This medication is available as a tablet. Take it on an empty stomach 1 hour before or 2 hours after meals.

What to do if you miss a dose

If you take this medication regularly and you miss a dose, take it as soon as possible. However, if it's almost time for your next dose, skip the missed dose and go back to your regular schedule. Don't take double doses.

What to do about side effects

You may experience headaches, drowsiness, nervousness, dry mouth, dizziness, nausea, or diarrhea. Contact your primary health care provider if these symptoms persist or become severe.

What you must know about alcohol and other drugs

Check with your primary health care provider before drinking alcoholic beverages because the combined effects of alcohol and this medication may increase the risk of drowsiness.

   If you're taking this medication regularly, be sure to tell your primary health care provider if you're taking large amounts of aspirin at the same time (for example, for arthritis). This medication may mask the warning signs — such as ringing in the ears — that you're taking too much aspirin. Also, tell your primary health care provider about other drugs you may be taking.

Special directions

• Make sure you know how you react to this medication before you drive, use machinery, or perform other activities that require alertness.
• Inform the primary health care provider that you're taking this medication before you have skin tests for allergies because this medication may affect the test results.

✔ Keep in mind

• Tell your primary health care provider if you're breast-feeding or you become pregnant while taking this medication.
• Be aware that children and older adults are especially sensitive to the effects of astemizole.
• Tell your primary health care provider if you have other medical problems, especially asthma, an enlarged prostate, urinary tract blockage or difficulty urinating, or glaucoma. They may affect the use of astemizole.

Additional instructions

_____
_____
_____
_____
_____
_____
_____
_____
_____
_____
_____
_____

Taking atenolol

Dear Patient,

Atenolol is used to treat high blood pressure, relieve chest pain caused by angina, and prevent another heart attack in recent heart attack victims. The brand name is Tenormin.

How to take atenolol
Swallow the tablet whole—don't crush, break, or chew it.

Your primary health care provider may tell you to check your pulse rate before and after taking atenolol. If it's much slower than usual, call him before the next dose.

Try not to miss doses. Some conditions become worse when this medication isn't taken regularly.

What to do if you miss a dose
Take it as soon as possible. However, if it's within 8 hours of your next dose, skip the missed dose and resume your regular schedule. Don't take double doses.

What to do about side effects
Contact the primary health care provider *immediately* if you have trouble breathing, swollen ankles, or a sudden weight gain of 3 pounds or more (signs that you're retaining water) or if your blood pressure rises.

You may feel light-headed and extremely tired and have a slow pulse rate. If these symptoms persist or become severe, contact your primary health care provider.

What you must know about other drugs
Tell your primary health care provider if you're taking other medications. If you're taking other medications to lower your blood pressure, atenolol may lower your blood pressure too much. If you're taking digoxin (Lanoxin), your pulse rate may become dangerously slow. Indomethacin (Indocin) may make atenolol less effective.

If you're taking an antidiabetic medication or insulin, check your blood glucose level carefully because atenolol can hide low blood glucose levels.

Special directions
• Avoid activities that require alertness.
• You may be especially sensitive to cold while taking atenolol, especially if you have blood circulation problems.
• Don't suddenly stop taking this medication because your condition may worsen. Your primary health care provider may reduce the amount you're taking gradually.
• Before surgery (including dental surgery), emergency treatment, or medical tests, tell the primary health care provider or dentist that you're taking atenolol.
• Check with your health care provider before taking nonprescription medications.

✓ Keep in mind
• Tell your primary health care provider of other medical problems, especially breathing problems, diabetes, kidney or liver disease, depression, or thyroid problems. Call your health care provider if you become pregnant while taking this medication.
• If you have allergies to medications, foods, preservatives, or dyes, this medication may worsen allergic reactions and make them harder to treat.
• Older adults are more sensitive to atenolol and likely to experience side effects.
• If you're an athlete, you should know that atenolol use is banned by the National Collegiate Athletic Association and the U.S. Olympic Committee.

Additional instructions
_____
_____

Taking atorvastatin

Dear Patient,

Your primary health care provider has prescribed atorvastatin because you have high cholesterol. This medication will improve your condition by limiting the production of cholesterol by your body. The brand name of this drug is Lipitor.

How to take atorvastatin
This medication is available as a tablet. It may be taken either with or without food.

What to do if you miss a dose
If you miss a dose, take it as soon as you remember. However, if it's close to your next dose, skip the missed dose. Don't take double doses.

What to do about side effects
You may experience headache, muscle pain, flatulence (gas), indigestion, a rash, or trouble sleeping while taking this drug. Contact your primary health care provider if these side effects become severe.

What you must know about alcohol and other drugs
Don't drink alcohol while on this medication because it can cause liver damage.

Tell your primary health care provider or pharmacist if you're taking antifungal drugs, such as fluconazole, cyclosporine, and erythromycin, or fibrates such as gemfibrozil or clofibrate, as these combinations may cause severe muscle damage.

If you are taking digoxin or birth control pills, tell your primary health care provider, as the doses may have to be adjusted while on atorvastatin.

Special directions
• Your cholesterol will need to be tested every 3 to 6 months, or on a regular basis.
• Notify your primary health care provider immediately if you have muscle pain, fatigue, or fever.
• Modifying your diet, exercising, and losing weight (if needed) may help improve your condition.

✔ Keep in mind
• Don't breast-feed or become pregnant while on this drug.
• Let your primary health care provider know if you have a liver or kidney disease.

Additional instructions

_____
_____
_____
_____
_____
_____
_____
_____
_____
_____
_____

Taking atropine

Dear Patient,

Your primary health care provider has prescribed atropine to relieve your stomach and intestinal cramps or spasms. It's also used with antacids or other medications to treat peptic ulcer.

The ophthalmic (eye) form of atropine is used to dilate (enlarge) the pupil and to treat certain eye inflammations. Your container may be labeled Atropisol or Ocu-Tropine.

How to take atropine

Atropine is available in tablet form and also as an ophthalmic solution and an ophthalmic ointment. Carefully check your prescription label. Follow the directions exactly.

Take *tablets* 30 minutes to 1 hour before meals, unless your primary health care provider instructs otherwise.

If you're using *eyedrops,* wash your hands first. With your middle finger, apply pressure to the inner corner of the eye (continue applying pressure with this finger for 2 to 3 minutes after using the medication). Tilt your head back and, with the index finger of the same hand, pull the lower eyelid away from the eye to form a pouch. Squeeze the drops into the pouch and gently close the eye. Don't blink. Keep the eye closed for 1 to 2 minutes so the medication will be absorbed.

If you're applying *eye ointment,* wash your hands, then pull the lower eyelid away from the eye to form a pouch. Squeeze a thin strip of ointment into the pouch. Gently close your eyes, and keep them closed for 1 to 2 minutes to allow the medication to be absorbed.

Wash your hands immediately after using eyedrops or ointment. And if you gave this medication to an infant or a child, also wash his hands and any other place the medication may have touched. Don't let any of the medication enter his mouth.

To keep the medication germ-free, don't let the applicator tip touch any surface. Also keep the container tightly closed.

What to do if you miss a dose

If you forget to take your tablet or to use your ophthalmic atropine, do so as soon as you remember. But if it's almost time for your next dose, skip the missed dose and resume your normal schedule. Don't take or apply double doses.

What to do about side effects

If you're taking the *tablet* form, make sure family members know to contact the primary health care provider *immediately* if you become so sleepy that you can't be roused.

More common side effects (with the tablet form) include difficulty sleeping, dizziness, rapid pulse rate, palpitations, chest pain, dry mouth, constipation, and blurred vision. If these symptoms persist or worsen, call the primary health care provider.

Common side effects associated with the *ophthalmic* form include blurred vision and sensitivity to light. If these symptoms persist or worsen, contact your primary health care provider.

What you must know about other drugs

Tell the primary health care provider about other medications you're taking. Atropine taken with methotrimeprazine (Levoprome) can cause involuntary body movements, such as twitching, changes in muscle tone, and abnormal posture.

Don't take oral atropine within 2 to 3 hours of taking antacids or diarrhea medications. Taking these medications too close together may prevent atropine from working properly.

(continued)

Taking atropine (continued)

Special directions

For oral atropine

! *Warning:* If you think you may have taken an overdose, get emergency help at once.

• Make sure you know how you react to this medication before driving or performing activities that require alertness.

• Because you may sweat less while taking oral atropine, your body temperature may increase. Take extra care not to become overheated during exercise or in hot weather because it may result in heatstroke. Also, hot baths or saunas may make you feel dizzy or faint while you're taking atropine.

• If you feel dizzy, light-headed, or faint when getting up from a bed or chair, rising slowly may lessen this problem.

• To relieve mouth dryness, use sugarless hard candy or gum, ice chips, or a saliva substitute. If dryness persists for more than 2 weeks, check with your primary health care provider or dentist. Continuing mouth dryness increases the risk of dental disorders.

• Check with your primary health care provider before you begin using new medications (prescription or nonprescription) or if you develop new medical problems while taking atropine.

• Check with your primary health care provider before you stop using atropine. The primary health care provider may want you to reduce your dosage gradually. Stopping atropine abruptly may cause unpleasant withdrawal effects, such as vomiting, sweating, and dizziness.

For ophthalmic atropine

• Make sure you know how you react to this medication before driving or performing other activities requiring alertness and clear vision.

• Protect light-sensitive eyes by wearing sunglasses and avoiding bright lights.

• Blurred vision and light sensitivity may last for several days after you stop using this medication. If these effects persist longer, notify your primary health care provider.

✔ Keep in mind

• If you're breast-feeding, be aware that oral atropine may reduce milk flow and that ophthalmic atropine can cause such side effects as rapid pulse rate, fever, or dry skin in breast-feeding infants. Discuss these possibilities with your primary health care provider.

• Children (especially those with blond hair and blue eyes) and older adults are especially sensitive to ophthalmic atropine and its side effects.

Additional instructions

_____

_____

_____

_____

_____

_____

_____

_____

_____

_____

Taking attapulgite

Dear Patient,

Attapulgite is used to relieve diarrhea. It works by absorbing the germs or bacteria that may be causing the diarrhea and by decreasing water losses. The brand names of this drug are Donnagel, Kaopectate, and Parepectolin.

How to take attapulgite
This medication is available as tablets, chewable tablets, and liquid.

What to do if you miss a dose
This medication should be taken after each unformed stool until diarrhea subsides. If you miss taking a dose, do so as soon as you remember.

What to do about side effects
Constipation is the only side effect. If this occurs, stop taking the medication.

What you must know about other drugs
If possible, don't take any other medications within 24 hours of taking attapulgite because the effectiveness of these medications may be decreased.

Special directions
• If your diarrhea doesn't improve in 48 hours, call your primary health care provider.

Warning: If you notice blood or mucus in your stool, stop taking the medication and call your primary health care provider.

✔ Keep in mind
• To replace the fluids you're losing from your body, drink plenty of clear liquids and eat bland foods. Check with your primary health care provider if your urination decreases or dizziness, light-headedness, dry mouth, or increased thirst occurs.

Additional instructions
_____
_____
_____
_____
_____
_____
_____
_____
_____
_____
_____

Taking azathioprine

Dear Patient,

Also called Imuran, azathioprine decreases the body's natural immunity. This helps to prevent a rejection reaction after organ transplantation. It's also used to treat rheumatoid arthritis.

How to take azathioprine
Check the label on your prescription bottle; follow the directions exactly.

What to do if you miss a dose
If your dosing schedule is once a day, don't take the dose you missed and don't double the next dose. Instead, resume your normal dosing schedule and check with your primary health care provider.

If you're taking more than one dose a day, take the missed dose as soon as you remember it. If it's time for your next dose, take both doses together, then resume your usual schedule. If you miss more than one dose, notify your primary health care provider.

If you vomit after taking a dose, notify your primary health care provider, who will instruct you either to take the dose again or to wait until the next scheduled dose.

What to do about side effects
Notify your primary health care provider *immediately* if you have a fever, chills, wet cough, or other symptoms of infection; black stools; bloody urine; unusual bruising or bleeding; or increased tiredness or weakness.

What you must know about other drugs
Tell your primary health care provider about other medications you're taking. If you're taking allopurinol (Zyloprim), you'll need a lower azathioprine dose.

Special directions
• Tell your primary health care provider if you have other medical problems. They may affect the use of azathioprine.
• Schedule regular checkups so that your primary health care provider can monitor azathioprine therapy and check for side effects.
• Don't stop taking azathioprine without first consulting your primary health care provider.
• During and after azathioprine therapy, don't receive any vaccinations unless your primary health care provider approves. Azathioprine increases your risk of getting the infection that the vaccine prevents.

Warning: Caution close associates who receive the oral polio vaccine that they could pass the polio virus to you. If you can't avoid people who have received this vaccine, wear a protective mask over your nose and mouth.

Warning: Because azathioprine increases your risks of infection and bleeding, take these precautions:
–Avoid people with known infections.
–Call your primary health care provider immediately if you think you're getting sick.
–Be careful not to cut yourself using a toothbrush, dental floss, or a razor.
–Avoid touching your eyes or nose.
–Avoid contact sports or other activities in which bruising or injury can occur.

✔ Keep in mind
• If you become pregnant, stop taking azathioprine and notify your primary health care provider. Also, don't breast-feed while taking this medication.

Additional instructions

Taking azithromycin

Dear Patient,

Your primary health care provider has prescribed azithromycin because you have an infection. This medication will improve your condition by interfering with bacterial growth. The brand name of this drug is Zithromax.

How to take azithromycin
This medication is available as a tablet, an oral liquid, and an injection. The oral medication should be taken 1 hour before or 2 hours after meals with 8 ounces of water.

What to do if you miss a dose
If you miss a dose, take it as soon as you remember. However, if it's close to the time for your next dose, skip the missed dose. Don't take double doses.

What to do about side effects
If fever, rash, difficulty breathing, or swelling of your face, mouth, neck, hands, or feet occur, call your primary health care provider *immediately*. These are signs of an allergic reaction.

More common side effects of this medication include diarrhea, nausea, vomiting, stomach discomfort, dizziness, and headache.

What you must know about other drugs
Don't take antacids that contain aluminum or magnesium within 1 hour before or 2 hours after taking azithromycin because azithromycin will be less effective.

Tell your primary health care provider about all other medications you're taking, because several of them may affect azithromycin's ability to work properly.

Special directions
• Finish taking the medication even if you feel better.

✔ Keep in mind
• If you become pregnant while on this drug, notify your primary health care provider. Also tell him if you're breast-feeding.
• Tell your primary health care provider if you have liver disease.

Additional instructions

_____
_____
_____
_____
_____
_____
_____
_____
_____
_____
_____

Taking aztreonam

Dear Patient,

Aztreonam is used to treat bacterial infections. The medication label may read Azactam.

How to take aztreonam

Aztreonam is available in a vial and must be injected into a muscle. Carefully check the label on your prescription vial, and follow the directions exactly. This label tells you how much medication to inject and when to inject it. If you don't know how to give yourself an intramuscular injection, have someone who is skilled in giving an injection give you your medication.

Inject the drug deeply into a large muscle mass, such as the upper outer quadrant of your buttock or the outer side portion of your thigh.

To help clear up your infection completely, you must finish the full course of prescribed aztreonam therapy, even if you begin to feel better after a few days.

For this medication to be most effective, it must be administered at evenly spaced times as directed.

What to do if you miss a dose

If you miss a dose of your medication, contact your primary health care provider for instructions.

What to do about side effects

Stop using the medication and tell the primary health care provider *immediately* if you develop pain, swelling, or redness at the injection site; difficulty breathing; wheezing; a tight feeling in your chest; difficulty swallowing; hives; a rash; or itching. These symptoms indicate that you may be having an allergic reaction to aztreonam.

Some common side effects of aztreonam include abdominal or stomach cramps, nausea, vomiting, and diarrhea. If these symptoms persist or become severe, notify your primary health care provider.

What you must know about other drugs

Tell your primary health care provider about other medications you're taking. Furosemide (Lasix) or probenecid (Benemid) may raise the amount of aztreonam in your blood.

Special directions

• Check with your primary health care provider before you begin taking any new prescription or nonprescription medication.
• Contact your primary health care provider if you develop new medical problems while using aztreonam.

✔ Keep in mind

• Tell your primary health care provider if you have other medical problems, especially liver or kidney disease. These and other medical problems may affect your use of aztreonam.

Additional instructions

_____
_____
_____
_____
_____
_____
_____
_____
_____
_____
_____

Taking baclofen

Dear Patient,

Baclofen is used to relax certain muscles and relieve the spasms, cramping, and tightness caused by disorders such as multiple sclerosis or some spinal injuries. A brand name for baclofen is Lioresal.

How to take baclofen

Baclofen comes in tablet form. Read your medication label carefully, and follow the directions exactly. To prevent possible stomach upset, take baclofen with milk or meals.

What to do if you miss a dose

Take the dose as soon as you remember, as long as it's within about an hour of the scheduled dose. If you don't remember until later, skip the dose you missed and resume your normal dosing schedule. Don't take double doses.

What to do about side effects

Contact your primary health care provider *immediately* if you have seizures or blurred vision. Other side effects include drowsiness, dizziness, weakness, fatigue, and nausea. Call the primary health care provider if these side effects persist or worsen.

What you must know about alcohol and other drugs

Tell your primary health care provider if you drink alcoholic beverages and take other medications that depress the central nervous system (antidepressants, antihistamines, and barbiturates, for example). These increase baclofen's side effects.

Special directions

● Make sure you know how you react to this medication before you drive, operate machinery, or do anything else that requires full alertness and good vision.

! *Warning:* Don't abruptly stop taking this medication; unwanted side effects may occur. Ask your primary health care provider how to gradually reduce your dosage before stopping completely.

✔ **Keep in mind**

● Tell your primary health care provider if you have other medical problems, particularly diabetes, seizure disorder, kidney disease, mental or emotional problems, stroke, and brain disorders.
● If you have diabetes, baclofen may raise your blood glucose level. Check your blood glucose level carefully, and if you notice a change, tell your primary health care provider.
● If you're breast-feeding or you become pregnant while taking this medication, contact your primary health care provider.
● If you're an older adult, you may be especially sensitive to baclofen and may experience more side effects.
● If you're an athlete, you should know that baclofen is banned by the National Collegiate Athletic Association and the U.S. Olympic Committee. Its use may disqualify you from certain amateur athletic events.

Additional instructions

_____
_____
_____
_____
_____
_____
_____
_____
_____
_____

Taking beclomethasone

Dear Patient,

Beclomethasone oral inhalant is used to prevent or reduce the frequency or severity of asthma attacks. Keep in mind that it can't relieve an asthma attack that has already started.

The nasal form of beclomethasone helps to relieve the stuffy nose and irritation related to hay fever, other allergies, and other nasal problems. It also helps to prevent nasal polyps from growing back after they've been surgically removed.

How to take beclomethasone
Beclomethasone comes in an aerosol form for oral inhalation (brand names: Beclovent and Vanceril) and in aerosol or spray form for nasal use (brand names: Beconase and Vancenase).

Before using your medication, carefully read the directions that come with the container. Follow them exactly. If you don't understand the directions or aren't sure how to use the medication, check with your primary health care provider or pharmacist.

For this medication to work, you must take it every day at regular intervals as your primary health care provider prescribes. Keep in mind that up to 4 weeks may pass before you feel the medication's full effects.

What to do if you miss a dose
Take the dose as soon as you remember. But if it's almost time for your next dose, skip the missed dose and resume your normal dosing schedule. Don't take double doses.

What to do about side effects
Nasal beclomethasone may cause mild, transient nasal burning and stinging. If this persists or becomes severe, contact your primary health care provider.

Special directions
For the oral inhalant
• Notify your primary health care provider if you experience unusual stress; if you have an asthma attack that doesn't improve after you take a bronchodilator; if signs of mouth, throat, or lung infection occur; if your symptoms don't improve; or if your condition worsens.
• Carry a medical identification card stating that you're taking beclomethasone and may need additional medication in an emergency situation, during a severe asthma attack or other illness, or when you're under unusual stress.
• Before surgery (including dental surgery) or emergency treatment, tell the primary health care provider or dentist that you're taking beclomethasone.
• If you're also using a bronchodilator inhalation aerosol, such as albuterol, use it first and then wait about 5 minutes before taking beclomethasone, unless directed otherwise by your primary health care provider.
For the nasal form
• If you're taking this medication for more than a few weeks, see your primary health care provider regularly.
• Check with your health care provider if you develop signs of a nasal, sinus, or throat infection; if your symptoms don't improve within 3 weeks; or if your condition worsens.

✔ Keep in mind
• Tell your primary health care provider if you have other medical problems, particularly lung disease or infections of the mouth, nose, sinuses, throat, or lungs.

Additional instructions

_____

_____

Taking benazepril

Dear Patient,

Your primary health care provider has prescribed benazepril because you have high blood pressure. It will lower your blood pressure by interfering with salt and water retention. The brand name of this drug is Lotensin.

How to take benazepril

This medication is available as tablets. It may be taken either with or without food.

What to do if you miss a dose

Take the dose as soon as you remember. But if it's almost time for your next dose, skip the missed dose and resume your normal dosing schedule. Don't take double doses.

What to do about side effects

Call your primary health care provider *immediately* if you have a sore throat, fever, or rash, difficulty breathing, or swelling of your face, mouth, neck, hands or feet. These are signs of a possible allergic reaction to the medication.

Other side effects include nausea, dizziness, headache, impaired taste perception, and a dry cough that lasts throughout your course of treatment. If the cough becomes worse or the other side effects persist, call your primary health care provider.

What you must know about other drugs

Tell your primary health care provider if you're taking diuretics (water pills) or other medications for high blood pressure, as this combination may lower your blood pressure too much. If you're taking potassium or potassium-sparing diuretics, this may raise your potassium too much.

Take antacids 1 hour before or 2 hours after taking benazepril to keep benazepril's effectiveness from decreasing. If you're taking digoxin or lithium, the primary health care provider may need to change the dosages of these medications because their levels in your blood will increase. If you're also taking allopurinol, you have a higher risk of side effects from benazepril.

Special directions

- When you first start taking benazepril, rise slowly to avoid light-headedness.
- Don't use salt substitutes as these may contain potassium.
- Don't stop benazepril suddenly unless your primary health care provider says it's safe to do so.
- Tell your primary health care provider if you're also taking diuretics. Taking them along with benazepril may cause your blood pressure to drop too much at the start of therapy.
- Be aware that you need periodic blood tests to check your liver and kidney function as well as potassium level.

✔ Keep in mind

- Tell your primary health care provider if you're breast-feeding or if you become pregnant while taking this medication.
- Tell the primary health care provider if you have liver or kidney disease.

Additional instructions

_____
_____
_____
_____
_____
_____
_____

Taking benztropine

Dear Patient,

Benztropine relieves symptoms of Parkinson's disease and controls reactions to medications that cause Parkinson-like symptoms. The brand name is Cogentin.

How to take benztropine

Follow the directions on your prescription exactly. To lessen stomach upset, take benztropine with meals, unless your primary health care provider directs otherwise.

What to do if you miss a dose

Take the dose as soon as you remember, unless it's within 2 hours of your next scheduled dose. If this happens, skip the missed dose and resume your normal dosing schedule. Don't take double doses.

What to do about side effects

Common side effects include constipation and dry mouth. If these effects persist or worsen, contact your primary health care provider.

What you must know about alcohol and other drugs

Check with your primary health care provider before drinking alcoholic beverages or taking nonprescription medications. Also tell your primary health care provider about other medications you're taking. Amantadine (Symadine, Symmetrel); phenothiazines, such as chlorpromazine (Thorazine); and tricyclic antidepressants, such as imipramine (Tofranil), may increase your risk of benztropine side effects.

Don't take benztropine within 1 hour of taking antacids or medication for diarrhea. Doing so may reduce benztropine's effectiveness.

Special directions

• Tell your primary health care provider if you have other medical problems. They may affect the use of benztropine.

Warning: If you think you've taken an overdose of benztropine, get help *at once.*

• If your eyes are sensitive to light, wear sunglasses and avoid bright lights.
• Make sure you know how you react to benztropine before performing activities that require clear vision and alertness.
• If you feel dizzy or light-headed when arising, get up slowly.
• Avoid becoming overheated because benztropine may make you sweat less and thus increase your body temperature.
• To relieve dry mouth, use sugarless hard candy or gum, ice chips, or a saliva substitute. Consult your dentist if dryness persists because it increases the risk of tooth decay and other disorders.
• Have regular checkups, especially during the first few months you're taking benztropine, so that your health care provider can adjust the dosage to meet your needs.
• Don't stop taking benztropine abruptly. Check with your primary health care provider, who may direct you to gradually reduce the dosage.

✔ Keep in mind

• If you're breast-feeding, check with your primary health care provider before taking benztropine.
• Children and older adults may be especially sensitive to benztropine and more likely to experience side effects.

Additional instructions

_____

_____

Taking bethanechol

Dear Patient,

Bethanechol is used to treat certain bladder or urinary tract disorders. It stimulates urination and complete bladder emptying. The label may read Duvoid or Urecholine.

How to take bethanechol
Bethanechol comes in tablet form. Carefully follow the directions for how much medication to take and when to take it.

Unless your primary health care provider directs otherwise, take bethanechol on an empty stomach (either 1 hour before or 2 hours after meals) to minimize possible nausea and vomiting.

What to do if you miss a dose
If you forget to take your medication and you remember within an hour or so of the scheduled dosing time, take it right away. But if you don't remember until 2 or more hours after your scheduled dosing time, skip the dose you missed and resume your normal dosing schedule. Don't take double doses.

What to do about side effects
Although it's uncommon, bethanechol can cause shortness of breath and wheezing. If you have breathing problems, call your primary health care provider *immediately.* You may be having an allergic reaction to the medication.

Common side effects include abdominal cramps and diarrhea. If these symptoms persist or become severe, contact your primary health care provider.

Besides breathing problems, less common side effects include tearing, headache, flushing, and sweating.

What you must know about other drugs
Tell your primary health care provider about other medications you're taking. For example, anticholinergic agents — such as atropine or propantheline (Pro-Banthine), procainamide (Pronestyl), and quinidine (CinQuin) — may decrease bethanechol's effectiveness.

Special directions
• Inform your primary health care provider if you have other medical problems because bethanechol may aggravate some disorders.
• You may feel dizzy, light-headed, or faint, especially when arising from a lying or sitting position. To minimize this problem, get up slowly.

✔ Keep in mind
• Contact your primary health care provider if you become pregnant while taking bethanechol.

Additional instructions

_____
_____
_____
_____
_____
_____
_____
_____
_____
_____
_____

Taking bisacodyl

Dear Patient,

Bisacodyl is used to relieve constipation. Brand names include Dulcolax and Fleet Bisacodyl.

How to take bisacodyl

Bisacodyl is available in tablet, enema, powder for rectal solution, and suppository forms.

Follow your primary health care provider's instructions. Also follow the manufacturer's package directions exactly if you're using the Fleet enema, powder for rectal solution, or suppository form.

Whichever bisacodyl form you use, drink six to eight 8-ounce glasses of liquid daily to help soften your stools.

Take the *tablet* on an empty stomach for rapid effect. Because the tablets are specially coated to prevent stomach irritation, don't chew, crush, or take them within an hour of drinking milk or taking antacids. You may want to take tablets at bedtime to produce results the next morning.

If you're using a *suppository* and it's too soft to insert, chill it for 30 minutes or run cold water over it before removing the foil wrapper. To insert it, first wash your hands, then remove the wrapper and moisten the suppository with cold water. Lie on your side and use your finger to gently push the suppository into your rectum.

To use the *enema,* first lubricate your anus with petroleum jelly (Vaseline). Then lie on your side and gently insert the rectal tip of the enema applicator. Squeeze all the solution from the enema bottle.

What to do about side effects

Notify the primary health care provider if you notice rectal bleeding, blistering, pain, severe burning, itching, or other irritation you didn't have before using this medication.

Common side effects include nausea, vomiting, abdominal cramps and, with the suppository, a burning sensation in the rectum. If these symptoms persist or worsen, contact your primary health care provider.

Special directions

• If you have other medical problems, check with your primary health care provider before using bisacodyl.
• Don't use bisacodyl or other laxatives if you have stomach or lower abdominal pain, cramping, bloating, soreness, nausea, or vomiting. Instead, notify your primary health care provider as soon as possible.

Warning: Don't use bisacodyl within 2 hours of taking other medications; doing so can reduce other medications' effects.

• Never use bisacodyl for more than 1 week unless your primary health care provider prescribes it.
• If a change in bowel function persists longer than 2 weeks or keeps returning, check with your primary health care provider before using bisacodyl.
• Don't use bisacodyl unless you need it. Overusing laxatives may damage bowel structures, foster dependence, and cause weakness, poor coordination, dizziness, and light-headedness.

Keep in mind

• Don't use bisacodyl in children under age 6 unless prescribed by a primary health care provider.

Additional instructions

_____
_____
_____
_____

Taking blood pressure-lowering medications

Dear Patient,

Your primary health care provider has prescribed antihypertensives because you have high blood pressure. In general, these drugs lower your blood pressure by slowing down your heart rate, opening up your blood vessels and lowering resistance in them, or affecting chemicals in your body that may be causing high blood pressure.

How to take antihypertensives

This medication is available as a tablet, an injection, and a patch that is put on the skin. The tablets are generally taken on a regular basis one to several times daily. The patch is changed weekly. Some antihypertensives work better if they're taken with food, so check with your primary health care provider or pharmacist.

What to do if you miss a dose

Try not to miss any doses, but if you do, take the dose as soon as you remember. However, if it's almost time for your next dose (within 4 to 8 hours for long-acting antihypertensives), skip the missed dose. Don't take double doses.

What to do about side effects

If you have chest pain, a slow heartbeat, trouble breathing, fainting, a rash, no desire to eat, pain around your midsection, darkened urine, flulike symptoms, or sudden weight gain, call your primary health care provider at once. You may be having an allergic reaction to this medication.

More common side effects include diarrhea, nausea, abdominal pain, vomiting, dizziness, fatigue, headache, drowsiness, and a decrease in sexual function. If these problems become troublesome, call your primary health care provider.

What you must know about other drugs

Tell your primary health care provider if you're taking quinidine, fluoxetine, paroxetine, or propafenone because they may increase the level of antihypertensives in your system. Antihypertensives may also lower blood sugar, so tell your primary health care provider if you're on insulin or other diabetes medications because these doses may need to be adjusted. Also inform him if you're taking more than one antihypertensive—this might lower your blood pressure too much.

Also inform your primary health care provider if you're taking digoxin (he may need to adjust your digoxin dose); if you're taking rifampin or cimetidine (they may lower or raise the level of the antihypertensive in your system); and if you're taking reserpine or a class of drugs known as monoamine oxidase (MAO) inhibitors (they may lower your pressure and heart rate too much).

Special directions

! *Warning:* Don't stop this drug suddenly. The primary health care provider will probably tell you to taper the dose gradually over 1 to 2 weeks.
• You may be asked to take your pulse daily before your dose. If your heart rate feels lower, or if your pulse is less than what your primary health care provider said it should be, call him.
• Get up slowly from a lying or sitting position until you know how this medication affects you. Otherwise, you may feel lightheaded or even faint.

✔ Keep in mind

• Tell your primary health care provider if you're breast-feeding or if you become pregnant.

(continued)

Taking blood pressure-lowering medications *(continued)*

• Tell your primary health care provider if you have liver or kidney disease.
• If you're a diabetic and your blood sugar changes, call your primary health care provider.
• If you're an older adult, you may be more sensitive to the drug's effects and may need lower doses.
• If you wear contact lenses, your eyes may be drier than usual with some antihypertensives.

Additional instructions

_____
_____
_____
_____
_____
_____
_____
_____
_____
_____
_____

Taking bromocriptine

Dear Patient,

By regulating certain hormones, bromocriptine treats menstrual problems, enhances fertility in some women, and stops breast milk production. It's also used for Parkinson's disease, acromegaly (overproduction of growth hormone), and pituitary disorders. The label may read Parlodel.

How to take bromocriptine
This medication comes in capsules and tablets. Carefully read the medication label, and follow the directions exactly. If bromocriptine upsets your stomach, try taking it with meals or milk.

What to do if you miss a dose
Take it as soon as you remember, as long as it's within 4 hours of the scheduled dosing time. After a longer time, skip the missed dose and resume your normal schedule. Don't take double doses.

What to do about side effects
Contact your primary health care provider if you suddenly become short of breath or have chest pain, blurred vision, headache, or severe nausea and vomiting.

Common side effects include dizziness, headache, abdominal cramps, and light-headedness. If these symptoms persist or become severe, call the primary health care provider.

What you must know about alcohol and other drugs
Avoid alcoholic beverages when taking bromocriptine. The combination may cause unwanted side effects. Also tell your health care provider about other prescription and nonprescription medications you're taking. Other drugs may intensify or decrease bromocriptine's effect or require dosage changes.

Special directions
• Have regular checkups so your primary health care provider can monitor your condition and bromocriptine's effects.
• Know how you react to this medication before you perform activities requiring alertness.
• If you feel dizzy or faint when arising from bed or a chair, get up slowly.
• To relieve dry mouth, use sugarless hard candy or gum, ice chips, or a saliva substitute. Persistent dryness increases the risk of tooth decay and other mouth disorders.
• Bromocriptine may take several weeks to become effective. Don't stop the drug or reduce your dosage without consulting your primary health care provider.
• When treating infertility, your primary health care provider may advise birth control measures (other than oral contraceptives) at first. Later, you can determine when to stop using birth control.

✓ Keep in mind
• If you're pregnant or breast-feeding, consult your primary health care provider before taking bromocriptine.
• Older adults may be more sensitive to this drug and its side effects.
• Tell your primary health care provider if you have other medical problems, particularly uncontrolled high blood pressure, liver disease, or emotional illness. They may affect the use of bromocriptine.

Additional instructions

_____
_____
_____
_____
_____

Taking brompheniramine with phenylpropanolamine

Dear Patient,

This medication relieves a stuffy or runny nose and sneezing from colds and allergies. Brand names include Bromatap, Bromatapp, and Dimetapp.

How to take this drug

This medication comes in tablet, extended-release tablet, and elixir forms. Carefully read the medication label, and follow the directions exactly. Take the medication with food, milk, or water to reduce stomach upset.

Swallow an extended-release tablet whole; don't break, crush, or chew it. If you can't swallow it, consult the primary health care provider, nurse, or pharmacist.

What to do if you miss a dose

Take the dose as soon as you remember. If it's almost time for your next dose, skip the dose you missed and resume your normal dosing schedule. Never take double doses.

What to do about side effects

Call the primary health care provider *immediately* if you have a rapid or irregular heartbeat, a tight chest, sore throat, fever, unusual tiredness or weakness, or unusual bleeding or bruising.

Common side effects include a dry mouth, thick phlegm, drowsiness and, possibly, nervousness, restlessness, and insomnia. If these effects persist, call your primary health care provider.

What you must know about alcohol and other drugs

Tell your primary health care provider about other medications you're taking. Taking this medication with alcoholic beverages and other medications that depress the central nervous system (such as antihistamines and pain and seizure medications) increases the side effects of all the medications. And taking this drug with appetite suppressants increases the risk of overdose. Signs of overdose include difficulty breathing, severe drowsiness, persistent headache, and seizures.

Special directions

• Know how you respond to this medication before you drive or perform other activities requiring alertness.
• If you have trouble sleeping, take the day's last dose a few hours before bedtime.
• Relieve dry mouth with ice chips or sugarless gum or hard candy.

✔ Keep in mind

• If you're pregnant or breast-feeding, consult your primary health care provider about using this medication.
• Use this medication cautiously in young children and older adults.
• Inform the primary health care provider if you have asthma, heart or blood vessel disease, high blood pressure, glaucoma, diabetes, an overactive thyroid, or urinary problems. Also report any allergic or unusual reactions to antihistamines.
• If you're an athlete, you should know that the National Collegiate Athletic Association and the U.S. Olympic Committee disqualify athletes from competitions if urine samples contain excess phenylpropanolamine.

Additional instructions

_____
_____
_____
_____
_____

Taking bumetanide

Dear Patient,

Bumetanide stimulates urination and reduces water in your body. The label may read Bumex.

How to take bumetanide
Carefully check your medication label. Follow the directions exactly. So that urination doesn't interrupt your sleep, take your single daily dose in the morning after breakfast. If you're taking more than one dose a day, take the last dose before 6 p.m. unless directed otherwise by your primary health care provider.

What to do if you miss a dose
Take it as soon as you remember unless it's almost time for your next dose. Then you should skip the dose you missed and resume your normal dosing schedule. Don't take double doses.

What to do about side effects
Common side effects include fatigue, dizziness, light-headedness, and fainting. If these symptoms persist or become severe, contact your primary health care provider.

What you must know about other drugs
Tell your primary health care provider about other medications you're taking. Taking some antibiotics with bumetanide increases your risk of hearing problems. Probenecid (Probalan), indomethacin (Indocin), and some analgesics may decrease bumetanide's effects.

Special directions
• Before taking bumetanide, inform your primary health care provider if you have other medical problems.
• Because this medication may reduce electrolytes needed by your body (such as potassium, chloride, sodium, calcium, and magnesium), have your blood tested regularly.
• To replace lost potassium, eat foods and drink beverages containing potassium (for example, citrus fruits and orange juice). Or take a potassium supplement or other medication prescribed by your primary health care provider to minimize potassium loss.
• To prevent excessive water and potassium loss, call your primary health care provider if you experience persistent vomiting or diarrhea.
• To help relieve dizziness or light-headedness, get up slowly from bed or a chair, limit the amount of alcoholic beverages you drink, and take care not to get overheated. If the problem persists or worsens, tell your primary health care provider.
• Before surgery (including dental surgery) or emergency treatment, inform the primary health care provider or dentist that you're taking bumetanide.

✓ Keep in mind
• If you have diabetes, check your blood glucose levels carefully and notify your primary health care provider if you note any changes.
• If you become pregnant while taking bumetanide, tell your primary health care provider promptly.
• Older adults are especially sensitive to this medication and its side effects.
• If you're an athlete, be aware that the National Collegiate Athletic Association and the U.S. Olympic Committee ban the use of bumetanide.

Additional instructions

_____

_____

Taking buspirone

Dear Patient,

This medication (also called BuSpar) is used to treat certain anxiety disorders and to relieve anxiety symptoms.

How to take buspirone

Carefully check your medication label. Follow the directions exactly. Be aware that you may not feel buspirone's full effects until 1 to 2 weeks after you begin taking it.

What to do if you miss a dose

If you forget to take your medication, take it as soon as you remember. But if it's almost time for your next dose, skip the dose you missed and resume your regular dosing schedule. Never take double doses.

What to do about side effects

Common side effects include drowsiness and dizziness. If these symptoms persist or worsen, notify your primary health care provider.

What you must know about alcohol and other drugs

Tell your primary health care provider about other medications you're taking. Buspirone taken with alcoholic beverages and other central nervous system depressants, such as sleeping pills, some cold or allergy medications, and tranquilizers, can cause drowsiness. When taken with monoamine oxidase (MAO) inhibitors, such as isocarboxazid (Marplan), buspirone may raise your blood pressure.

Special directions

• Inform your primary health care provider about your medical history, especially drug abuse or dependency or kidney or liver disease. These and other medical problems may affect the use of buspirone.

• If you're taking this medication regularly for a long time, schedule regular checkups so your primary health care provider can monitor your progress and buspirone's effects.

• Make sure you know how you react to this medication before you drive, operate machinery, or perform other activities requiring physical coordination and alertness.

Warning: If you think you may have taken an overdose of this medication, get emergency help at once.

✓ Keep in mind

• If you're an athlete, be aware that the National Collegiate Athletic Association and the U.S. Olympic Committee ban the use of buspirone in certain competitions.

Additional instructions

_____
_____
_____
_____
_____
_____
_____
_____
_____
_____
_____

Taking captopril

Dear Patient,

Captopril helps control high blood pressure and heart failure. The label may read Capoten.

How to take captopril

Carefully read the medication label. Follow the directions exactly. Take captopril 1 hour before meals unless your primary health care provider directs otherwise.

What to do if you miss a dose

Take the dose as soon as you remember. But if it's almost time for your next scheduled dose, skip the dose you missed and take your next dose at the scheduled time. Don't take double doses.

What to do about side effects

Contact your health care provider *immediately* and stop taking this medication if you have a fever, chills, hoarseness, sudden trouble swallowing or breathing, or swelling of your face, mouth, hands, or feet. These symptoms may indicate an allergic reaction.

A common side effect is a dry, continuing cough. If it persists or worsens, notify your primary health care provider.

What you must know about other drugs

Tell the primary health care provider about other medications you're taking. Some antacids and analgesics may decrease captopril's effectiveness. Captopril taken with digoxin (Lanoxin) can increase the risk of toxic effects. And taking potassium supplements with captopril increases your risk for having too much potassium.

Special directions

• See your primary health care provider regularly to monitor captopril's effectiveness and to check for side effects.

• Don't stop taking this medication on your own even if you feel better. Although high blood pressure may not produce symptoms, you may still need ongoing treatment.
• Remember to follow any prescribed special diet that will help this medication lower your blood pressure.
• Don't take new medications (prescription or nonprescription) without first consulting your primary health care provider.
• Dizziness, light-headedness, or even fainting may follow the first dose of this medication, especially if you have been taking a diuretic (water pill). These side effects may also follow heavy sweating, which depletes body water and lowers blood pressure. Avoid becoming overheated.

Warning: Notify your primary health care provider promptly if you become sick while taking this medication, especially if you have severe or continuing vomiting or diarrhea, which can cause rapid body water loss and low blood pressure.
• Before medical tests, surgery (including dental surgery), or emergency treatment, tell the primary health care provider or dentist that you're taking captopril.

✔ Keep in mind

• If you become pregnant while taking captopril, tell your primary health care provider, who may change your prescription to another blood pressure medication. If you're breast-feeding, discuss the use of captopril with your primary health care provider.

Additional instructions

_____

_____

_____

_____

Taking carbamazepine

Dear Patient,

This medication controls some types of seizures. It's also used to treat trigeminal neuralgia pain. The label may read Epitol or Tegretol.

How to take carbamazepine

Carbamazepine comes in oral suspension, tablet, and chewable tablet forms. Carefully read your medication label. Follow the directions exactly. Take carbamazepine with meals.

What to do if you miss a dose

Take the dose as soon as you remember. If it's almost time for your next dose, skip the dose you missed and take the next dose at the scheduled time. Never take double doses. If you miss more than one dose a day, check with your primary health care provider.

What to do about side effects

Consult the primary health care provider *at once* if you have abnormal blood test results or signs of infection (fever, chills, cough) or unusual bleeding (bruises or bloody urine or stools).

Common side effects include dizziness, drowsiness, clumsiness, nausea, vertigo (sensation that objects are spinning), mouth sores, and rash. If these symptoms persist or worsen, notify your primary health care provider.

What you must know about alcohol and other drugs

Be sure to tell your primary health care provider about other medications you're taking. Alcoholic beverages and central nervous system depressants (such as sleeping pills and cold remedies) may reduce alertness and coordination. Some drugs may decrease or increase carbamazepine's effects and the effects of other drugs you take.

Special directions

• As a pain reliever, carbamazepine works only for certain kinds of pain. Don't take it for other discomfort.
• If you're taking carbamazepine for seizures, don't stop using it without consulting your primary health care provider, who may reduce the dosage gradually.
• Have regular checkups to monitor your progress and make dosage changes.
• Know how you react to carbamazepine before driving or performing other activities requiring alertness.
• Your sensitivity to sunlight may increase, especially at first. Protect yourself from the sun. If you have a severe reaction, notify your primary health care provider.
• Before medical tests, surgery, dental work, or emergency treatment, tell the primary health care provider that you're taking carbamazepine.
• Carry an identification card or bracelet that states you're taking carbamazepine.

✅ Keep in mind

• If you have diabetes, carbamazepine may affect your urine glucose level.
• If you're pregnant or breast-feeding, consult the primary health care provider before taking carbamazepine.
• Children and older adults may be especially sensitive to this medication.
• If you're an athlete, you should know that carbamazepine is banned by the National Collegiate Athletic Association and the U.S. Olympic Committee.

Additional instructions

_____

_____

Taking carisoprodol

Dear Patient,

This medication relaxes your muscles and relieves the pain and discomfort of strains, sprains and other muscle injuries. The label may read Soma.

How to take carisoprodol

Carisoprodol comes in tablet form. Carefully read your medication label. Follow the directions exactly.

What to do if you miss a dose

If you forget to take your medication and remember within an hour or so of the scheduled dosing time, take the dose you missed right away. But if you don't remember until later, skip the missed dose and resume your normal dosing schedule. Don't take double doses.

What to do about side effects

Common side effects include drowsiness, dizziness, and skin changes. If these symptoms persist or worsen, call your primary health care provider. If dizziness occurs, avoid sudden changes in posture. Use caution when climbing stairs.

What you must know about alcohol and other drugs

Tell your primary health care provider if you're taking other medications. Avoid taking carisoprodol with alcoholic beverages or other drugs that depress the central nervous system (such as sleeping pills and cold remedies). Doing so can cause increased drowsiness and dizziness.

Special directions

- Before you start to take carisoprodol, tell your primary health care provider if you have other medical problems. They may affect the use of this medication.
- If you're taking this medication for more than a few weeks, see your primary health care provider regularly to check your progress.
- Know how you react to carisoprodol before you drive, operate machinery, or perform other activities requiring alertness and coordination.

✔ Keep in mind

- If you become pregnant while taking carisoprodol, tell your primary health care provider.
- If you're breast-feeding, be aware that carisoprodol passes into breast milk and can cause drowsiness and stomach upset in breast-feeding infants; discuss its use with your primary health care provider.
- If you're an athlete, be aware that carisoprodol is banned by the National Collegiate Athletic Association and the U.S. Olympic Committee. Its use could result in your disqualification from amateur athletic competitions.

Additional instructions

_____
_____
_____
_____
_____
_____
_____
_____
_____
_____

Taking carvedilol

Dear Patient,

Your primary health care provider has pre-scribed carvedilol because you have high blood pressure or a condition known as heart failure. This medication will lower your blood pressure by slowing your heart rate and relieve heart failure by opening up your blood vessels and lowering resistance in them. The brand name of this drug is Coreg.

How to take carvedilol
This medication is available as tablets. It should be taken with food.

What to do about side effects
Notify your primary health care provider im-mediately if you have chest pain, trouble breathing, a rash, no desire to eat, pain around your midsection, darkened urine, or unexplained flulike symptoms.

Common side effects include diarrhea, nausea, abdominal pain, vomiting, dizzi-ness, or headache. If they become trouble-some, call your primary health care provider.

What you must know about other drugs
If you're taking quinidine, fluoxetine, paroxe-tine, or propafenone, tell your primary health care provider immediately because these medications may increase the level of carvedilol in your system. Since carvedilol may lower blood sugar, tell your primary health care provider if you're on insulin or diabetic medications because these may need to be adjusted.

Report to your primary health care provider if you also take clonidine, because this combination may drop your blood pres-sure too much. Reserpine and drugs known as monoamine oxidase (MAO) inhibitors may also lower your blood pressure and heart rate too much. If you take digoxin, the primary health care provider may need to adjust your digoxin dose. Taking rifampin or cimetidine may lower or raise the amount of carvedilol in your system. Also report if you're taking a calcium channel blocker be-cause your blood pressure and heart rate may need to monitored periodically.

Special directions
• Don't stop taking this drug suddenly. The primary health care provider will probably have you taper the dose gradually over 1 to 2 weeks.
• If you sense that your heart rate has de-creased, or if you take your blood pressure and it measures less than 55 beats per minute, call your primary health care provider.

✔ Keep in mind
• If you're a diabetic and your blood sugar changes, call your primary health care provider.
• If you wear contact lenses, your eyes may be drier than usual.
• Tell your primary health care provider if you're breast-feeding or become pregnant while on this medication.
• If you're an older adult, you may be more sensitive to this medication's effects and may need lower doses.

Additional instructions
_____
_____
_____
_____
_____
_____
_____
_____

Taking cefaclor

Dear Patient,

Cefaclor is used to treat infections caused by bacteria. The label may read Ceclor.

How to take cefaclor
Carefully check the label on your prescription bottle, which contains either capsules or a liquid.

Follow the directions exactly. Take your daily doses at evenly spaced times over 24 hours, as your primary health care provider prescribes. If this medication upsets your stomach, you may take it with food. If you're taking the liquid, shake the bottle well. Then use a medicine dropper or a measuring spoon to pour each dose accurately.

What to do if you miss a dose
If you forget to take your medication and your dosing schedule is one dose a day, space the missed dose and the next scheduled dose 10 to 12 hours apart. If you're taking two doses a day, space the missed dose and the next dose 5 to 6 hours apart. If you're taking three or more doses a day, space the missed dose and the next dose 2 to 4 hours apart. After taking the dose you missed, resume your normal dosing schedule.

What to do about side effects
Common side effects include diarrhea, nausea, and a rash. If these persist or worsen, contact your primary health care provider.

What you must know about other drugs
Tell your primary health care provider if you're taking other medications. Probenecid (Benemid) may increase cefaclor's effects.

Special directions
• Before starting to take cefaclor, inform your primary health care provider if you have other medical problems. They may affect the use of this medication.
• To help clear up your infection completely, take the medication for the full course of treatment, even if you begin to feel better after a few days. If you stop taking it too soon, your infection may recur.
• If your symptoms don't improve within a few days or if you feel worse, notify your primary health care provider.
• If you have mild diarrhea, you may take a diarrhea medication containing kaolin or attapulgite (Kaopectate or Diasorb) — but no other type. Another type may increase or prolong diarrhea. Severe diarrhea is a serious side effect; if it occurs, check with your primary health care provider before taking any more diarrhea medication.

✔ Keep in mind
• If you have diabetes, be aware that cefaclor may cause false results with some urine glucose tests. Check with your primary health care provider before changing your diet or the dosage of your diabetes medication.
• If you're breast-feeding, consult your primary health care provider before using cefaclor.

Additional instructions
_____
_____
_____
_____
_____
_____
_____

Taking cefadroxil

Dear Patient,

Your primary health care provider has prescribed cefadroxil because you have an infection. This medication will improve your condition by killing bacteria or preventing their growth. The brand name of this medication is Duricef.

How to take cefadroxil

This medication is available as capsules, tablets, or an oral liquid. It can be taken either with or without food, but if it upsets your stomach, taking it with food may help.

Take cefadroxil exactly as directed on the label, spacing out doses as evenly as you can. If the dosage schedule interferes with your everyday routine, call your primary health care provider or pharmacist for advice. Keep the liquid medication refrigerated, and don't use it after the expiration date on the label.

What to do if you miss a dose

If you miss a dose and it's not time for your next dose, take the missed dose as soon as you remember. If it's close to your next dose, skip the missed dose. Don't take double doses.

What to do about side effects

If you have bloody diarrhea; a rash; trouble breathing; swelling of your face, mouth, neck, hands, or feet; or seizures, call your primary health care provider *at once.*

More common side effects are diarrhea, nausea, vomiting , stomach cramps, dizziness, and headache. On rare occasions, women have vaginal itching or discharge.

What you must know about other drugs

If you're also taking probenecid, cefadroxil will remain in your system longer.

Special directions

● Finish taking all your prescription even if you start to feel better.
● Tell your primary health care provider if you're allergic to penicillin because cefadroxil may cause a similar reaction.

✔ Keep in mind

● If you're a diabetic, this medication may cause false-positive results in urine glucose tests. Ask your pharmacist what test strip to use while on cefadroxil.
● Tell your primary health care provider if you're breast-feeding or if you become pregnant.
● Tell your primary health care provider if you have kidney disease. He may need to adjust your cefadroxil dose.

Additional instructions

_____
_____
_____
_____
_____
_____
_____
_____
_____
_____

Taking cefixime

Dear Patient,

Your primary health care provider has prescribed cefixime because you have an infection. This medication will improve your condition by killing bacteria or preventing their growth. The brand name of this drug is Suprax.

How to take cefixime

Cefixime is available as tablets or an oral liquid. It can be taken either with or without food, but if it upsets your stomach, taking it with food may help.

Take cefixime exactly as directed on the label. Space out doses as evenly as you can, but if this interferes with your everyday routine, call your primary health care provider or pharmacist. Don't use the liquid form after the expiration date on the label. The liquid doesn't need refrigeration.

What to do if you miss a dose

If you miss a dose and it's not time for your next dose, take the missed dose as soon as you remember. If it's close to your next dose, skip the missed dose. Don't take double doses.

What to do about side effects

If you have bloody diarrhea; a rash; difficulty breathing; swelling of your face, mouth, neck, hands or feet; or seizure, call your primary health care provider *immediately.*

More common side effects include diarrhea, nausea, vomiting, dizziness, headache, and stomach cramps. Women may rarely experience vaginal itching or discharge.

What you must know about other drugs

If you're also taking probenecid, cefixime will remain in your system longer.

Special directions

- Take all of your prescription, even if you start to feel better.
- Tell your primary health care provider if you're allergic to penicillin because cefixime may cause a similar reaction.

✔ Keep in mind

- If you're a diabetic, this medication may cause false-positive results in urine glucose tests. Ask your pharmacist what test strip to use while on this medication.
- Tell your primary health care provider if you're breast-feeding or if you become pregnant.
- Tell your primary health care provider if you have kidney disease. He may need to adjust your cefixime dose.
- If you have phenylketonuria, report this to your primary health care provider or pharmacist because the oral suspension contains phenylalanine.

Additional instructions

_____
_____
_____
_____
_____
_____
_____
_____
_____
_____
_____

Taking cefprozil

Dear Patient,

Your primary health care provider has prescribed cefprozil because you have an infection. This medication will improve your condition by killing bacteria or preventing their growth. The brand name of this medication is Cefzil.

How to take cefprozil

This medication is available as tablets or an oral liquid. It can be taken either with or without food, but if it upsets your stomach, taking it with food may help. Take this medication exactly as directed on the label, spacing out doses as evenly as possible. If this interferes with your everyday routine, call your primary health care provider or pharmacist. Don't use the liquid after the expiration date on the label, and keep it refrigerated.

What to do if you miss a dose

If you miss a dose and it's not time for your next dose, take the missed dose as soon as you remember. If it's close to your next dose, skip the missed dose. Don't take double doses.

What to do about side effects

If you have bloody diarrhea; a rash; difficulty breathing; swelling of your face, mouth, neck, hands, or feet; or seizures, call your primary health care provider *immediately.*

More common side effects include diarrhea, nausea, vomiting, stomach cramps, dizziness, and headache. Women may rarely have vaginal itching or discharge.

What you must know about other drugs

If you're also taking probenecid, cefprozil will remain in your system longer.

Special directions

• Finish your entire prescription, even if you start to feel better.
• Tell your primary health care provider if you're allergic to penicillin because cefprozil may cause a similar reaction.

✔ Keep in mind

• If you're a diabetic, this medication may cause false-positive results in urine glucose tests. Ask your pharmacist what test strip to use while on cefprozil.
• Tell your primary health care provider if you have kidney disease. He may need to adjust the cefprozil dose.
• Tell your primary health care provider if you're breast-feeding or if you become pregnant.

Additional instructions

_____
_____
_____
_____
_____
_____
_____
_____
_____
_____
_____
_____
_____

Taking cefuroxime axetil

Dear Patient,

This medication is an antibiotic used to treat various infections, but not colds or flu. The label may read Ceftin.

How to take cefuroxime axetil

This medication comes in tablet form. Carefully check your medication label, and follow the directions exactly. Take the medication on a full stomach. If you can't swallow the tablet, you may crush it and mix it with a small amount of food.

What to do if you miss a dose

If you forget to take your medication, take it as soon as you remember. If it's almost time for your next dose and your dosing schedule is two times a day, space the dose you missed and the next scheduled dose 5 to 6 hours apart. Then resume your normal dosing schedule.

What to do about side effects

Occasionally, this medication produces serious side effects, including allergic reaction, anemia, and colitis. If you have a fever, rash, itchy skin, restlessness, or difficulty breathing, stop taking the medication and *immediately* seek emergency medical care.

If you experience fatigue, weakness, pale skin, nausea, vomiting, appetite loss, and diarrhea, report these effects to your primary health care provider promptly.

What you must know about other drugs

Tell your primary health care provider about other medications you're taking. Probenecid (Benemid) may increase the amount of cefuroxime axetil in your blood.

Special directions

- Tell your primary health care provider if you're allergic to this medication or other medications, especially other antibiotics.
- Avoid taking diarrhea medication without first consulting your primary health care provider. Many diarrhea medications can increase or prolong diarrhea.
- Check with your primary health care provider before taking new medications (prescription or nonprescription) or if you develop new medical problems.
- To be sure that the infection clears up completely, take this medication for the entire time your primary health care provider prescribes, even if your symptoms subside.
- If your symptoms don't subside within a few days or if you feel worse, call your primary health care provider.

✓ Keep in mind

- If you're pregnant or breast-feeding, consult your primary health care provider before taking this medication.
- Inform your primary health care provider if you have kidney disease or other medical problems because he may need to adjust the medication dose.

Additional instructions

_____
_____
_____
_____
_____
_____
_____
_____
_____
_____
_____

Taking cephalexin

Dear Patient,

This antibiotic is used to treat various infections, but not colds or flu. Brand names include Keflex and Keftab.

How to take cephalexin

Cephalexin comes in tablets, capsules, and an oral suspension. Carefully check your medication label. This tells you how much to take at each dose and when to take it. Follow the directions exactly.

Take tablets or capsules with food or milk to decrease possible stomach upset.

Store the suspension in the refrigerator. Keep the bottle closed tightly and shake it well before using. Discard unused suspension after 14 days.

What to do if you miss a dose

Take it as soon as you remember. But if it's almost time for your next dose and your dosing schedule is three or more times a day, space the dose you missed and the next scheduled dose 2 to 4 hours apart. Then resume your normal dosing schedule.

What to do about side effects

Occasionally, this medication produces serious side effects, including allergic reaction, anemia, and colitis. If you experience a fever, rash, itching, restlessness, or difficulty breathing, stop taking the medication and seek emergency medical care *immediately*.

If you experience fatigue, weakness, pale skin, nausea, vomiting, loss of appetite, or diarrhea, report these effects to your primary health care provider promptly.

What you must know about other drugs

To ensure that you benefit from treatment, tell your primary health care provider about other medications you're taking. Probenecid (Benemid) may increase the effects of cephalexin.

Special directions

• Tell your primary health care provider if you're allergic to this medication or other medications, especially other antibiotics.
• Check with your primary health care provider before taking new medications (prescription or nonprescription) or if new medical problems develop.
• Avoid taking diarrhea medication without consulting your primary health care provider. Many diarrhea medications can increase or prolong diarrhea.
• To be sure that your infection clears up completely, take your medication for the entire time your primary health care provider prescribes, even if your symptoms subside.
• If symptoms don't subside in a few days or if they worsen, call your primary health care provider.

✓ Keep in mind

• If you're pregnant or breast-feeding, check with your primary health care provider before taking this medication.
• Inform your primary health care provider if you have kidney disease or other medical problems because he may need to adjust your medication dose.

Additional instructions

_____
_____
_____
_____
_____
_____
_____

Taking cetirizine

Dear Patient,

Your primary health care provider has prescribed cetirizine because you have hay fever or other allergies. This medication will improve your condition by preventing the effects of a substance called histamine. The brand name of this medication is Zyrtec.

How to take cetirizine
This medication is available as a tablet. It may be taken either with or without food. If it causes stomach upset, taking it with food may help.

What to do if you miss a dose
If you miss a scheduled dose, take it as soon as you remember if it's not close to your next scheduled dose. If it is close to your next dose, skip the missed dose and resume your normal dosing schedule. Don't take double doses.

What to do about side effects
Side effects include nervousness, increased appetite, and dryness of the mouth, nose, and throat. Sugarless candy, gum, or ice chips may help. Contact your primary health care provider if these effects become severe.

What you must know about alcohol and other drugs
Don't drink alcohol while taking cetirizine because it may cause severe drowsiness. Sedatives and tranquilizers will also cause severe drowsiness combined with cetirizine, so tell your primary health care provider or pharmacist if you're taking these medications.

Also inform your primary health care provider if you take aspirin regularly because the effects of too much aspirin, such as ringing in the ears, will be masked by cetirizine.

Special directions
• Know how you react to this drug before you drive, operate machinery, or participate in any activity that requires full alertness.
• Avoid prolonged exposure to the sun because this drug may make you more sensitive.
• Tell your primary health care provider if you're having skin testing for allergies because this medication will affect test results.

✔ Keep in mind
• Children and older adults are more sensitive to the effects of this medication.
• Tell your primary health care provider if you have glaucoma, peptic ulcer disease, or difficulty urinating before starting cetirizine. He may need to adjust the dose.
• Don't breast-feed or become pregnant while on this medication.

Additional instructions
_____
_____
_____
_____
_____
_____
_____
_____
_____
_____
_____
_____

Taking chloral hydrate

Dear Patient,

Chloral hydrate is used to help calm you and help you sleep. Brand names include Aquachloral Supprettes and Noctec.

How to take chloral hydrate
Chloral hydrate comes in capsule, syrup, and suppository forms. Follow directions on the label exactly. To aid sleep, take chloral hydrate 15 to 30 minutes before bedtime. Take the *capsule* form after meals. Swallow it whole, and drink a full glass (8 ounces) of liquid to minimize possible stomach upset. For the same reason, mix a *syrup* dose in half a glass of liquid before taking.

If you're using a *suppository* and it's too soft to insert, chill it briefly (30 minutes in the refrigerator) or run cold water over it before removing the foil wrapper. To insert it, first wash your hands, then remove the wrapper and moisten the suppository with cold water. Lie on your side and use your finger to gently push the suppository into your rectum.

What to do if you miss a dose
If you forget to take your medication, skip the missed dose. Take the next scheduled dose. Don't take double doses.

What to do about side effects
If you have serious side effects, such as extreme drowsiness, swallowing or breathing difficulties, or seizures, stop the medication and get emergency medical care *at once.*

Common side effects include drowsiness, dizziness, a hangover-like feeling, and nausea. If these effects persist or worsen, tell your primary health care provider.

What you must know about alcohol and other drugs
Don't drink alcoholic beverages while taking chloral hydrate. It can lead to an overdose.

Tell your primary health care provider about other medications you're taking. Certain drugs that cause drowsiness (for example, allergy and cold medications, pain relievers, muscle relaxants, and anesthetics) can increase chloral hydrate's effects. And chloral hydrate will increase the effects of anticoagulants (blood thinners).

Special directions
• Let your primary health care provider know if you've ever had allergic reactions to drugs or foods.
• Check with your primary health care provider before taking new medications or if you develop new medical problems.
• Know how you react to this medication before you drive or perform other activities that require alertness.

! Warning: Take this medication only as directed. Overuse can lead to dependency. Also, don't stop taking this medication without consulting your primary health care provider, who may adjust the dosage to prevent withdrawal effects.

✔ Keep in mind
• If you're pregnant or breast-feeding, check with your primary health care provider before taking this medication.
• Tell your primary health care provider if you have other medical problems, including drug dependency or heart, liver, stomach, intestinal, kidney, blood, and emotional disorders. They may affect the use of this medication.

Additional instructions
_____
_____
_____
_____

Taking chloramphenicol

Dear Patient,

Chloramphenicol treats specific severe infections. Because it may cause serious side effects, the primary health care provider prescribes it only when other antibiotics are ineffective. It is never used for minor infections or to prevent infection.

Common brand names include Ak-Chlor Ophthalmic, Chloromycetin Ophthalmic, Chloromycetin Otic, and Chloroptic S.O.P.

How to take chloramphenicol

Chloramphenicol comes in eardrops, eyedrops or eye ointment, and skin creams. Carefully read your medication label, and follow the directions exactly.

Wash your hands before and after applying medication to your eyes, ears, or skin. Keep eye, ear, and skin medications as germ-free as possible. Don't touch a dropper tip or let it touch anything, including your eye or ear. After using ointment, wipe the tip of the tube with a clean tissue. Keep all containers tightly closed.

To use *eardrops,* lie down or tilt your head so the infected ear is up. Gently pull your earlobe up and back (down and forward for children) to straighten the ear canal; then squeeze the drops into the ear canal. Keep your head tilted for 1 to 2 minutes. Then put a sterile cotton ball at the entrance to (but not in) your ear opening to hold the medication in.

To use *eyedrops* or *eye ointment,* gently clean any crusted matter from your eyes. Sit down, and if you're using eyedrops, tilt your head back. Gently pull down your lower lid to create a pocket. Carefully squeeze eyedrops or a thin strip of ointment into the pocket, then close your eyes gently. Don't blink. Keep your eyes closed for 1 to 2 minutes. After applying ointment, your vision may be blurred for a few minutes.

Before applying *skin cream,* wash the site with soap and water and dry it thoroughly.

What to do if you miss a dose

If you miss a dose of *ear, eye,* or *skin medication,* take it as soon as you remember. But if it's almost time for your next dose, skip the dose you missed and take your next dose at the scheduled time.

What to do about side effects

Serious blood problems (such as severe anemia, infections, and abnormal bleeding) may occur with all forms of this medication, but particularly with long-term use of the *cream form.* Promptly report fever, weakness, confusion, bleeding, sore throat, or mouth sores to your primary health care provider.

If you develop signs and symptoms of an allergic reaction—fever, rash, itching, restlessness, difficulty swallowing or breathing—stop taking the medication and seek emergency medical care *immediately.*

Also stop using the medication and seek emergency medical care *immediately* if you're giving this medication to an infant who develops a swollen abdomen, breathing difficulties, extreme sleepiness, or grayish skin.

When using *eye medication,* be alert for itching, swelling, or persistent burning. With *ear medication,* be alert for ear pain or fever. With *skin cream,* watch for a rash, itching, or burning. If these effects occur, stop taking the medication and call your primary health care provider.

What you must know about other drugs

Discuss other medications you're taking with your primary health care provider. Acetaminophen (Tylenol), for example, affects

(continued)

Taking chloramphenicol (continued)

the amount of chloramphenicol circulating in the blood, which may increase the drug's effects.

Special directions
• To ensure that your infection clears up completely, take this medication for the entire time prescribed, even when your symptoms subside.
• If you don't notice improvement in a few days, or if your symptoms worsen, notify your primary health care provider.
• Check with your primary health care provider before taking new medications (prescription or nonprescription) or if you develop new medical problems.
• Because of possible bleeding problems, be careful when brushing and flossing your teeth. If possible, delay dental procedures until you stop taking this medication.
• Don't share this medication with anyone. Also, use separate washcloths and towels to prevent spreading the infection.
• Report any allergic reactions to chloramphenicol or other medications or food.

✔ Keep in mind
• Before using chloramphenicol eardrops, tell the primary health care provider if you've ever had a punctured or ruptured eardrum.
• If you're pregnant or breast-feeding, tell your primary health care provider before taking chloramphenicol.
• Inform the primary health care provider if you have other medical problems, especially kidney or liver disease, bleeding problems, porphyria, or glucose-6-phosphate dehydrogenase (G6PD) deficiency.

Additional instructions

_____

_____

_____

_____

_____

_____

_____

_____

_____

_____

Taking chlordiazepoxide

Dear Patient,

Chlordiazepoxide is used to relieve mild to moderate anxiety and tension. Brand names may include Libritabs and Librium.

How to take chlordiazepoxide

This medication comes in tablets and capsules. Carefully read the medication label, and follow the directions exactly. Take this medication only as your primary health care provider prescribes. Taking too much may lead to dependency.

What to do if you miss a dose

Take it as soon as you remember. But if it's almost time for the next dose, skip the dose you missed and take your next dose at the regular time. Don't take double doses.

What to do about side effects

You may feel drowsy or have a hangover-like feeling. If these symptoms persist or worsen, tell your primary health care provider.

What you must know about alcohol and other drugs

Remember to tell your primary health care provider about other medications you're taking. And avoid using alcoholic beverages with this drug. Chlordiazepoxide increases the effects of alcohol and other drugs that depress the nervous system, including some allergy and cold remedies, seizure medications, and pain relievers.

Special directions

• Before starting chlordiazepoxide, inform the primary health care provider if you're allergic to other medications (such as other benzodiazepines).
• Know how you respond to this medication before driving or performing other activities requiring alertness.

• If you think that this drug isn't helping you after a few weeks, consult your primary health care provider. Don't increase the dosage on your own.

! *Warning:* If you're taking this medication for a long time, don't suddenly stop taking it; unpleasant withdrawal symptoms may occur. Consult your primary health care provider to help you gradually reduce the dosage before completely stopping chlordiazepoxide.

✔ Keep in mind

• If you're pregnant or breast-feeding, tell your primary health care provider before taking chlordiazepoxide.
• Children and older adults who take chlordiazepoxide may experience more side effects.
• Inform the primary health care provider about your medical history because certain disorders may affect chlordiazepoxide therapy. For example, a brain disease increases the risk for side effects, and sleep apnea may worsen with this medication.
• If you're an athlete, you should know that the National Collegiate Athletic Association and the U.S. Olympic Committee ban the use of chlordiazepoxide. Taking it may disqualify you from amateur athletic competitions.

Additional instructions

_____
_____
_____
_____
_____
_____
_____
_____

Taking chlorpheniramine

Dear Patient,

This medication can relieve or prevent hay fever and other allergy symptoms. Common brand names include Aller-Chlor and Chlor-Trimeton.

How to take chlorpheniramine
This medication comes in tablet, chewable tablet, timed-release tablet or capsule, and syrup forms. Carefully read the medication label. Follow the directions exactly. To reduce possible stomach upset, you can take this medication with food or a full glass of milk or water.

If you're taking the timed-release tablets or capsules, swallow them whole — don't break, chew, or crush them. If you have trouble swallowing, consult your primary health care provider, nurse, or pharmacist.

What to do if you miss a dose
If you forget to take your medication, take it as soon as you remember. If it's almost time for the next dose, skip the dose you missed, and take your next dose at the regular time. Don't take double doses.

What to do about side effects
You may feel jittery or drowsy, and your mouth may be dry. If these symptoms persist or worsen, tell your primary health care provider.

What you must know about alcohol and other drugs
Tell your primary health care provider about other medications you're taking. Avoid taking chlorpheniramine with alcoholic beverages, medications that depress the nervous system (some allergy and cold remedies, seizure medications, and pain relievers), and monoamine oxidase (MAO) inhibitors, such as isocarboxazid (Marplan). Doing so increases unwanted side effects. Keep in mind, too, that chlorpheniramine may hide unwanted side effects of high-dose aspirin therapy (for arthritis, for example), such as ringing in the ears.

Special directions
• Before you undergo allergy tests, tell the primary health care provider that you're taking this medication. Chlorpheniramine may affect test results.
• Relieve a dry mouth with ice chips or sugarless gum or hard candy.
• Know how you respond to this medication before you drive or perform other activities requiring alertness.

✔ Keep in mind
• If you're breast-feeding, tell your primary health care provider before taking this medication.
• Children and older adults are especially sensitive to this medication's side effects.

Additional instructions
_____

Taking chlorpromazine

Dear Patient,

Chlorpromazine is used to treat persistent hiccups, mild withdrawal from alcohol, tetanus, and certain mental and emotional disorders. The label may read Thorazine.

How to take chlorpromazine

Chlorpromazine comes in tablet, sustained-release capsule, concentrate, syrup, and suppository forms. Carefully read the medication label. Follow the directions exactly. You may take oral forms of this medication with food, milk, or water to minimize stomach upset.

Swallow a sustained-release capsule whole. Don't crush, chew, or break it.

Mix the concentrated form in 2 to 4 ounces of water, soda, juice, milk, pudding, or applesauce.

What to do if you miss a dose

If you forget to take your medication and you're taking one dose a day, take it as soon as you remember that day. If you don't remember it until the next day, skip the dose you missed and take your next regular dose.

If you're taking more than one dose a day and you remember it within an hour or so of the scheduled time, take it right away. If you don't remember it until later, skip the missed dose and take your next dose at the regular time.

What to do about side effects

If you have a persistent fever, sore throat, joint pain, or unusual bruising or bleeding, stop taking this medication and call the primary health care provider *at once.*

Other possible side effects include unusual movements, such as lip smacking or jumpy arms and legs, blurred vision, dry mouth, constipation, inability to urinate, and sensitivity to sunlight. If any of these symptoms persist or worsen, call your primary health care provider.

What you must know about alcohol and other drugs

Avoid alcoholic beverages or other drugs that depress the central nervous system because chlorpromazine intensifies their effect.

Tell the primary health care provider about other medications you're taking because chlorpromazine may change their effects. For example, it decreases the effects of medications that lower blood pressure and prevent blood clots.

Special directions

- Check with your primary health care provider before taking new medications (prescription or nonprescription).
- Before surgery, dental work, or emergency treatment, tell the primary health care provider or dentist that you're taking this drug.
- Be sure of your response to this medication before performing activities requiring alertness and clear vision.
- If you become extra sensitive to light, protect yourself from direct sunlight.
- To relieve dry mouth, use ice chips or sugarless gum or hard candy.

✔ Keep in mind

- If you're pregnant or breast-feeding, tell your primary health care provider before using chlorpromazine.
- Children and older adults are especially sensitive to side effects from chlorpromazine.

Additional instructions

_____

_____

_____

Taking chlorpropamide

Dear Patient,

Because you have diabetes, your primary health care provider has prescribed chlorpropamide to lower your blood glucose level. Brand names for this drug include Diabinese.

How to take chlorpropamide
Chlorpropamide comes in tablets. Take it exactly as ordered. Don't take more or less of it. And take it at the same time each day.

What to do if you miss a dose
Take it as soon as possible. But if it's almost time for your next dose, skip the missed dose and take the next one on schedule. Don't take two doses together.

What to do about side effects
Tell your primary health care provider if you develop a rash, facial flushing, swelling, or shortness of breath because these symptoms may signal an allergic reaction.

Low blood glucose may occur while you use this medication. Watch for symptoms, such as cool pale skin, difficulty concentrating, shakiness, headache, cold sweats, or feelings of anxiety. If these occur, eat or drink something sugary, such as glucose tablets or fruit juice. If you don't feel better within 15 minutes, eat or drink more sugary food and call your health care provider *right away*.

Also tell your health care provider if you experience nausea, vomiting, or heartburn.

What you must know about alcohol and other drugs
Avoid drinking alcohol, except in amounts your primary health care provider permits, because combined use of chlorpropamide and alcohol may make you ill or cause your blood glucose level to drop.

Talk to your health care provider before taking other prescription or nonprescription medications. Many medications can react with chlorpropamide to make your blood glucose too high or too low. You need to avoid certain antidepressants; sulfonamides (sulfa medications); chloramphenicol (Chloromycetin), an antibiotic; blood thinners; steroids; glucagon (a hormone); and water pills.

Also, taking chlorpropamide with certain medications for high blood pressure may cover up symptoms of low blood glucose or make a bout of low blood glucose last longer. Aspirin-containing products and appetite-control, cough, or cold medications may also alter your blood glucose control.

Special directions
• Carefully follow your special plan regarding meals, exercise, avoiding infection, and personal hygiene. Following your special meal plan is the most important part of controlling your diabetes. It's also necessary for chlorpropamide to work well.
• Test for glucose in your blood or urine as your primary health care provider directs. Regular testing lets you know your diabetes is under control, and warns you when it's not.
• Your sensitivity to sunlight may be increased, so limit your exposure to the sun.

✔ Keep in mind
• If you're pregnant, check with your health care provider before taking this medication.
• Don't use chlorpropamide if you're breastfeeding.
• If you're an older adult, you may be especially prone to chlorpropamide's side effects.
• Tell your health care provider of other medical problems, especially if you're a diabetic or have a heart, liver, or kidney condition.

Additional instructions

_____

_____

Taking cholesterol-lowering medications

Dear Patient,

Your primary health care provider has prescribed a cholesterol-lowering medication because you have high levels of cholesterol or other fats in your blood. In general, these drugs work by limiting the production of cholesterol by your body, or by removing bile acids, which combine with cholesterol and are eliminated from the body through bowel movements.

How to take these drugs

These medications are available as tablets, capsules, granules, or powders. Most may be taken either with or without food; however, lovastatin should be taken with meals.

What to do if you miss a dose

If you miss a dose, take it as soon as possible. However, if it's almost time for your next dose, skip the missed dose and then go back to your regular dosing schedule. Don't take double doses.

What to do about side effects

Notify your primary health care provider *immediately* if fatigue, fever, or severe or constant muscle pain occur. You may experience headache, mild muscle pain, flatulence (gas), indigestion, a rash, constipation, and dizziness while taking this drug. Contact your primary health care provider if these become severe.

What you must know about alcohol and other drugs

Don't drink alcohol while on this medication — liver damage may result. Tell your primary health care provider or pharmacist if you're taking antifungal drugs (such as fluconazole, cyclosporine, or erythromycin), fibrates (such as gemfibrozil or clofibrate), or niacin because these combinations may cause severe muscle damage.

Also tell your primary health care provider if you're taking digoxin or birth control pills because the doses of these drugs may have to be adjusted. Cholesterol-lowering medications may also decrease the effects of anticoagulant medications and the absorption and blood levels of many other medications. Check with your primary health care provider or pharmacist.

Special directions

- Your cholesterol level needs to be checked every 3 to 6 months, or on a regular basis. You'll also need liver function tests and other laboratory tests.
- Modifying your diet, exercising more, and losing weight (if necessary) may help your condition.
- Tell your primary health care provider or dentist that you're taking this drug before you have surgery or a medical procedure.

✔ Keep in mind

- Don't breast-feed or become pregnant while on this drug.

Additional instructions

_____
_____
_____
_____
_____
_____
_____
_____
_____
_____

Taking cholestyramine

Dear Patient,

Your primary health care provider has prescribed cholestyramine to lower your blood cholesterol level and to remove substances called bile acids from your body. Other names for this medication include Questran and Questran Light.

How to take cholestyramine

Cholestyramine comes as a chewable bar and a powder.

If you're taking the *powder* form of this medication, follow these steps:
• First, mix the medication with liquid. Never take it in its dry form because you might choke.
• Place the prescribed dose in 2 ounces of any beverage and stir thoroughly.
• Add an additional 2 to 4 ounces of beverage and again mix thoroughly (it won't dissolve). Drink the liquid.
• After drinking all the liquid, rinse the glass with a little more liquid and drink that also.

You may also mix the powder with milk in hot or regular breakfast cereals or in thin soups. Or add it to pulpy fruits, such as crushed pineapple or fruit cocktail.

If you're taking the *chewable bar* form of this medication, chew each bite well before swallowing.

Don't stop taking cholestyramine without first checking with your primary health care provider.

What to do if you miss a dose

Take the dose as soon as possible. But if it's almost time for your next dose, skip the missed dose and take the next dose on schedule. Don't double dose.

What to do about side effects

You may experience constipation, nausea, or rashes. Check with your primary health care provider if these symptoms persist or become bothersome.

What you must know about other drugs

Tell your primary health care provider about other medications you're taking. Many medications may not be absorbed well if taken at the same time as cholestyramine. Examples include acetaminophen (Tylenol), certain blood thinners, beta blockers, corticosteroids, digoxin (Lanoxin), fat-soluble vitamins (A, D, E, and K), iron preparations, some water pills, and thyroid hormone. If possible, take cholestyramine 2 hours before or after taking other medication to prevent this problem.

Special directions

• Because cholestyramine can make certain medical problems worse, tell your primary health care provider if you have gallbladder disease or a history of constipation or digestive problems.
• Also let your primary health care provider know if you're allergic to tartrazine (a yellow food dye) because the powder form of this medication contains tartrazine.
• This medication may not work well if you're very overweight, so you may be advised to go on a reducing diet. However, check with your primary health care provider before starting any diet.

✔ Keep in mind

• If you're pregnant or breast-feeding, check with your primary health care provider before taking this medication.
• If you're an older adult, you may be especially prone to side effects.

Additional instructions

_____

_____

Taking cimetidine

Dear Patient,

This medication treats ulcers and may prevent their return. It may also be used to treat Zollinger-Ellison disease, an illness in which the stomach makes too much acid. The medication label may read Tagamet.

How to take cimetidine

Cimetidine is available as an oral solution or tablets. Carefully check the prescription label, and follow the directions as ordered. If you're taking this medication once a day, take it at bedtime, unless otherwise directed. If you're taking two doses a day, take one in the morning and one at bedtime. If you're taking more than two doses a day, take them with meals and at bedtime for best results.

What to do if you miss a dose

Take the dose as soon as possible. But if it's almost time for your next dose, skip the missed dose and take your next dose as scheduled. Don't double dose.

What to do about side effects

A common side effect is mild, temporary diarrhea. If this symptom doesn't go away or if it becomes severe, call your primary health care provider.

What you must know about other drugs

Tell your primary health care provider about other medications you're taking. Antacids may interfere with the absorption of cimetidine.

Also, cimetidine can interfere with the breakdown of other medications in your body, including warfarin (Coumadin), a blood thinner; phenytoin (Dilantin), a seizure medication; some sedatives; theophylline (Theo-Dur), an asthma medication; and propranolol (Inderal), a heart and high blood pressure medication.

Special directions

- Realize that several days may pass before cimetidine begins to relieve your stomach pain. In the meantime, you may take antacids, unless your primary health care provider has told you not to use them. Wait 30 minutes to 1 hour between taking the antacid and cimetidine.
- Tell the primary health care provider that you're taking this medication before you have skin tests for allergies or tests to determine how much acid your stomach produces.
- Avoid cigarette smoking because it reduces the effectiveness of cimetidine.
- Notify your primary health care provider *immediately* if you've been told that your complete blood count is abnormal or you develop signs and symptoms of infection or bleeding.
- Contact your primary health care provider if your ulcer pain continues or gets worse while taking cimetidine.

✔ Keep in mind

- If you're pregnant or breast-feeding, talk to your primary health care provider before you use this medication.
- If you're an older adult, you may be especially prone to cimetidine's side effects.
- If you have kidney or liver disease or another medical problem, tell your primary health care provider.

Additional instructions

_____
_____
_____
_____
_____
_____

Taking ciprofloxacin

Dear Patient,

Your primary health care provider has ordered ciprofloxacin to treat a bacterial infection in your body. The label may read Cipro.

How to take ciprofloxacin

This medication is available in tablets.

Carefully check the label on your prescription, and follow the directions exactly. Take your dose with a full glass of water. You may take it with meals or on an empty stomach. Take this medication at evenly spaced times, day and night, to keep a constant amount in your body.

Keep taking ciprofloxacin for the full time of treatment, even if you begin to feel better after a few days. If you stop taking it too soon, your symptoms may return.

What to do if you miss a dose

Take the dose as soon as possible. But if it's almost time for your next dose, skip the missed dose and take your next dose on schedule. Don't double dose.

What to do about side effects

Call your primary health care provider *right away* if you have a seizure while taking this medication. Check with your primary health care provider if you have nausea, diarrhea, or a rash.

What you must know about other drugs

Tell your primary health care provider about other medications you're taking. Antacids containing magnesium hydroxide or aluminum hydroxide may decrease the absorption of ciprofloxacin. Therefore, if you take these antacids, take them 2 hours before or after taking ciprofloxacin. Probenecid (Benemid), a gout medication, may increase the risk of side effects from ciprofloxacin. Ciprofloxacin may increase the blood levels of theophylline (Theo-Dur), an asthma medication, which could lead to side effects.

Special directions

● Drink several extra glasses of water every day while taking this medication, unless your primary health care provider gives you other directions. Drinking extra water will help to prevent side effects.
● If your symptoms don't improve within a few days or if they become worse, check with your primary health care provider.
● Ciprofloxacin may make you more sensitive than usual to sunlight, so limit your exposure to direct sun. Use sunblock with an SPF of at least 15 if prolonged exposure to sun occurs.
● This medication may make you dizzy or drowsy. Make sure you know how you react to it before you drive, use machines, or perform other activities that require full alertness.

✔ Keep in mind

● Before taking ciprofloxacin, tell your primary health care provider if you have other medical problems, especially conditions that cause seizures. Also reveal if you've ever had an allergic reaction to ciprofloxacin or another medication.
● Don't take this medication if you're pregnant or breast-feeding unless instructed by your primary health care provider.
● Don't give this medication to infants, children, or adolescents unless instructed by your primary health care provider.

Additional instructions

_____
_____
_____
_____

Taking cisapride

Dear Patient,

Cisapride is used to increase the movements or contractions of the stomach and intestines. This medication treats symptoms such as heartburn caused by a backward flow of stomach acid into the esophagus, a condition known as gastroesophageal reflux disease (GERD). The label may read Propulsid.

How to take cisapride

This medication is available in tablet and liquid forms. Take it 15 minutes before meals and at bedtime.

What to do if you miss a dose

If you miss a dose, take it as soon as you remember. However, if it's close to your next scheduled dose, skip the missed dose and then return to your regular schedule. Don't take double doses.

What to do about side effects

This medication may cause abdominal cramping, constipation, diarrhea, drowsiness, headache, nausea, unusual tiredness, or weakness. Contact your primary health care provider if these become severe.

What you must know about alcohol and other drugs

Warning: Don't take cisapride with antifungal remedies, erythromycin-like medications, medications for depression or other emotional problems, or certain drugs that regulate your heart. The effects of cisapride may be altered and serious side effects may occur.

Tell your primary health care provider if you currently take a medication for abdominal cramps because it may alter cisapride's effects. Cimetidine or ranitidine may also be affected by cisapride. If you take Coumadin, inform your primary health care provider because you may need periodic blood tests to check the effects of Coumadin.

Cisapride may cause your body to absorb alcohol more quickly, so you'll notice alcohol's effects sooner. Inform your health care provider if you plan to drink alcohol.

Special directions

• Check with your primary health care provider if your symptoms don't improve within a few days or if they get worse.
• Tell your primary health care provider about your medical history and what medications you're taking. Certain conditions, including heart and kidney disease, can prevent you from taking cisapride safely.

✓ Keep in mind

• Tell your primary health care provider if you're breast-feeding or if you become pregnant.
• Older adults are especially sensitive to the effects of this medication, so doses may need to be adjusted.

Additional instructions

_____
_____
_____
_____
_____
_____
_____
_____
_____
_____
_____

Taking clarithromycin

Dear Patient,

Your primary health care provider has prescribed clarithromycin because you have an infection. This antibiotic kills the bacteria causing your infection, but it doesn't work on colds or the flu virus. It's also used along with other medications to treat ulcers caused by a bacteria. The brand name of this drug is Biaxin.

How to take clarithromycin

This medication is available as a tablet and an oral liquid suspension. It can be taken either with or without food. If you're taking the liquid suspension, be sure to shake the bottle well before measuring a dose. Use a specially marked medication spoon to make sure you get the right amount in each dose. To keep a constant amount of this medication in your blood, space doses evenly.

What to do if you miss a dose

If you miss a dose of clarithromycin, take it as soon as you remember. If it's near the time of the next scheduled dose, skip the missed dose and go back to your regular schedule. Don't take double doses.

What to do about side effects

If you have shortness of breath, rash, itching, or yellow eyes or skin, contact your primary health care provider *immediately.* These may be signs of an allergic reaction.

You may also experience nausea, vomiting, headache, or diarrhea when taking this medication. These side effects often go away as your body adjusts to the medication. You may also experience a bad taste in your mouth. Contact your primary health care provider if any of these side effects continue or are bothersome.

What you must know about other drugs

Check with your primary health care provider before taking this medication if you are on theophylline (Theo-Dur, Slo-bid) for asthma, carbamazepine (Tegretol) for seizures, digoxin (Lanoxin) for heart problems, or warfarin (Coumadin) for blood clotting problems. Clarithromycin can cause abnormally high levels of these medications in your body and may cause more side effects.

Check with your primary health care provider before taking this medication if you're on zidovudine (Retrovir). Zidovudine blood levels can become too low when you're on clarithromycin.

Special directions

• Continue taking clarithromycin for the full treatment time, even if you start to feel better.
• Don't store the liquid suspension in the refrigerator. Store both the suspension and the tablet forms at room temperature, away from heat, light, and humidity.
• Tell the primary health care provider about your medical history, including allergies to erythromycin.

✔ Keep in mind

• Tell the primary health care provider if you're breast-feeding or if you become pregnant while taking this medication.
• People with liver or kidney problems or allergies to erythromycin may need a lower dose of clarithromycin or a different type of antibiotic.

Additional instructions

_____

_____

_____

Taking clemastine

Dear Patient,

Your primary health care provider has pre-scribed clemastine to relieve your hay fever or other allergy. If you're taking the *syrup* form, the label may read Tavist. If you're tak-ing the *tablets,* the label may read Tavist-1.

How to take clemastine
Carefully check the prescription label, and take the medication exactly as ordered. Take it with food, water, or milk to lessen stomach irritation.

What to do if you miss a dose
If you take this medication regularly and you miss a dose, take it as soon as possible. But if it's almost time for your next dose, skip the missed dose and take your next dose on schedule. Don't double dose.

What to do about side effects
This medication may make you feel drowsy or cause dryness of your mouth. Call your primary health care provider if these symp-toms persist or become severe.

What you must know about alcohol and other drugs
Don't drink alcoholic beverages while taking this medication. Doing so could cause you to become oversedated.

Tell your primary health care provider about other medications you're taking. De-pressants (medications that slow down your central nervous system) may increase the sedative effect of clemastine. Don't use clemastine if you take monoamine oxidase (MAO) inhibitors.

Also let your primary health care provider know if you take large amounts of aspirin, such as for arthritis pain. Clemastine may cover up warning signs of aspirin overdose.

Special directions
• This medication can aggravate certain conditions, so tell your primary health care provider about other medical problems.
• Inform the primary health care provider that you're taking this medication before you have skin tests for allergies because clemastine may alter the test results.
• Know how you react to clemastine before you drive, use machines, or perform other activities that require alertness.
• Call your primary health care provider *im-mediately* if you've been told your complete blood count is abnormal or if you develop a fever, shortness of breath, or bleeding.
• If you experience dry mouth with this med-ication, try using sugarless hard candy or gum, ice chips, or a saliva substitute. If your dry mouth lasts for more than 2 weeks, check with your primary health care provider or dentist.

✓ Keep in mind
• If you're pregnant or breast-feeding, don't use clemastine unless your primary health care provider instructs you otherwise.
• Children and older adults are especially sensitive to the effects of clemastine and are more likely to develop side effects.
• Tell your primary health care provider if you have asthma, glaucoma, an enlarged prostate, bladder problems, difficulty urinat-ing, heart disease, an overactive thyroid, di-abetes, or stomach ulcers. Clemastine can aggravate these conditions.

Additional instructions

_____

_____

_____

_____

Taking clindamycin

Dear Patient,

Your primary health care provider has prescribed clindamycin to treat your bacterial infection. If you're taking the *oral* form of this medication, such as a capsule or liquid, the label may read Cleocin. If you're applying *topical* clindamycin to your skin, the label may read Cleocin T Gel, Cleocin T Lotion, or Cleocin T Topical Solution.

How to take clindamycin

If you're taking *capsules*, take them with a full glass (8 ounces) of water or with meals. If you're using the *oral solution,* measure your dose with a specially marked measuring spoon, not a household teaspoon.

Before you apply topical clindamycin, wash the affected skin and pat dry. If you're using the *gel* or *lotion*, apply a thin film of medication.

If you're using the *topical solution,* wait 30 minutes after washing or shaving before applying this medication because the alcohol it contains may sting. Avoid getting this medication in your eyes, nose, or mouth.

What to do if you miss a dose

If you miss an *oral* dose, take it as soon as possible. But if it's almost time for your next dose (and you take three or more doses a day), space the missed dose and the next dose 2 to 4 hours apart. Then go back to your regular dosing schedule.

If you miss a *topical* dose, apply it as soon as possible. But if it's almost time for your next dose, skip the missed dose and apply your next dose on schedule.

What to do about side effects

Call your primary health care provider *right away* if you have severe, bloody diarrhea; abdominal pain, with vomiting; black, tarry, or bloody stools; signs of an allergic reaction, such as chest tightness, wheezing, hives, itching, or a rash.

Also check with your primary health care provider if you have nausea, mild diarrhea, or difficulty swallowing.

What you must know about other drugs

Tell your primary health care provider about other medications you're taking. Erythromycin (another antibiotic) may prevent clindamycin from working properly. Also avoid the use of kaolin (an ingredient in some diarrhea medications) because it decreases the absorption of clindamycin.

Special directions

• Keep taking this medication for the full time of treatment, even if you feel better.
• Tell your primary health care provider if you have other medical problems because this medication may aggravate them.
• Before having surgery (including dental surgery) with a general anesthetic, tell the primary health care provider or dentist that you're taking clindamycin.

✔ Keep in mind

• If you're pregnant or breast-feeding, check with your primary health care provider before using this medication.
• People with asthma, allergies, or diseases of the liver, kidney, stomach or intestines may find that these conditions are aggravated by taking clindamycin.

Additional instructions

_____
_____
_____
_____
_____

Taking clonazepam

Dear Patient,

Your primary health care provider has prescribed this medication to help your condition. Clonazepam acts on the nervous system to prevent seizures. A common brand name for clonazepam is Klonopin.

How to take clonazepam

Clonazepam is available in tablet form. Carefully check the prescription label, and follow the directions exactly. Don't take more than the prescribed amount.

Take this medication faithfully every day in regularly spaced doses.

What to do if you miss a dose

If you're taking this medication regularly and you miss a dose, take it as soon as possible. However, if it's almost time for your next dose, skip the missed dose and take your next dose on schedule. Don't double dose.

What to do about side effects

Get emergency help *at once* if you have the following signs of overdose: slurred speech, confusion, severe drowsiness, and staggering.

Also call your primary health care provider *at once* if this medication starts to slow your breathing or makes breathing difficult. Check with your primary health care provider if you become drowsy, your mouth starts to water, or you notice odd changes in your behavior.

What you must know about alcohol and other drugs

Tell your primary health care provider about other medications you're taking. Don't drink alcoholic beverages while taking clonazepam because the combination may cause over-sedation. For the same reason, avoid other central nervous system depressants (that slow down your nervous system) while using clonazepam. Examples of depressants include sleeping pills, tranquilizers, narcotic painkillers, and many cold and flu medications.

Special directions

• Tell your primary health care provider about your medical history, especially if you have liver or lung disease, kidney problems, or glaucoma.
• See your primary health care provider regularly to determine if you need to continue taking this medication because it may become habit-forming.
• Your primary health care provider may want you to carry medical identification stating that you're taking this medication.
• Before any medical tests, tell the primary health care provider that you're taking clonazepam because it may alter the test results.
• Because this medication can make you drowsy, make sure you know how you react to it before you drive, use machines, or perform other hazardous activities that require alertness.

✔ Keep in mind

• If you're pregnant or breast-feeding, check with your primary health care provider before taking this medication.
• If you're an athlete, you should know that use of clonazepam is banned by the National Collegiate Athletic Association and the U.S. Olympic Committee.

Additional instructions

_____
_____
_____
_____

Taking clonidine

Dear Patient,

Clonidine is usually prescribed to treat high blood pressure. The brand name for the *tablet* form is Catapres. The brand name for the *skin patch* is Catapres-TTS.

How to take clonidine

If you're taking the *tablets,* take them at the same times each day. Even if you feel well, continue to take clonidine exactly as directed.

If you're using the *skin patch,* apply it to a clean, dry, hairless area on your upper arm or chest. Change the patch every 7 days or as often as your health care provider orders. Place the patch at a different site every week to prevent skin irritation. Be sure to read the instructions that come with the patches.

What to do if you miss a dose

Take it as soon as you remember. Then go back to your regular dosing schedule.

If you miss two or more tablet doses in a row or if you miss changing the skin patch for 3 or more days, check with your health care provider right away. If you go too long without clonidine, your blood pressure may rise, possibly causing unpleasant effects.

What to do about side effects

Call your primary health care provider *at once* if you have a severe headache, visual changes, or extreme dizziness. Also call if you become drowsy or constipated or your mouth feels dry.

If you're using the skin patch, you may experience itching or a rash. If these symptoms persist or become severe, call your primary health care provider.

What you must know about alcohol and other drugs

Don't drink alcoholic beverages, except in amounts permitted by your primary health care provider, while taking clonidine because the combination may cause oversedation. Similarly, central nervous system depressants, such as sleeping pills and tranquilizers, may cause oversedation when used with clonidine.

If you're taking clonidine with propranolol (Inderal) or other beta blockers, these medications may raise your blood pressure when taken together. Also, clonidine may not work properly when taken with certain antidepressants.

Special directions

• Keep all appointments for follow-up visits, so your primary health care provider can check your progress.
• Keep the skin patch on while showering, bathing, or swimming. If it loosens, cover it with the extra adhesive provided.
• Because clonidine may make you drowsy, make sure you know how you react to it before you drive, use machines, or perform other hazardous activities that require alertness.
• Use care when getting up from a lying or sitting position, to avoid light-headedness.

✔ Keep in mind

• If you're pregnant or breast-feeding, check with your primary health care provider before taking this medication.
• If you're an older adult, this medication may make you dizzy or faint. Take care to prevent falls.
• If you have other medical problems (especially heart or kidney disease, diabetes, or depression), tell your health care provider.

Additional instructions

_____
_____
_____

Taking clorazepate

Dear Patient,

Your primary health care provider has prescribed clorazepate to help your condition. This medication is used to prevent seizures in people with seizure disorders and to relieve extreme feelings of nervousness or tension. Brand names include Gen-XENE, Tranxene-SD, and Tranxene T-Tab.

How to take clorazepate
This medication comes in tablet or capsule form.

Follow your primary health care provider's instructions exactly. Don't take more, and don't take it more often or longer than the label directs because this medication can be habit-forming.

If you're taking clorazepate for a seizure disorder, take it every day in regularly spaced doses, as ordered.

What to do if you miss a dose
Take the dose as soon as possible. But if it's almost time for your next dose, skip the missed dose and take your next dose on schedule. Don't double dose.

What to do about side effects
Get emergency help *at once* if you have these symptoms of an overdose: slurred speech, confusion, severe drowsiness, and staggering. Check with your primary health care provider if this medication makes you feel drowsy, lethargic, or like you have a hangover.

What you must know about alcohol and other drugs
Tell your primary health care provider about other medications you're taking. Avoid alcoholic beverages and other central nervous system depressants (medications that slow down your nervous system) while taking clorazepate because this combination may cause oversedation. Cimetidine (Tagamet), an ulcer medication, may also cause increased drowsiness when used with clorazepate.

Special directions
• Tell your primary health care provider of other medical problems, especially glaucoma, myasthenia gravis, Parkinson's disease, kidney or liver disease, or a history of mental illness or drug abuse.
• If you're taking this medication for a long time, don't stop taking it without first checking with your primary health care provider.
• If you're taking clorazepate for a seizure disorder, your primary health care provider may want you to carry medical identification stating that you're taking it.
• Before you have medical tests, tell the primary health care provider that you're taking clorazepate because this drug may alter the test results.
• Because this medication can make you drowsy, make sure you know how you react to it before you drive, use machines, or perform other hazardous activities that require alertness.

✔ Keep in mind
• If you're pregnant or breast-feeding, check with your primary health care provider before taking this medication.
• If you're an older adult, you may be especially prone to side effects.
If you're an athlete, you should know that clorazepate use is banned by the National Collegiate Athletic Association and the U.S. Olympic Committee.

Additional instructions

_____

_____

Taking clotrimazole

Dear Patient,

Your primary health care provider has prescribed clotrimazole to treat your fungal infection. If you're taking clotrimazole *lozenges,* the label may read Mycelex Troches. If you're using a *topical lotion, cream,* or *solution* on your skin, the medication may be called Lotrimin or Mycelex. If you're taking this medication for a *vaginal* infection, the label may read Gyne-Lotrimin.

How to take clotrimazole

If you're taking the *lozenge* form, hold the lozenge in your mouth and allow it to dissolve slowly and completely. This may take 15 to 30 minutes. Try not to swallow your saliva during this time. Don't chew the lozenges or swallow them whole.

If you're applying *topical* clotrimazole to your skin, apply enough to cover the area, and rub it in gently. Avoid getting it in your eyes. Don't put a bandage over the treated area unless instructed by your primary health care provider.

If you're using the *vaginal* form, fill the applicator with cream to the level indicated or unwrap a tablet, wet it with lukewarm water, and place it on the applicator. To insert the medication, follow the directions on the package.

Continue to take your medication, even if your symptoms clear up in a few days. Otherwise, your infection may return. Because fungal infections may be slow to clear up, you may need to take your medication every day for several weeks or more.

What to do if you miss a dose

Take it as soon as possible. However, if it's almost time for your next dose, skip the missed dose and take your next dose on schedule.

What to do about side effects

If you're using the *lozenges,* check with your primary health care provider if you experience nausea and vomiting.

If you're applying the *topical* form of this medication, call your primary health care provider if redness, blistering, or swelling occurs. Also call if the treated area burns or stings.

If you're using the *vaginal* form, check with your primary health care provider if you feel burning or irritation in your vagina.

Special directions

• Tell your primary health care provider if you have other medical problems, especially liver disease. Also mention if you're allergic to this medication.
• If you're using the lozenges and your symptoms don't go away within 1 week or they become worse, check with your primary health care provider. If you're using clotrimazole for a skin infection, check with your primary health care provider if your symptoms haven't gone away within 4 weeks.
• If you're using the lozenges, tell the primary health care provider before you have liver tests; this medication may alter the test results.

☑ Keep in mind

• Don't give clotrimazole lozenges to children under age 5. They may be too young to use them safely.
• If you're pregnant, don't use the vaginal form of this medication without first checking with your primary health care provider.

Additional instructions

_____

_____

Taking cloxacillin

Dear Patient,

Your primary health care provider has prescribed cloxacillin (a form of penicillin) to treat your bacterial infection. Brand names include Cloxapen and Tegopen.

How to take cloxacillin
This medication comes in capsules and an oral solution. If you're taking the *capsules,* don't break, chew, or crush them — swallow them whole. If you're taking the *oral* solution, use a dropper or specially marked measuring spoon to measure each dose accurately.

Take your dose with a full glass (8 ounces) of water on an empty stomach, either 1 hour before or 2 hours after meals, unless your primary health care provider tells you otherwise. Don't take your dose with fruit juice or carbonated drinks; doing so may prevent cloxacillin from working.

Keep taking your medication, even after you start to feel better. Stopping too soon may allow your infection to return.

What to do if you miss a dose
Take the dose as soon as possible. But if it's almost time for your next dose, adjust your dosing schedule as follows.

If you take two doses a day, space the missed dose and the next dose 5 to 6 hours apart.

If you take three or more doses a day, space the missed dose and the next dose 2 to 4 hours apart.

Then resume your regular dosing schedule.

What to do about side effects
Call your primary health care provider *at once* if you develop symptoms of an allergic reaction to this medication, such as difficulty breathing, skin rash, hives, itching, or wheezing.

If you develop nausea, heartburn, or diarrhea, check with your primary health care provider, especially if these symptoms persist or become severe.

What you must know about other drugs
Tell the primary health care provider about other medications you're taking. If you're taking probenecid (Benemid), a gout medication, your blood levels of cloxacillin may increase. This may or may not be a beneficial effect; check with your primary health care provider.

If you develop severe diarrhea, don't take any diarrhea medications without first checking with your primary health care provider. Some of these medications may make your diarrhea worse.

Special directions
• Tell your primary health care provider about your medical history, especially if you're allergic to other antibiotics, including penicillins, cephalosporins, and griseofulvin. Also reveal if you have kidney disease.
• If you become allergic to cloxacillin, carry medical identification stating this.
• Before you have medical tests, tell the primary health care provider that you're taking cloxacillin because this medication may interfere with some test results.

✔ Keep in mind
• If you're pregnant or breast-feeding, check with your primary health care provider before using this medication.

Additional instructions
_____
_____
_____
_____

Taking colestipol

Dear Patient,

Your primary health care provider has prescribed colestipol to lower your blood cholesterol level. The label may read Colestid.

How to take colestipol
This medication comes in powder form.

Never take colestipol in its dry form because it might cause choking. Instead, follow these steps:
- Add the proper amount of colestipol to at least 3 ounces of your favorite drink. However, if you use a carbonated drink, slowly mix the powder in a large glass to prevent excess foaming.
- Stir until the medication is completely mixed (it won't dissolve). Then drink.
- After drinking all the liquid, rinse the glass with a little more liquid and drink that also, to make sure you get all the medication.

You may also mix colestipol with thin soups, milk in hot or cold cereals, or pulpy fruits, such as crushed pineapple, pears, or fruit cocktail.

What to do if you miss a dose
Take the dose as soon as possible. But if it's almost time for your next dose, skip the missed dose and go back to your regular dosing schedule. Don't double dose.

What to do about side effects
Constipation is the most common side effect of this medication. If it persists or becomes severe, check with your primary health care provider about decreasing your dosage of colestipol.

What you must know about other drugs
Tell your primary health care provider about other medications you're taking. Colestipol may decrease the absorption of any medication that you take by mouth. Therefore, if you take another oral medication, take it at least 1 hour before or 4 hours after you take colestipol. Also, certain drugs for diabetes may prevent this medication from working properly.

Special directions
- Tell your primary health care provider about your medical history, especially if you have problems with your liver, gallbladder, or digestive tract.
- Carefully follow the special diet your primary health care provider has given you, which is necessary for colestipol to work properly.
- See your primary health care provider regularly so that he can check your cholesterol level and decide if you should continue to take this medication.
- If constipation develops, eat more fiber-rich foods, such as fruits, vegetables, and whole-grain cereals. Also, check with your primary health care provider about using a stool softener.

! *Warning:* Don't stop taking colestipol without first checking with your primary health care provider. When you stop taking it, your blood cholesterol level may rise again. Your primary health care provider may want you to follow a special diet to help prevent this from happening.

✔ Keep in mind
- If you're pregnant, check with the health care provider before taking this medication.
- If you're an older adult, you may be especially sensitive to side effects from colestipol.

Additional instructions
_____
_____
_____

Taking co-trimoxazole

Dear Patient,

Your primary health care provider has prescribed this antibiotic medication to treat your bacterial infection. Brand names include Bactrim, Cotrim, and Septra.

How to take co-trimoxazole

Co-trimoxazole is available in tablets and an oral suspension. Take the tablets or oral suspension with a full glass (8 ounces) of water.

If you have trouble swallowing the *tablet* form, you may crush it and take it with water. If you're taking the *oral suspension,* shake the bottle well before using. Use a specially marked spoon or dropper, not a household teaspoon, to measure the correct dose.

Keep taking co-trimoxazole, even after you begin to feel better. If you stop too soon, the infection may return.

What to do if you miss a dose

Take the dose as soon as possible. However, if it's almost time for your next dose, adjust your schedule as follows.

If you're taking two doses a day, space the skipped dose and the next dose 6 hours apart.

If you're taking three or more doses each day, space the skipped dose and the next dose 2 to 4 hours apart.

Then resume your regular schedule.

What to do about side effects

Get emergency help *at once* if you have symptoms of an allergic reaction, such as difficulty breathing, wheezing, or hives.

Stop taking this medication and call your primary health care provider *right away* if you have a persistent fever, a sore throat, or joint pain; feel extremely tired; start to bleed; or start to bruise easily. Check with your primary health care provider if you experience skin problems, nausea, vomiting, or diarrhea.

What you must know about other drugs

Taking co-trimoxazole can increase the effects of certain medications, especially blood thinners and certain drugs for diabetes. Certain anticonvulsant medications (for seizures), when used with co-trimoxazole, can increase the chance of side effects. Co-trimoxazole may also prevent birth control pills from working well. Use another form of birth control.

Special directions

● Tell your primary health care provider about your medical history, especially if you have kidney or liver problems, porphyria, severe allergies, asthma, or acquired immunodeficiency syndrome (AIDS). Also reveal if you're allergic to this medication or other sulfa drugs.
● Drink extra water — up to 3 to 4 quarts daily — to prevent side effects, such as kidney stones, from this medication.
● Co-trimoxazole may make you more sensitive to sunlight, so try to avoid exposure to direct sunlight. If you will experience excessive exposure to the sun, use a sunblock with a skin protection factor (SPF) of at least 15.

✔ Keep in mind

● If you're pregnant or breast-feeding, talk to your primary health care provider before using this medication.
● If you have diabetes and take co-trimoxazole, you may need to test your urine glucose with a glucose enzymatic test, such as Clinistix or Tes-Tape, because copper sulfate tests may give false-positive results.

Additional instructions

_____

_____

Taking cromolyn

Dear Patient,

Cromolyn is used to prevent asthma attacks, to relieve allergies, and to treat a rare condition called mastocytosis. Cromolyn comes in several forms: oral capsules (Gastrocrom), nasal solution or powder (Nasalcrom), inhalation (Intal), or eyedrops (Opticrom).

How to take cromolyn

If you're taking the *oral capsules,* dissolve the capsule contents in 4 ounces of hot water. Stir until the powder completely dissolves and the solution is clear. Add an equal amount of cold water to the solution. Don't mix your dose with fruit juice, milk, or foods. Doing so may prevent your medication from working well.

If you're using the *inhalation aerosol,* read the directions before using. Keep the spray away from your eyes.

If you're using *capsules for inhalation,* never swallow them. Read the directions before using the special inhaler.

If you're using the *solution for inhalation,* use this medication only in a power-operated nebulizer with an adequate flow rate and a face mask or mouthpiece. Make sure you understand exactly how to use it. Hand-operated nebulizers aren't used with this medication.

If you're using the *nasal* forms, first clear your nasal passages by blowing your nose. To use the nasal forms, you need special spray devices. Read the package instructions.

To use the *eyedrops,* wash your hands, then tilt your head back and pull the lower eyelid away from the eye to form a pouch. Squeeze the drops into the pouch and close the eye. Don't blink. Keep the treated eye closed for 1 to 2 minutes. Don't touch the applicator tip to any surface.

Don't use cromolyn more often than your primary health care provider ordered. It may take at least 1 week before you feel better if you have hay fever. If you have chronic allergic rhinitis, it may take up to 1 month.

What to do if you miss a dose

Take the dose as soon as possible. Then take any remaining doses for that day at regularly spaced intervals. Don't double dose.

What to do about side effects

If you're using the powder form for nasal inhalation, *call for emergency help* if you start to wheeze and have difficulty breathing after using this medication.

Any form of this medication may make you cough or cause soreness or dryness of the mouth and throat. If these symptoms persist, call your primary health care provider.

What you must know about other drugs

If you have asthma, you may be taking cromolyn along with an adrenocorticoid, such as cortisone (Cortone Acetate) or prednisone (Deltasone). If so, don't stop taking the adrenocorticoid, even if your asthma seems better, unless your primary health care provider tells you to do so.

Special directions

• Tell your health care provider if you have other medical problems, especially asthma or diseases of the heart, kidney, or liver.
• If your mouth or throat feels dry or irritated after using cromolyn, gargle after each dose.

✓ Keep in mind

• If you're pregnant or breast-feeding, check with your primary health care provider before taking this medication.

Additional instructions

_____

_____

Taking cyclobenzaprine

Dear Patient,

This medication is a muscle relaxant. It's given to relieve muscle pain, stiffness, and discomfort caused by strains, sprains, or injuries. The label may read Flexeril.

How to take cyclobenzaprine
Cyclobenzaprine comes in tablet form. Carefully check the label on your prescription bottle, which tells you how much medication to take. Follow the directions exactly as ordered.

What to do if you miss a dose
If you remember within an hour or so of the missed dose, take it right away. Then go back to your regular dosing schedule. But if you don't remember until later, skip the missed dose and take your next dose on schedule. Don't take two doses together.

What to do about side effects
Drowsiness is the most common side effect of cyclobenzaprine. If it persists or becomes severe, call your primary health care provider. Also check with your primary health care provider if you develop constipation, heartburn, or abdominal pain, or if your mouth feels dry.

What you must know about alcohol and other drugs
Avoid drinking alcohol while you're taking cyclobenzaprine because the combination may cause oversedation. For the same reason, avoid using other central nervous system depressants (medications that slow your nervous system), such as tranquilizers, sedatives, sleeping aids, and many medications for hay fever, colds, and flu.

Check with your primary health care provider before you take other prescription or nonprescription medications.

Special directions
• Tell your primary health care provider if you have other medical problems, especially heart, kidney, or liver disease; an overactive thyroid gland; glaucoma; or difficulty urinating.
• Because cyclobenzaprine can cause drowsiness, make sure you know how you react to it before you drive, use machines, or perform other activities that require alertness.
• If this medication makes your mouth feel dry, you may use sugarless hard candy or gum, ice chips, or a saliva substitute. However, if your dry mouth lasts for more than 2 weeks, check with your primary health care provider or dentist. Continuing dryness of the mouth may increase the chance of tooth decay, gum disease, and fungal infections.
• If you're constipated from using cyclobenzaprine, try drinking several extra glasses of water daily. If that doesn't help, check with your primary health care provider about using a stool softener.

✓ Keep in mind
• If you're an athlete, be aware that use of this medication is banned in biathlon and modern pentathlon events by the U.S. Olympic Committee.

Additional instructions
_____
_____
_____
_____
_____
_____
_____

Taking cyclosporine

Dear Patient,

To keep your transplant functioning normally, your primary health care provider has prescribed cyclosporine. This medication is also known as Neoral or Sandimmune.

How to take cyclosporine

Cyclosporine comes in liquid or capsules. If you take the *liquid* form, measure your dose precisely. Each milliliter of liquid contains 100 milligrams of cyclosporine. Store the liquid at room temperature to prevent it from becoming too thick.

If you wish, mix your dose in a glass container with fruit juice (preferably at room temperature) or milk to make it taste better. Stir it well and drink it immediately. Then rinse the glass with a little more liquid and drink that also to make sure you take all the medication. Don't mix cyclosporine with grapefruit juice, and don't mix Neoral with milk, because the taste may be harsh.

If you take the *capsules,* you should know that they come in two strengths: 25 milligrams and 100 milligrams. You may be taking some of both strengths to obtain an exact dose. Swallow the capsules whole. Don't chew or open them.

Take your dose at the same time each day, preferably in the morning. Take it with meals if it causes nausea.

What to do if you miss a dose

If you forget to take a dose or if you vomit soon after taking it, call your primary health care provider *right away.* Follow his instructions for getting back on schedule. Never skip a dose or take two doses together.

What to do about side effects

Call your primary health care provider *right away* if you have chills or a fever, need to urinate frequently, notice your heart beating irregularly, feel unusually weak or tired or your legs feel unusually heavy or weak, see blood in your urine, have a seizure, or have breathing problems.

Also check with your primary health care provider if you have diarrhea or stomach pain with nausea and vomiting; swollen, tender, or bleeding gums; headaches or dizziness (indicating a rise in blood pressure); shaky or trembling hands; or a change in hair texture or growth.

What you must know about other drugs

Check with your primary health care provider before you take other medications, including nonprescription preparations. Also tell your primary health care provider before you have any immunizations (vaccinations) while you're being treated with cyclosporine and after you stop taking it.

Special directions

• Tell your primary health care provider if you have other medical problems, especially high blood pressure or liver or kidney disease.
• If cyclosporine causes unwanted hair growth, remove the hair with a depilatory.
• Keep all appointments for follow-up tests so your primary health care provider can detect side effects early.
• See your dentist regularly, and inform him that you're taking cyclosporine.

✔ Keep in mind

• If you're pregnant or breast-feeding, check with your primary health care provider before taking cyclosporine.

Additional instructions

_____

_____

Taking danazol

Dear Patient,

Your primary health care provider has prescribed this medication to treat your condition. Danazol helps treat many medical problems, including endometriosis, breast cysts, and a rare condition called hereditary angioedema. The label may read Danocrine.

How to take danazol

Carefully check the prescription label and follow the directions exactly. For danazol to help you, you must take it regularly for the full time of treatment ordered by your primary health care provider.

What to do if you miss a dose

Take it as soon as possible. However, if it's almost time for your next dose, skip the missed dose and take your next dose on schedule. Don't double dose.

What to do about side effects

If you're female, tell your primary health care provider right away if you develop any masculinizing side effects while taking danazol. These effects include weight gain, increased hair growth on your body, a decrease in breast size, voice deepening, and oiliness of your skin or hair.

Special directions

• Tell your primary health care provider if you have other medical problems, especially kidney, heart, or liver disease. If you're female, also reveal if you have a history of abnormal vaginal bleeding.
• Go for regular checkups to make sure that danazol doesn't cause unwanted effects.
• If you're taking this medication for endometriosis or breast cysts, your menstrual period may be irregular, or you may not have a menstrual period while you're taking danazol. This is to be expected. However, if

regular menstruation doesn't begin within 60 to 90 days after you stop taking this medication, check with your primary health care provider.
• If you're female, don't use birth control pills while taking danazol. Select a birth control method that doesn't contain hormones, such as condoms or a diaphragm.
• If you're taking danazol for breast cysts, examine your breasts regularly. Check with your primary health care provider right away if you detect unusual changes in how your breasts feel.
• Danazol may increase your sensitivity to sunlight, so limit your exposure to the sun. If out in the sun for prolonged periods, use sunblock with at least a skin protection factor (SPF) of 15.

✔️ Keep in mind

• If you're pregnant or think you may be, don't take danazol. Continued use of danazol during pregnancy may cause male-like changes in female babies. For the same reason, check with your primary health care provider before you use this medication if you're breast-feeding.
• If you have diabetes, danazol may affect your glucose levels. If you notice a change in the results of your blood or urine glucose test, call your primary health care provider.
• If you're an older man, taking danazol may increase your risk of developing prostate enlargement or cancer.
• If you're an athlete, you should know that the use of danazol is banned by the U.S. Olympic Committee.

Additional instructions

_____

_____

_____

Taking dantrolene

Dear Patient,

Your primary health care provider has prescribed a muscle relaxant called dantrolene to help your condition. Dantrolene relieves muscle spasms, cramping, and tightness caused by multiple sclerosis, cerebral palsy, stroke, and other conditions. The label may read Dantrium.

How to take dantrolene

If you're taking the *capsule* form, take your dose with milk or meals to help prevent digestive upset.

If you have trouble swallowing the capsules, follow these steps:
• Empty the number of capsules needed for one dose into a small amount of fruit juice or other liquid.
• Stir gently to mix the powder with the liquid. Then drink right away.
• Rinse the glass with a little more liquid and drink that also to make sure you've taken the entire dose.

What to do if you miss a dose

If you remember within an hour or so of the missed dose, take it right away. Then go back to your regular dosing schedule. But if you don't remember until later, skip the missed dose and take your next dose on schedule. Don't double dose.

What to do about side effects

Call your primary health care provider at once if your skin or eyes start to turn yellow, if you develop a fever, or if your skin feels itchy. These symptoms could be signs of hepatitis, a liver disorder. Also call if you feel dizzy or drowsy or have muscle weakness, diarrhea, or constipation.

What you must know about alcohol and other drugs

Don't drink alcohol while taking dantrolene because the combination may lead to oversedation. For the same reason, avoid other central nervous system depressants (medications that slow your nervous system), such as sleeping pills, tranquilizers, muscle relaxants, narcotic pain relievers, and many cold, flu, and allergy remedies.

Special directions

• Tell your primary health care provider if you have other medical problems, especially lung, heart, or liver disease.
• Go for regular checkups, especially if you're taking dantrolene for a long time. You may need to have certain blood tests to check for unwanted side effects.
• Because dantrolene can make you drowsy or dizzy, make sure you know how you react to it before you drive, use machines, or perform other activities that could be dangerous if you're not alert.

✔ Keep in mind

• If you're pregnant or breast-feeding, check with your primary health care provider before using dantrolene.
• If you're an athlete, you should know that dantrolene is banned by the National Collegiate Athletic Association and the U.S. Olympic Committee.

Additional instructions

_____
_____
_____
_____

Taking desipramine

Dear Patient,

Your primary health care provider has prescribed desipramine to help relieve your depression. Brand names include Norpramin and Pertofrane.

How to take desipramine

Desipramine comes in capsules and tablets. Follow your primary health care provider's instructions exactly. Don't take more of it or take it more often or longer than directed. Take your dose with food, even for a bedtime dose, unless your health care provider has told you to take it on an empty stomach. Don't stop taking this medication suddenly; check with your health care provider first.

What to do if you miss a dose

If you miss a dose, adjust your dosing schedule as follows. If you take one dose a day at bedtime, don't take the missed dose in the morning. It may cause disturbing side effects during waking hours. Instead, check with your primary health care provider.

If you take more than one dose a day, take the missed dose as soon as possible. However, if it's almost time for your next dose, skip the missed dose and take your next dose on schedule. Don't double dose.

What to do about side effects

Check with your primary health care provider if you feel drowsy, dizzy, or light-headed, especially when you get up suddenly from a lying or sitting position. Also call if you experience an irregular or fast heartbeat, blurred vision, dry mouth, constipation, difficulty urinating, or unusual sweating.

What you must know about alcohol and other drugs

Check with your primary health care provider about drinking alcoholic beverages while taking desipramine. Also tell your primary health care provider if you're taking other medication. Desipramine may not work well if taken with barbiturates (sedatives). Taking the ulcer medication cimetidine (Tagamet) may increase the risk of side effects from desipramine.

Other medications that you may need to avoid while taking this medication are methylphenidate (Ritalin), epinephrine (Adrenalin), and certain medications used to treat depression and other psychiatric disorders.

Special directions

- Tell your primary health care provider if you have other medical problems, especially heart, liver, or kidney disease; breathing problems; an overactive thyroid; diabetes; or an enlarged prostate.
- Don't drive, use machines, or perform other activities that require alertness until you know how desipramine affects you.
- If desipramine makes you feel faint when you get up from a sitting or lying position, get up slowly.
- Before you have any medical tests, tell your primary health care provider in charge that you're taking desipramine because the medication may affect some test results.

✔ Keep in mind

- If you're pregnant or breast-feeding, check with your primary health care provider before you take desipramine.
- If you have diabetes, this medication may affect your glucose levels. If you notice a change in the results of your blood or urine glucose test, call your health care provider.

Additional instructions

_____

_____

Taking desmopressin

Dear Patient,

Your primary health care provider has prescribed a hormone called desmopressin to help your condition. Desmopressin is used to prevent or control symptoms associated with diabetes insipidus, such as frequent urination, increased thirst, and water loss. Brand names include DDAVP and Stimate.

How to take desmopressin

If you're using the nasal solution form, first read the patient directions in the package. Before you administer your dose, gently blow your nose to clear your nasal passages.

If you're using the injection form, follow your primary health care provider's instructions.

What to do if you miss a dose

If you miss a dose, adjust your dosing schedule as follows.

If you take one dose a day, take the missed dose as soon as possible. Then go back to your regular dosing schedule. But if you don't remember the missed dose until the next day, skip the missed dose and go back to your regular dosing schedule.

If you take more than one dose a day, take the missed dose as soon as possible. Then go back to your regular dosing schedule. However, if it's almost time for your next dose, skip the missed dose and take your next dose on schedule. Don't double dose.

What to do about side effects

Generally, desmopressin causes few side effects. But check with your primary health care provider if you experience any unwanted effects, such as headache, runny nose, nausea, or skin flushing, especially if these symptoms persist or seem severe.

Special directions

• Tell your primary health care provider if you have other medical problems, especially heart or blood vessel disease, high blood pressure, or a stuffy nose caused by a cold or an allergy.
• If you're using the nasal solution form, check with your primary health care provider if you develop a runny nose from a cold or an allergy. Nasal congestion can interfere with the absorption of this medication.
• If you experience a mild headache from taking this medication, you may take aspirin or acetaminophen (Tylenol), unless your primary health care provider gives you other instructions.
• Your primary health care provider may ask you to check your weight daily to determine if your body is holding enough water.

✔️ Keep in mind

• If you're pregnant or breast-feeding, check with your primary health care provider before taking this medication.
• If you're an older adult, you may be especially prone to desmopressin's side effects.

Additional instructions

_____
_____
_____
_____
_____
_____
_____
_____
_____

Using ophthalmic dexamethasone

Dear Patient,

Your primary health care provider has prescribed dexamethasone to treat your eye problem. If you're using dexamethasone eyedrops, the medication label may read Maxidex Ophthalmic Suspension. If you're using the eye cream or ointment, the label may read Decadron Phosphate Ophthalmic or Maxidex Ophthalmic.

How to use dexamethasone

If you're using eyedrops, follow these steps.
• First, wash your hands. Shake your bottle of eyedrops.
• Tilt your head back, and pull the lower eyelid away from the eye to form a pouch.
• Squeeze the correct number of drops into the pouch and gently close your eye. Don't blink.
• Repeat on the other eye, if directed.
• Keep your eyes closed for 1 to 2 minutes to allow the medication to be absorbed. If you think you didn't get a drop into your eye, use another drop.

If you're using eye cream or ointment, follow the steps above given for eyedrops, but don't tilt your head back to use the cream or ointment.

Try to keep your medication as germ-free as possible. Don't touch the applicator tip to any surface, including your eye. Keep the container tightly closed between uses.

What to do if you miss a dose

Administer the medication as soon as possible. Then use any remaining medication for that day at regularly spaced intervals. But if it's almost time for your next dose, skip the missed one and go back to your regular schedule.

What to do about side effects

Stop using the medication and call your primary health care provider right away if you notice any changes in vision. Tell your primary health care provider if you develop further problems with your eyes, such as blurred vision, burning, stinging, redness, or wateriness.

Special instructions

• Tell your primary health care provider if you have other medical problems with your eyes, such as a corneal abrasion or glaucoma. Also tell him if you're allergic to this or other medications.
• Once your eye infection is cured, don't save your medication and use it for a new eye infection. Always check with your primary health care provider first.
• Don't share this medication with family members, even if they have symptoms that resemble yours. If a family member has the same symptoms, call your primary health care provider.
• Don't rub or scratch around your eye area while taking this medication. You might accidentally hurt your eye.
• Keep all appointments for follow-up visits with your primary health care provider.

Additional instructions

_____
_____
_____
_____
_____
_____
_____
_____

Taking oral dexamethasone

Dear Patient,

Your primary health care provider has prescribed oral dexamethasone to treat your condition. The label may read Decadron, Hexadrol, or Dexone.

How to take dexamethasone

Dexamethasone comes in tablet, oral solution, and elixir forms. Carefully check the label on your prescription bottle, and follow the directions exactly. Don't take dexamethasone more often than ordered.

Take your medication with food to prevent stomach irritation. If you're taking only one dose daily, take it in the morning for best results.

Don't stop taking dexamethasone suddenly. Check with your primary health care provider first.

What to do if you miss a dose

Take it as soon as possible. Then take any remaining doses for that day at regularly spaced intervals. But if it's almost time for your next dose, skip the missed one and take the next one on schedule. Don't double dose.

What to do about side effects

Call your primary health care provider at once if you have trouble breathing or start to retain water. The medication may be causing a serious heart problem.

Also call if you experience mood changes, difficulty sleeping, weakness, unusual thirst, frequent urination, or weight loss despite eating regularly.

What you must know about other drugs

Tell your primary health care provider about other medications you're taking, including nonprescription ones. He may want you to avoid certain pain relievers, such as aspirin, because they can increase the risk of stomach problems.

Your primary health care provider also may need to adjust your dose of dexamethasone if you take barbiturates (found in some sleeping pills and medications for seizure disorders) or certain other medications. Also, check with him before you have any vaccinations.

Special directions

• Tell your primary health care provider if you have other medical problems, especially a fungal infection, ulcers, high blood pressure, diabetes, or diseases of the kidney, liver, blood, bones, or other organs.
• Keep all appointments for follow-up visits.
• Your primary health care provider may want you to carry a medical identification card stating that you're using this medication and that you may need additional medication during an emergency, a severe asthma attack, or other illness, or unusual stress.

✔ Keep in mind

• If you're pregnant or breast-feeding, check with your primary health care provider before using dexamethasone.

Additional instructions

_____
_____
_____
_____
_____
_____
_____
_____
_____
_____

Applying topical dexamethasone

Dear Patient,

Your primary health care provider has prescribed dexamethasone to treat your skin or scalp problem. The brand names for this medication include Decaderm, Decaspray, and Decadron.

How to apply dexamethasone
Topical dexamethasone is available in spray, gel, and cream forms. First, read the patient instructions provided in your medication package. Follow the directions exactly as ordered. Before applying your medication, wash the affected skin gently.

If you're using the gel or cream, apply a thin coat of medication. Rub in the gel or cream gently to avoid injuring your skin. If you're treating a hairy area, part the hair and apply the medication directly to the affected area. Keep the medication away from your eyes, mouth, nose, and other mucous membranes.

If you're using the spray, shake the can well. Then spray while moving the nozzle over the affected area. Take care not to get the spray in your eyes or inhale it.

If you've used your fingers to apply your medication, be sure to wash your hands when you're finished.

Don't wrap the treated skin with a bandage or other tight dressing, unless your primary health care provider has told you to do so.

What to do if you miss a dose
Apply the medication as soon as possible. But if it's almost time for your next application, skip the missed one and apply the next one on schedule.

What to do about side effects
Check with your primary health care provider if you experience skin reactions to this medication, including a rash, itching, burning, redness, or dryness. Also report signs of skin infection, such as redness, pain, and oozing.

Special directions
• Tell your primary health care provider if you have other medical problems, especially poor circulation.
• Keep all appointments for follow-up visits, so your primary health care provider can check your progress and detect unwanted side effects early.
• If you're using this medication to treat diaper rash in a young child, don't cover the child's bottom with a tight-fitting diaper or plastic pants.

✔ Keep in mind
• Check with your primary health care provider before applying this medication on children.

Additional instructions

_____

Taking diabetes medications

Dear Patient,

These medications are used to treat diabetes by lowering your blood sugar. Diabetes is a condition that may cause serious kidney, eye, nervous system, and other problems if it's not carefully watched and controlled.

This information sheet contains general information about antidiabetic medications. It's not meant to take the place of a sheet describing the particular medication you're taking.

How to take diabetes medications

Medications that lower blood sugar may be taken orally (by mouth) or by injection. The diabetes medication given by injection is called insulin.

There are different types of insulin that act in the body for short or long periods of time. Your primary health care provider will select and prescribe the type and amount of insulin that is right for your type of diabetes.

Someone will teach you how to take the insulin out of the vial and inject it into your body. Listen and follow these instructions carefully. Don't be afraid to ask questions or voice concerns. It's extremely important that you understand how to measure the amount of insulin in a syringe and inject it properly.

Diabetes medications taken by mouth include chlorpropamide (Diabinese), glyburide (DiaBeta, Micronase), glipizide (Glucotrol), glimepiride (Amaryl), acarbose (Precose), metformin (Glucophage), troglitazone (Rezulin), miglitol (Glyset), and repaglinide (Prandin).

Some of these medications are taken once a day before breakfast; others are taken twice or three times a day before meals.

What to do if you miss a dose

Missing an injection of insulin can be dangerous. If this happens, check your blood sugar immediately. If it's high, call your primary health care provider for guidance on how much insulin to inject. Don't try to guess.

Some providers give their patients detailed written instructions on what to do if blood sugar is high. If you don't have instructions, call your primary health care provider if you have symptoms of high blood sugar (listed later), even if your blood sugar is normal or only slightly high when you test it.

If you miss an oral dose of diabetes medication, take it as soon as you remember. If it's near the time of the next scheduled dose, skip the missed dose and go back to your regular schedule. Don't take double doses.

What to do about side effects

Many side effects are possible with diabetic medications, depending on which you're taking. The most serious side effects are caused by taking too little or too much of the medication, which causes fluctuations in blood sugar. Untreated, these fluctuations can be deadly—so be sure you understand and follow your primary health care provider's instructions.

Taking too much medication causes low blood sugar. Although different people react differently to low blood sugar, some common side effects are anxiety, blurred vision, confusion, cold sweats, extreme hunger, nausea, headache, shakiness, and tiredness.

When symptoms first occur, eat a quick-acting sugar—such as honey, fruit juice, or table sugar—or take the prescription medication glucagon, if your primary health care provider prescribes it. If side effects persist, contact your primary health care provider immediately.

Taking too little medication causes high blood sugar. These symptoms come on slower than those of low blood sugar and

(continued)

Taking diabetes medications *(continued)*

include blurred vision, fruit-like breath odor, dry mouth, unusual thirst, trouble breathing, flushed and dry skin, increased urination, and loss of appetite. Contact your primary health care provider immediately if you notice symptoms of high blood sugar. He'll instruct you on how to decrease your blood sugar level.

What you must know about alcohol and other drugs
Alcohol can interact with some oral diabetes medications, resulting in flushing, shakiness, nausea, and vomiting. Alcohol may also change the way your body handles blood sugar control. Every patient is different, so ask your primary health care provider if you can drink alcohol in moderation or if you should avoid it.

Special directions
• If you're taking insulin, store it between 36° and 80° F. Unopened vials can be stored in the refrigerator. Never freeze insulin or leave it in sunlight.
• If your insulin looks cloudy, gently roll the vial between your hands before withdrawing the dose with a syringe.
• If you're mixing different types of insulins in the same syringe before injecting them, always put the insulins into the syringe in the same order.
• Ask your primary health care provider for written instructions to follow if you become ill or can't eat.
• Monitor your blood sugar or urine sugar exactly as instructed. Knowing these levels at different times during the day or when you're having side effects can help your primary health care provider manage your medication doses better.
• Wear a medication alert bracelet or necklace at all times.

• Carry a source of sugar with you at all times in case you get symptoms of low blood sugar.
• Some oral diabetes medications can cause sun sensitivity. Check with your primary health care provider or pharmacist to see if your medication fits into this category.

✔ Keep in mind
• Oral diabetes medications are not recommended for children.

Additional instructions
_____

Taking diazepam

Dear Patient,

Your primary health care provider has prescribed diazepam to help your condition. Because diazepam causes relaxation, it's helpful for treating severe tension or anxiety as well as muscle spasms. It's also used to prevent seizures. The label may read Valium, Valrelease, or Zetran.

How to take diazepam

Diazepam comes in extended-release capsules, an oral solution, and tablets. Carefully check the prescription label, and follow the directions exactly as ordered. Don't increase your dose. If you're taking the extended-release capsules, don't crush, break, or chew them — swallow them whole.

If you're taking diazepam regularly, don't suddenly stop taking it without first checking with your primary health care provider.

What to do if you miss a dose

Take it right away if you remember within an hour or so of the missed dose. However, if you don't remember until later, skip the missed dose and take your next dose on schedule. Don't double dose.

What to do about side effects

Get emergency help *at once* if you suddenly start to feel very unwell and experience difficulty breathing, faintness, or a dramatic change in your heart or pulse rate.

Check with your primary health care provider if this medication makes you feel drowsy, lethargic, or like you have a hangover. Also call if you start to stagger when you walk.

What you must know about alcohol and other drugs

Don't drink alcoholic beverages while taking diazepam because the combination may cause oversedation. For the same reason, avoid other central nervous system depressants (medications that slow down your nervous system), such as sleeping pills, tranquilizers, and many cold and flu medications. Taking diazepam with the ulcer medication cimetidine (Tagamet) may also lead to increased drowsiness.

Special directions

• Tell your primary health care provider if you have other medical problems, such as glaucoma, myasthenia gravis, Parkinson's disease, and liver or kidney problems. Also mention if you have a history of drug addiction or psychological problems.
• See your primary health care provider regularly to determine if you need to continue taking this medication because if you take too much, it may become habit-forming.
• Before you have medical tests, tell your health care provider that you're taking diazepam because it may alter the test results.
• Make sure you know how you react to diazepam before you drive, use machines, or perform other activities that could be dangerous if you're not fully alert.

✔ Keep in mind

• If you're pregnant or breast-feeding, check with your primary health care provider before taking this medication.
• If you're an older adult, realize that you may be especially prone to diazepam's side effects.
• If you're an athlete, you should know that diazepam is banned by the National Collegiate Athletic Association and the U.S. Olympic Committee.

Additional instructions

_____

_____

Taking diclofenac

Dear Patient,

Diclofenac is given to relieve joint pain, swelling, and stiffness caused by arthritis. The label may read Voltaren.

How to take diclofenac

Take this medication with milk, meals, or a full glass (8 ounces) of water. Also, avoid lying down for about 15 to 30 minutes after taking this medication. This helps prevent irritation of your esophagus (food tube). Swallow the tablets whole — don't chew or break them.

What to do if you miss a dose

Take the dose as soon as possible. However, if it's almost time for your next dose, skip the missed dose and take your next dose on schedule. Don't double dose.

What to do about side effects

Get emergency help if you are having an allergic reaction, (wheezing, difficulty breathing, hives, itching, or a rash). Also call your primary health care provider right away if you hear ringing or buzzing in your ears.

Be aware that diclofenac can cause serious bleeding from the digestive tract, including ulcers. Stop taking this medication and check with your primary health care provider *at once* if you have any of these warning signs: severe abdominal or stomach pain; black, tarry stools; severe, continuing nausea or heartburn; or vomiting of blood or material that looks like coffee grounds.

Check with your primary health care provider if you feel drowsy or have a headache, abdominal discomfort, or diarrhea.

What you must know about alcohol and other drugs

Avoid alcoholic beverages while taking diclofenac because stomach problems are more likely to occur.

Tell your primary health care provider about other medications you're taking. If you take blood thinners, taking diclofenac may increase your risk of bleeding. Also, don't take aspirin or acetaminophen (Tylenol) for more than a few days while taking this medication, unless your primary health care provider tells you otherwise.

Diclofenac may increase the toxicity of certain medications, including cyclosporine (Sandimmune or Neoral), an antibiotic; digoxin (Lanoxin), a heart medication; lithium (Lithane), a medication for manic-depressive disorder; and methotrexate (Mexate), a cancer medication.

Diclofenac may also interfere with the effects of water pills. If you have diabetes, your primary health care provider may need to adjust your medications for this disease.

Special directions

• Tell your primary health care provider if you have other medical problems, especially ulcers, porphyria, or liver or kidney disease. Also tell him if you're allergic to diclofenac, aspirin, or other medications.
• Know how you react to diclofenac before you drive, use machines, or perform other activities that could be dangerous if you're not fully alert.

✓ Keep in mind

• If you're pregnant or breast-feeding, don't take this medication without your primary health care provider's consent.
• If you're an older adult, you may be especially prone to side effects from diclofenac.

Additional instructions

_____

_____

_____

Taking dicloxacillin

Dear Patient,

Your primary health care provider has prescribed dicloxacillin to treat your bacterial infection. The label may read Dycill, Dynapen, or Pathocil.

How to take dicloxacillin
This antibiotic medication comes in capsule and oral suspension forms.

If you're taking the capsule form, don't break, chew, or crush the capsule — swallow it whole.

If you're taking the oral suspension, use a dropper or specially marked measuring spoon to measure each dose accurately.

Take your medication with a full glass (8 ounces) of water on an empty stomach, either 1 hour before or 2 hours after meals, unless otherwise directed by your primary health care provider.

Continue to take your medication, even after you start to feel better. Stopping too soon may allow your infection to return.

What to do if you miss a dose
Take it as soon as possible. But if it's almost time for your next dose, adjust your dosage schedule as follows.

If you take two doses a day, space the missed dose and the next dose 5 to 6 hours apart.

If you take three or more doses a day, space the missed dose and the next dose 2 to 4 hours apart. Then resume your regular dosing schedule.

What to do about side effects
Call your primary health care provider *at once* if you develop any of the following signs of an allergic reaction: difficulty breathing, a rash, hives, itching, or wheezing.

Check with your primary health care provider if you experience nausea, heartburn, or diarrhea, especially if these symptoms persist or become severe.

What you must know about other drugs
Tell your primary health care provider about other medications you're taking. Probenecid (Benemid), a gout medication, may increase the effects of dicloxacillin. This effect may or may not be beneficial; check with your primary health care provider.

Special directions
• Tell your primary health care provider if you have a history of kidney problems or if you're allergic to this medication or other antibiotics.
• If you become allergic to this medication, you should carry a medical identification card or wear a medical identification bracelet stating this.

Warning: If you develop severe diarrhea, don't take any diarrhea medication without first checking with your primary health care provider. Diarrhea medications may make your diarrhea worse or last longer. For mild diarrhea, you may take a diarrhea medication containing kaolin or attapulgite.
• Tell your primary health care provider that you're taking dicloxacillin before you have medical tests because this medication may alter test results.

✓ Keep in mind
• If you're pregnant or breast-feeding, check with your primary health care provider before taking this medication.

Additional instructions
_____
_____

Taking dicyclomine

Dear Patient,

Your primary health care provider has prescribed dicyclomine to relieve your digestive cramps or spasms. This medication is often part of the treatment for stomach ulcers. The label may read Antispas, Bentyl, or Dibent.

How to take dicyclomine

Dicyclomine comes in capsule, syrup, and tablet forms. Carefully read the instructions on the prescription label and follow them exactly. Take this medication 30 minutes to 1 hour before meals, unless your primary health care provider directs otherwise.

If you're taking dicyclomine in the capsule form, don't break, chew, or crush it — swallow it whole.

Check with your primary health care provider before you stop using this medication. He may want to reduce your dosage gradually to prevent unwanted effects.

What to do if you miss a dose

Take the dose as soon as possible. But if it's almost time for your next dose, skip the missed dose and take your next dose on schedule. Don't double dose.

What to do about side effects

Check with your primary health care provider if you have any of the following side effects: headache, dizziness, palpitations, constipation, difficulty urinating, or impotence.

What you must know about other drugs

Don't take dicyclomine within 2 to 3 hours of taking antacids or medication for diarrhea because these medications may make dicyclomine ineffective.

Special directions

- Tell your primary health care provider if you have other medical problems, especially GI, heart, liver, or kidney disease; glaucoma; or an overactive thyroid. Also mention if you have a history of urinary problems.

! *Warning:* Because you may not sweat as much while taking dicyclomine, your body temperature may increase. Therefore, take care not to become too hot during exercise or hot weather because overheating could cause heatstroke. For the same reason, hot baths or saunas may make you dizzy or faint while you're taking dicyclomine.

- Make sure you know how you react to dicyclomine before you drive, use machines, or perform other activities that could be dangerous if you're not fully alert.
- If this medication makes your mouth feel dry, use sugarless hard candy or gum, ice chips, or a saliva substitute. If your mouth dryness lasts for more than 2 weeks, check with your primary health care provider or dentist.

✔ Keep in mind

- If you're pregnant or breast-feeding, check with your primary health care provider before taking this medication.
- If you're an older adult, you may be especially prone to side effects from dicyclomine.

Additional instructions

_____

_____

_____

_____

Taking didanosine

Dear Patient,

Your primary health care provider has prescribed didanosine. It's used to treat human immunodeficiency virus (HIV). This medication keeps HIV from reproducing and also seems to slow down immune system destruction. The brand name of this medication is Videx.

How to take didanosine

This medication is available as a tablet, an oral liquid solution, and an oral liquid suspension. It should be taken on an empty stomach, at least 2 hours before or 2 hours after you eat.

If you're taking the tablets, crush or chew them completely before swallowing them. If you find the tablets too hard to chew, mix them in at least 1 ounce of water and stir well until they break apart completely. Then take the mixture at once. No matter how you take them, the tablets contain special buffers to prevent stomach acid from destroying the medication. Remember: Always take two tablets at once to get the right amount of buffer in your system.

If you're giving didanosine to an infant 6 to 12 months old, one tablet will contain enough buffer.

If you are taking the oral solution, open the powder packet and pour the entire contents into a half-glass (4 ounces) of water. Don't use fruit juice or other acid-containing drinks (such as cola) to make the solution. Stir the mixture for 2 to 3 minutes until the powder dissolves completely; then drink all the solution.

If you are taking the liquid suspension, shake the bottle well before measuring out a dose. To keep a constant amount of this medication in your blood, space doses evenly.

Store the tablets and unopened oral solution packets at room temperature, away from heat, light, and humidity. Store the liquid suspension in the refrigerator.

What to do if you miss a dose

If you miss a dose of didanosine, take it as soon as you remember. If it's almost time for the next scheduled dose, skip the missed dose and go back to your regular schedule. Don't take double doses.

What to do about side effects

If you have nausea, vomiting, abdominal pain, or pain or numbness in your hands or feet, contact your primary health care provider *immediately.*

More common side effects are diarrhea, sleeping difficulty, mouth dryness, headache, and irritability. Often, these side effects will go away as your body adjusts to the medication. If they continue or worsen, contact your primary health care provider.

What you must know about alcohol and other drugs

Check with your primary health care provider before taking this medication if you are also taking trimethoprim (Proloprim, Trimpex). You'll probably be instructed to take this medication at least 2 hours before or after didanosine to allow both to work properly.

Also inform your primary health care provider if you're on dapsone (Avlosulfon), zalcitabine (Hivid), stavudine (Zerit), or isoniazid (Nydrazid). These medications may increase your chance of having pain, numbness, or tingling in your hands and feet. Many other medications have the same effect, so be sure to tell your primary health care provider and pharmacist about all prescription and nonprescription medications you're taking.

(continued)

Taking didanosine *(continued)*

Special directions

- If you've ever had an unusual reaction to didanosine, tell your primary health care provider.
- Didanosine contains a large amount of sodium, which can be of concern to patients on low sodium or other special diets.
- The tablet form contains phenylalanine, which can be a problem for patients with a disease called phenylketonuria.
- Tell your primary health care provider about your medical history, especially if you have kidney, heart, liver, or pancreas problems; high blood cholesterol; or are an alcoholic.

✔ Keep in mind

- Tell your primary health care provider if you're pregnant or considering breast-feeding, or if you become pregnant while taking this medication. Using birth control is important if you're infected with HIV, because the baby may also be HIV infected.
- Avoid any sexual activity that may cause body fluids to be exchanged with another person. If you do have vaginal, oral, or anal sex, you or your partner should wear a latex condom at all times.

Additional instructions

_____

_____

_____

_____

_____

_____

_____

_____

_____

_____

Taking diflunisal

Dear Patient,

Your primary health care provider has pre-scribed diflunisal to relieve your pain. This medication, which is similar to aspirin, is of-ten used to treat osteoarthritis symptoms, such as joint swelling, stiffness, and pain. The label may read Dolobid.

How to take diflunisal
Diflunisal comes in tablet form. Take diflu-nisal with food or an antacid and a full glass (8 ounces) of water. Don't crush or break the tablet—swallow it whole.

Also, don't lie down for about 15 to 30 minutes after taking your dose. This helps to prevent irritation of your esophagus (food tube).

What to do if you miss a dose
Take the dose as soon as you remember. However, if it's almost time for your next dose, skip the missed dose and take your next dose on schedule. Never double the dose.

What to do about side effects
Call your primary health care provider *at once* if you have any of the following warn-ing signs of GI bleeding or ulcers: severe stomach or abdominal pain; black, tarry stools; and vomiting of blood or material that looks like coffee grounds.

Also check with your primary health care provider if you have dizziness, a headache, a rash, ringing in your ears, vision changes, nausea, heartburn, stomach or abdominal pain, or diarrhea.

What you must know about alcohol and other drugs
Don't drink alcoholic beverages while taking diflunisal because the combination increas-es the risk of stomach problems.

Tell your primary health care provider about other medications you're taking. Don't take aspirin, acetaminophen (Tylenol), or other aspirin-related medications together with diflunisal for more than a few days, un-less your primary health care provider gives you other directions, because doing so may cause unwanted side effects.

If you take blood thinners, be aware that diflunisal may increase your risk of bleeding. Antacids may decrease the effectiveness of this medication.

Special directions
• Tell your primary health care provider if you have other medical problems, especial-ly ulcers, a heart condition, or kidney dis-ease. Also inform him if you're allergic to di-flunisal, aspirin, or other medications.
• Before having any kind of surgery (includ-ing dental surgery), tell your primary health care provider or dentist that you're taking di-flunisal.
• Know how you react to this medication be-fore you drive, use machines, or perform other activities that require full alertness.

✔ Keep in mind
• If you're pregnant or breast-feeding, don't take this medication without your primary health care provider's approval.
• If you're an older adult, you may be espe-cially sensitive to side effects from diflunisal.

Additional instructions
_____
_____
_____
_____
_____
_____

Taking digoxin

Dear Patient,

Your primary health care provider has prescribed digoxin to treat your heart condition. Digoxin helps to improve the strength and efficiency of the heart or to control an irregular heartbeat. Brand names for digoxin include Lanoxin and Lanoxicaps.

How to take digoxin

This medication is available as capsules, elixir, and tablets. Carefully check the label on your prescription bottle and follow the directions exactly as ordered. If you're taking the *elixir*, measure your dose only with the specially marked dropper.

Ask your primary health care provider about checking your pulse rate. If he wants you to, you should check your pulse rate before each dose. If it's much slower or faster than your usual rate (or less than 50 beats per minute), or if it changes rhythm or force, check with your primary health care provider. Such changes may mean side effects are occurring.

Don't stop taking digoxin without first checking with your primary health care provider. Stopping suddenly may cause a serious change in your heart's function.

What to do if you miss a dose

If you remember the missed dose within 12 hours, take it as soon as you remember. However, if you don't remember until later, skip the missed dose and take your next dose on schedule. Don't double dose.

What to do about side effects

Call your primary health care provider *right away* if you develop increased shortness of breath; sudden weight gain (3 or more pounds in 1 week); swelling of your ankles or fingers; visual changes, such as blurred vision, double vision, light flashes, or the appearance of yellow-green halos around images; digestive problems, such as loss of appetite, nausea, vomiting, or diarrhea; changes in your pulse rate; or hallucinations.

Also check with your primary health care provider if this medication makes you feel tired, weak, or agitated.

What you must know about other drugs

Tell your primary health care provider about other medications you're taking because many prescription and nonprescription medications can interact with digoxin. For example, digoxin may become toxic if taken with many medications, including certain antibiotics, heart medications, steroids, and water pills.

Other medications can decrease the absorption of digoxin, including cholesterol-lowering medications, antacids, and some diarrhea medications.

Special directions

- Tell your primary health care provider if you have other medical problems, especially kidney, liver, or lung disease or a history of rheumatic fever.
- Before having any kind of surgery (including dental surgery) or emergency treatment, tell your primary health care provider or dentist that you're taking digoxin.

✔ Keep in mind

- If you're pregnant or breast-feeding, check with your primary health care provider before using this medication.
- If you're an older adult, you may be especially prone to unwanted effects from digoxin.

Additional instructions

_____

_____

Taking diltiazem

Dear Patient,

This medication is used to relieve and control angina (chest pain) and high blood pressure. If you're taking the *tablet* form of diltiazem, the label may read Cardizem. If you're taking the *sustained-release capsules,* the label may read Cardizem CD, Cardizem SR, or Dilacor XR.

How to take diltiazem
Carefully check the label on your prescription bottle, and follow the directions exactly as ordered.

If you're taking the capsule form, don't crush or chew it — swallow it whole.

If you have been taking diltiazem regularly for several weeks, don't suddenly stop taking it. Your primary health care provider may want to reduce your dose gradually before you stop completely.

If you have high blood pressure, you may not notice any symptoms of this disorder. Even so, it's essential that you take diltiazem exactly as directed.

What to do if you miss a dose
Take the dose as soon as possible. However, if it's almost time for your next dose, skip the missed dose and take your next dose on schedule. Don't double dose.

What to do about side effects
Check with your primary health care provider if you feel nauseous, tired, or drowsy or have a headache or an irregular heartbeat. Also call if your feet and ankles become swollen or if you suddenly gain unexpected weight (more than 3 lbs in 1 week).

What you must know about other drugs
Tell your primary health care provider about other medications you're taking, so harmful interactions can be avoided. For example, Taking diltiazem with the ulcer medication cimetidine (Tagamet) can lead to toxic effects. If you take digoxin (Lanoxin) for a heart condition, diltiazem may cause an unwanted buildup of digoxin. Taking propranolol (Inderal) or other beta blockers (for high blood pressure) with diltiazem could lead to heart problems.

Special directions
• Tell your primary health care provider if you have other medical problems, especially severe high blood pressure, heart disease, or a liver or kidney condition.
• Keep appointments with your primary health care provider, so he can check your progress and adjust your dosage, if needed.
• Talk to your primary health care provider about how to exercise safely without overdoing it, to improve your condition.
• Ask your primary health care provider how to count your pulse rate. While you're taking diltiazem, check your pulse rate regularly. If it's much slower than your usual rate or less than 50 beats/minute, check with your primary health care provider. A pulse rate that is too slow may cause circulation problems.

✔ Keep in mind
• If you're pregnant or breast-feeding, check with your primary health care provider before using this medication.
• If you're an older adult, you may be especially sensitive to side effects from diltiazem.

Additional instructions
_____
_____
_____
_____
_____

Taking dimenhydrinate

Dear Patient,

Dimenhydrinate is used to relieve nausea and vomiting and to prevent or treat motion sickness. Brand names for this medication include Calm-X, Dimetabs, and Dramamine.

How to take dimenhydrinate

Dimenhydrinate comes in the form of tablets, chewable tablets, capsules, and syrup.

Carefully check the label on your prescription bottle, and follow the directions exactly as ordered.

If you're taking dimenhydrinate to prevent motion sickness, take it at least 1 to 2 hours before traveling. If this isn't possible, take it at least 30 minutes before traveling.

Take this medication with food or a glass of milk or water to lessen stomach irritation, if necessary.

What to do about side effects

Dimenhydrinate may make you feel drowsy. Occasionally, this medication causes headache, palpitations, blurred vision, and mouth dryness. If these side effects persist or become severe, call your primary health care provider.

What you must know about alcohol and other drugs

Check with your primary health care provider before drinking alcoholic beverages or taking other medications because the combined effects may make you overly drowsy.

Special directions

• Check with your primary health care provider before you take this medication if you have glaucoma, asthma, an enlarged prostate, or a seizure disorder.
• Don't take dimenhydrinate if you're allergic to it or to theophylline (Theo-Dur), an asthma medication.

• Tell your primary health care provider that you're taking dimenhydrinate before you have any skin tests for allergies because it may affect the test results.
• Know how you react to this medication before you drive, use machines, or perform other activities that could be dangerous if you're not fully alert.
• If this medication makes your mouth feel dry, you may get temporary relief by using sugarless hard candy or gum, melting bits of ice in your mouth, or using a saliva substitute.
• If you're taking dimenhydrinate to control nausea and vomiting, make sure your primary health care provider knows that you're taking this medication if you should suddenly develop symptoms of appendicitis, such as stomach or lower abdominal pain, cramping, and soreness.

✓ Keep in mind

• If you're pregnant or breast-feeding, check with your primary health care provider before using dimenhydrinate.
• Be aware that children and older adults are especially sensitive to side effects from this medication.

Additional instructions

_____
_____
_____
_____
_____
_____
_____
_____
_____
_____

Taking diphenhydramine

Dear Patient,

Diphenhydramine is used to relieve symptoms of numerous conditions, including hay fever, stuffy nose, insomnia, motion sickness, and nonproductive cough. This medication has more than 45 brand names, but some of the more common ones are Benadryl, Compoz, and Sominex Formula 2.

How to take diphenhydramine

Diphenhydramine is available without a prescription in the form of capsules, tablets, elixir, and syrup. Carefully check the medication label, and follow the directions exactly. Take your dose with food or a glass of milk or water to lessen stomach irritation, if necessary.

If you're taking diphenhydramine to prevent motion sickness, take it at least 1 to 2 hours before traveling. If that's not possible, take it at least 30 minutes ahead of time.

What to do if you miss a dose

If you're taking this medication regularly and you miss a dose, take it as soon as possible. However, if it's almost time for your next dose, skip the missed dose and take your next dose on schedule. Don't double dose.

What to do about side effects

While taking this medication, you may feel drowsy or nauseated or experience dryness of your mouth. Check with your primary health care provider if these side effects bother you or become severe.

What you must know about alcohol and other drugs

Avoid drinking alcoholic beverages while taking diphenhydramine because the combination may make you overly drowsy.

For the same reason, avoid concurrent use of other medications that slow down the nervous system, including narcotic painkillers, tranquilizers, and many cold and flu remedies. If you take certain antidepressants, your primary health care provider may not want you to take diphenhydramine because of the increased risk of unwanted effects.

If you regularly take large doses of aspirin for arthritis, be aware that diphenhydramine can cover up signs of an aspirin overdose, such as ringing in your ears.

Special directions

• Tell your primary health care provider if you have other medical problems, especially asthma, glaucoma, bladder conditions, heart disease, high blood pressure, or an overactive thyroid.
• Inform the primary health care provider that you're taking diphenhydramine before you have skin tests for allergies because the medication may affect the test results.
• Make sure you know how you react to this medication before you drive, use machines, or perform other activities that could be dangerous if you're not fully alert.
• If diphenhydramine makes your mouth or throat feel dry, use sugarless hard candy or gum, ice chips, or a saliva substitute.

✔ Keep in mind

• If you're pregnant or breast-feeding, check with your primary health care provider before taking diphenhydramine.
• Children and older adults are especially prone to side effects from this medication.

Additional instructions

_____
_____
_____
_____

Taking diphenoxylate with atropine

Dear Patient,

This medication, commonly known as Lomotil or Logen, is used to treat diarrhea. It works by slowing down intestinal movements.

How to take diphenoxylate with atropine

This medication comes in tablet and liquid forms. Carefully read the label on the medication bottle to know how much to take and when.

If you're taking the *liquid* form, make sure to measure the correct amount by using a specially marked measuring spoon or dropper. Using a regular household teaspoon may give you an incorrect dose.

What to do if you miss a dose

If you're taking this medication on a regular schedule and you forget to take a dose, take it when you remember. However, if it's almost time for the next dose, skip the missed dose and take your next dose on schedule. Don't double dose.

What to do about side effects

Call your primary health care provider if this medication causes bloating, constipation, loss of appetite, or stomach pain with nausea and vomiting.

This medication also may make you feel sleepy or dizzy and can cause dry mouth. If these symptoms persist or become bothersome, call your primary health care provider.

Special directions

• Tell your primary health care provider if you have other medical problems, especially liver disease or glaucoma.
• To help replace the fluid lost in your stool, drink clear liquids, such as apple juice, broth, ginger ale, or tea. During the next 4 hours, eat bland foods, such as plain bread or crackers, cooked cereals, and applesauce.
• Avoid citrus fruits, tomatoes, tomato sauce, caffeine, and alcoholic beverages because these foods can make diarrhea worse.

Warning: Call your primary health care provider if your diarrhea continues after 2 days or you develop a fever.
• Know how you respond to this medication before you drive a car or perform activities that require mental alertness.
• Don't use this medication again if you have diarrhea in the future. It can make certain forms of diarrhea worse.

✔ Keep in mind

• If you're pregnant or breast-feeding, check with your primary health care provider before using this medication.
• If you're an older adult, you may be especially prone to side effects from diphenoxylate with atropine.
• Don't give this medication to a child age 2 or younger because of the high risk of side effects.

Additional instructions

_____
_____
_____
_____
_____
_____
_____
_____
_____
_____

Taking dipyridamole

Dear Patient,

Your primary health care provider has prescribed dipyridamole to treat your heart condition. This medication is used to prevent blood clots after surgery to replace a heart valve. But it's also prescribed for other heart and blood vessel problems. Brand names include Apo-Dipyridamole, Novodipiradol, and Persantine.

How to take dipyridamole

This medication comes in tablet form. Carefully check the label on your prescription bottle, and follow the directions exactly as ordered. Take this medication in regularly spaced doses, as directed by your primary health care provider.

Take your dose with a full glass (8 ounces) of water at least 1 hour before or 2 hours after meals. However, to lessen stomach upset, your primary health care provider may want you to take dipyridamole with food or milk.

What to do if you miss a dose

Take it as soon as possible. But if it's within 4 hours of your next scheduled dose, skip the missed dose and go back to your regular dosing schedule. Don't double dose.

What to do about side effects

Check with your primary health care provider *immediately* if you get a headache, rash, or chest pain. More common side effects are dizziness and nausea.

What you must know about other drugs

If you've been instructed to take aspirin together with dipyridamole, take only the amount of aspirin ordered by your primary health care provider. If you need a medication to relieve pain or a fever, your primary health care provider may not want you to

take extra aspirin. You may want to discuss this issue with him ahead of time.

Special directions

• Tell your primary health care provider if you have other medical problems, especially chest pain or low blood pressure.
• Keep all appointments for follow-up visits, so your primary health care provider can check your progress.
• If you visit a dentist or primary health care provider other than the one who prescribed dipyridamole, be sure to tell him that you take this medication. Also mention whether or not you're taking it with a blood thinner or aspirin.
• This medication may make you feel dizzy, light-headed, or faint, especially when you get up from a lying or sitting position. Getting up slowly may help. If this problem continues or gets worse, check with your primary health care provider.

✓ Keep in mind

• If you're pregnant or breast-feeding, check with your primary health care provider before taking dipyridamole.

Additional instructions

_____
_____
_____
_____
_____
_____
_____
_____
_____
_____

Taking disopyramide

Dear Patient,

Your primary health care provider has pre-scribed disopyramide to treat your heart condition. This medication is used to correct irregular heartbeats or to slow an overactive heart. If you're taking the *capsule* form of disopyramide, the label may read Norpace. The brand name for the *extended-release capsules* is Norpace CR.

How to take disopyramide

Check the label on your prescription bottle. Follow the directions exactly.

If you're taking the *extended-release capsule,* swallow it whole without breaking, crushing, or chewing it.

Don't stop taking disopyramide without first checking with your primary health care provider. Stopping suddenly may cause a serious change in heart function.

What to do if you miss a dose

Take the dose as soon as possible unless the next scheduled dose is in less than 4 hours. If so, skip the missed dose and take the next on schedule. Don't double the dose.

What to do about side effects

Call your primary health care provider *right away* if you experience increasing shortness of breath, sudden weight gain (3 pounds or more in 1 week), or swelling of your ankles or fingers. Check with your primary health care provider if you experience blurred vi-sion, constipation, or dryness of your eyes, nose, or mouth, especially if these symp-toms persist or become severe.

What you must know about alcohol and other drugs

Don't drink alcoholic beverages until you've checked with your primary health care provider. When taken with disopyramide, alcohol may make your glucose level drop dangerously low and make you faint or dizzy.

Tell your health care provider about other medications you're taking. Other medications used to correct irregular heartbeats or slow an overactive heart may alter the effects of disopyramide beyond a safe level. Phenytoin (Dilantin), a seizure medication, may reduce the effectiveness of disopyramide.

Special directions

• Tell your health care provider if you have other medical problems, especially myasthe-nia gravis, glaucoma, difficulty urinating, oth-er heart conditions, or liver or kidney disease.
• This medication may make you dizzy, light-headed, or faint, especially when you get up from a lying or sitting position. Get-ting up slowly may help.
• Know how you react to this medication be-fore you drive, use machines, or perform other activities that could be dangerous if you're not fully alert.
• Disopyramide may make you sweat less. To prevent becoming overheated, don't overdo exercise, especially during hot weather.

✓ Keep in mind

• If you're pregnant or breast-feeding, check with your primary health care provider be-fore taking disopyramide.

Warning: If you have diabetes or heart failure, be alert for symptoms of low blood glucose while taking this medication. Symptoms include headache, shakiness, cold sweats, excessive hunger, and weak-ness. If these occur, eat or drink a sugary food and call your primary health care provider *right away.*

Additional instructions

_____

_____

Taking diuretics

Dear Patient,

Your primary health care provider has prescribed diuretics (water pills) for you. These medications reduce the amount of water in your body by increasing the flow of urine. Diuretics also help reduce high blood pressure.

How to take diuretics

These medications are available in tablet form. If you're in a health care facility or a supervised home care setting, you may receive the medications by injection.

The *tablets* are usually taken one to several times a day. If you take the medication several times a day, ask your primary health care provider for a recommended schedule. Because these drugs increase urination, you want to avoid taking them too close to bedtime. They can be taken either with or without food, but most patients take them after meals as part of a routine. Some diuretics need to be supplemented with potassium-rich foods, such as bananas or orange juice, to replace the potassium lost through the urine.

What to do if you miss a dose

If you miss a dose, take it as soon as you remember. If it's almost time for your next dose, skip the missed dose and then return to your normal routine. Don't take double doses.

What to do about side effects

If you have severe nausea, vomiting, or diarrhea contact your primary health care provider *at once* because you may be losing too much fluid.

Other side effects include dry mouth, increased thirst, irregular heartbeat, muscle cramps, unusual tiredness, weak pulse, and increased sensitivity to the sun (use a sunblock). In hot weather, you may also feel dizzy or light-headed, especially when rising from a sitting or lying position. If these side effects become troublesome, call your primary health care provider.

What you must know about alcohol and other drugs

Alcohol combined with diuretics may cause dizziness or light-headedness. So check with your health care provider before drinking.

Also check with your primary health care provider if you're taking antihypertensives because your blood pressure may drop too much. If you're also taking digoxin or lithium, your digoxin or lithium dose may need to be adjusted. Taking colestipol or cholestyramine may lower the effectiveness of the diuretic. Taking angiotensin-converting enzyme inhibitors, cyclosporine, or potassium supplements may increase the risk of side effects.

Special directions

Warning: Don't stop this medication suddenly. Your health care provider will probably have you taper off gradually.
• Notify your primary health care provider immediately if you have shortness of breath, back pain, trouble urinating, or a sudden weight gain.
• Tell your primary health care provider if you have diabetes or liver or kidney disease.
• Arise slowly from a sitting or lying position until you know the effects of this medication.

Keep in mind

• If you're pregnant or breast-feeding, check with your primary health care provider before taking this medication.
• Older adults may be more sensitive to the effects of diuretics and may need lower doses.

Additional instructions

_____

_____

Taking divalproex

Dear Patient,

Your primary health care provider has prescribed divalproex (valproic acid) for you. This medication is used to control seizures and to treat migraine headaches and some conditions that require better emotional control. The label may read Depakote.

How to take divalproex

Divalproex comes in capsule form. Swallow the capsule whole, without breaking or chewing it. Take it with food or water to keep it from upsetting your stomach, but don't take it with milk. If you have trouble swallowing pills, open the capsule and sprinkle the contents on pudding or applesauce. Then swallow the mixture immediately.

What to do if you miss a dose

If you take one dose a day, take the missed dose as soon as possible. If you don't remember until the next day, skip the missed dose and take your next dose as scheduled. Never take two doses at once.

If you take two or more doses a day and you remember the missed dose within 6 hours, take it right away. Then equally space your remaining doses for the day, and return to your regular routine the next day. Never take two doses at once.

What to do about side effects

Call your health care provider *at once* if you develop unusual bleeding or bruising, extreme drowsiness or dizziness, appetite loss, continued nausea and vomiting, tiredness or weakness, yellow eyes or skin, trembling, fever, rash, abdominal pain, or facial swelling.

What you must know about alcohol and other drugs

Avoid drinking alcoholic beverages while taking this medication. Alcohol may decrease the effectiveness of the medication and cause oversedation.

Don't take antacids or aspirin without first talking with your primary health care provider. These medications can cause undesirable side effects when taken along with divalproex. Also tell your primary health care provider if you're taking a blood thinner or other medications to control seizures.

Special directions

Warning: If you're taking this medication for seizures, don't stop taking it suddenly — you may have a seizure.
- Tell your primary health care provider if you have a history of liver disease because it may affect your body's ability to break down divalproex.
- Don't drive or do anything that could be dangerous if you're not alert until you know how you respond to this medication.
- Divalproex can affect how quickly your blood clots, so try not to cut yourself. For example, use an electric razor and a soft toothbrush.

✓ Keep in mind

- If you have diabetes, this medication may make urine tests for ketones unreliable.
- If you're pregnant or breast-feeding, don't take this medication until you talk with your primary health care provider.
- If you're an athlete, you should know that divalproex is banned and in some cases tested for by the U.S. Olympic Committee and the National Collegiate Athletic Association.

Additional instructions

_____

_____

_____

_____

Taking docusate salts

Dear Patient,

This medication is a laxative used to treat constipation. Docusate salts may contain calcium, potassium, or sodium. If you're taking *docusate calcium,* the label may read Pro-Cal-Sof or Surfak. If you're taking *docusate potassium,* the label may read Dialose or Kasof. *Docusate sodium*'s label may read Colace or Dioeze.

How to take docusate salts

Docusate calcium and *docusate potassium* come in capsule form. *Docusate sodium* is available in tablet, capsule, oral liquid, and syrup forms.

If your primary health care provider prescribed this medication, follow his directions exactly. If you bought this medication without a prescription, carefully read the package directions before taking your first dose.

What to do about side effects

Although side effects aren't common, this medication may irritate your throat or leave a bitter taste in your mouth. You may also have mild abdominal cramping or diarrhea. If these symptoms persist or become severe, call your primary health care provider.

What you must know about other drugs

Don't take mineral oil while you're taking docusate salts because it may cause your body to absorb too much mineral oil, causing unwanted effects.

Don't take docusate salts within 2 hours of taking another medication because docusate salts may interfere with the desired actions of other medications.

Special directions

Warning: Don't use docusate salts (or any other laxative) if you have signs of appendicitis or inflamed bowel, such as stomach or lower abdominal pain, cramping, bloating, soreness, nausea, or vomiting. Instead, check with your primary health care provider as soon as possible.

- Drink at least 6 to 8 glasses of water or other liquids daily. This will help soften your stools and relieve constipation.
- Don't take docusate salts for more than 1 week unless your primary health care provider has prescribed or ordered a special schedule for you. This is true even if you continue to have constipation.
- If you notice a sudden change in your bowel habits or function that lasts longer than 2 weeks, or that occurs from time to time, check with your primary health care provider before using this medication. Your primary health care provider will need to find the cause of your problem before it becomes more serious.
- Don't overuse docusate salts. Otherwise, you may become dependent on this medication to produce a bowel movement. In severe cases, overuse of laxatives can damage the nerves, muscles, and other tissues of the bowel.

✔ Keep in mind

- If you're pregnant, check with your primary health care provider before taking docusate salts.
- Don't give this medication to children under age 6 unless prescribed by a primary health care provider.

Additional instructions

_____
_____
_____
_____
_____

Taking donepezil

Dear Caregiver,

Your patient's primary health care provider has prescribed donepezil to treat Alzheimer's disease. This medication increases the levels of certain chemicals in the brain. The brand name of this medication is Aricept.

How to take donepezil

This medication is available as a tablet. It should be taken in the evening, just before the patient goes to bed. It may be taken either with or without food.

Don't store the medication container in the refrigerator. Store it at room temperature, away from heat, light, and humidity.

What to do if you miss a dose

Give the missed dose as soon as you remember. If it's almost time for the next scheduled dose, skip the missed dose and go back to the regular schedule. Don't administer double doses.

What to do about side effects

Call the primary health care provider *at once* if the patient's stool becomes unusually dark, black, or tarry-looking.

Other side effects of donepezil include muscle cramps, diarrhea, headache, poor appetite, nausea, vomiting, and trouble sleeping. The patient may also be unsteady on his feet, so watch him carefully until you know how he reacts to this medication. Call the primary health care provider if any of these problems persist or become severe.

What you must know about other drugs

Avoid giving the patient ibuprofen (Motrin), naproxen sodium (Aleve), and other medications for pain and inflammation because they may cause stomach or intestinal problems.

Some medications such as benztropine (Cogentin) used to treat Parkinson's disease may counterbalance the effects of donepezil. Some medications used for seizure control, including barbiturates, phenytoin (Dilantin), and carbamazepine (Tegretol), may also decrease the effectiveness of donepezil.

Special directions

• Give donepezil exactly as instructed. Although the medication can't cure Alzheimer's disease, it can help slow down memory loss over time.
• Tell the primary health care provider about the patient's medical history, especially heart or stomach problems or unusual reactions to donepezil in the past.
• Donepezil is usually used for mild to moderate Alzheimer's disease. Because brain function in patients with advanced Alzheimer's disease declines, donepezil may not be as effective in patients with advanced disease.
• Keep regularly scheduled appointments with the health care provider to make sure the medication is working properly.
• Call the health care provider if the patient's condition worsens. Dosage adjustment or medication change may be needed.
• Tell the patient's dentist or other health care providers that he's taking donepezil. If surgery is needed, also tell the surgeon and the anesthesiologist.

✔ Keep in mind

• Keep this medication out of the reach of children and confused patients. Contact a poison control center immediately if an overdose is suspected. Signs of an overdose include nausea, vomiting, muscle weakness, slow heartbeat, seizures, increased sweating, and mouth watering.

Additional instructions

_____

_____

Taking dorzolamide

Dear Patient,

Your primary health care provider has prescribed dorzolamide because you have glaucoma. This medication slows down fluid production inside the eyeball and decreases the eye pressure that causes glaucoma. The brand name of this medication is Trusopt.

How to take dorzolamide

This medication is available as an eye drop. To administer this medication, follow these steps:

• Wash your hands. Tilt your head back and pull your lower eyelid away from your eye to make a pouch for the medicine.
• Drop the medicine into this pouch. Repeat with the other eye.
• Let go of your eyelid and close your eyes carefully. Try not to blink.
• With your eyes closed, take your finger and apply gentle pressure to the inner corner of your eye for 1 to 2 minutes. This allows the medication to be absorbed better.
• Wash your hands again.
• If you're also taking other eye drop medicines, wait at least 10 minutes after using dorzolamide to use those products.

What to do if you miss a dose

If you miss a dose, give it as soon as you remember. If it's almost time for the next scheduled dose, skip the missed dose and go back to your regular schedule. Don't double dose.

What to do about side effects

If you experience eye pain, itching, redness, or swelling, or have blurred vision that lasts for a long time, contact your primary health care provider *immediately.*

More common side effects include a bitter taste in your mouth, eye dryness, blurred vision, tearing, headache, and light sensitivity. Often, these side effects go away as your body adjusts to the medication. If they continue or are bothersome, contact your primary health care provider.

What you must know about other drugs

Check with your primary health care provider before taking this medication if you're taking any eye drops containing silver (such as silver nitrate). Used together, dorzolamide and silver products can cause a chemical reaction in the eye.

Special directions

• Tell your primary health care provider if you've had an unusual reaction to dorzolamide in the past; to a related medication, acetazolamide (Diamox); to sulfa medications, water pills, or oral diabetic medications; or to preservatives such as benzalkonium chloride.
• Continue taking this medication exactly as prescribed, even if you don't feel any different. There is no cure for glaucoma, and medication must be taken daily to keep it in check.
• Don't store the container in the refrigerator. Store it at room temperature, away from heat, light, and humidity.
• Tell your primary health care provider about your medical history, especially liver or kidney problems. Although chances are slim that eye drops will cause problems within the body, some of the medication is absorbed into your bloodstream.

✔ Keep in mind

• If you're pregnant or breast-feeding, don't use this medication without first telling your primary health care practitioner.

Additional instructions

Taking doxazosin

Dear Patient,

Your primary health care provider has prescribed this medication to treat your high blood pressure. The label may read Cardura.

How to take doxazosin

This medication comes in tablet form. Carefully check the label on your prescription bottle, which tells you how much medication to take and when. Follow the directions exactly as ordered.

What to do if you miss a dose

Before you start taking doxazosin, ask your primary health care provider for instructions on what you should do in case you forget a dose of your medication.

What to do about side effects

Call your primary health care provider *immediately* if you develop a rash, muscle or joint pain, or an irregular heartbeat.

This medication may lower your blood pressure, causing you to feel dizzy, light-headed, or faint when you get up from a sitting or standing position. Usually, this effect begins to go away after the first dose, but it may recur if you stop taking your medication for a few days or if your dosage is adjusted. If this problem persists or becomes severe, call your primary health care provider.

Check with your primary health care provider if doxazosin makes you feel sleepy or gives you a headache.

What you must know about other drugs

Don't take doxazosin with other medications to treat high blood pressure unless your primary health care provider has directed you to do so. Taking this combination of medications may cause dangerously low blood pressure, possibly leading to loss of consciousness.

Special directions

- Tell your primary health care provider if you have other medical problems, especially liver disease.
- Keep appointments for primary health care provider's visits. You'll need to see your primary health care provider at least every 2 weeks until your dosage is set properly, then at regular intervals so your progress can be checked.
- If doxazosin makes you feel dizzy, light-headed, or faint when you get up from a lying or sitting position, try to get up slowly.
- Because doxazosin can make you dizzy, make sure you know how you react to it before you drive, use machines, or perform other activities that could be dangerous if you're not fully alert.
- Your primary health care provider may teach you how to take your blood pressure at home. If so, check your blood pressure at regular intervals and call your primary health care provider if you detect any significant changes.

✓ Keep in mind

- If you're pregnant or breast-feeding, check with your primary health care provider before taking this medication.

Additional instructions

_____
_____
_____
_____
_____
_____
_____
_____
_____
_____

Taking doxepin

Dear Patient,

Your primary health care provider has prescribed doxepin to help relieve your depression. The label may read Adapin or Sinequan.

How to take doxepin

This medication is available in capsules or as an oral solution. Follow your primary health care provider's instructions exactly. Don't take more of it, and don't take it more often or longer than he directs. Take doxepin with food, even for a daily bedtime dose, unless your primary health care provider has told you to take it on an empty stomach.

If you're using the *oral solution,* use the dropper provided to measure the dose accurately. Just before you take each dose, dilute it in about 4 ounces of water, milk, or juice. Don't use grape juice or carbonated beverages because these liquids may decrease doxepin's effectiveness.

Don't stop taking doxepin suddenly without first calling your health care provider.

What to do if you miss a dose

If you miss a dose, adjust your dosing schedule as follows.

If you take one dose a day at bedtime, check with your primary health care provider. Don't take the missed dose in the morning because it may cause disturbing side effects during waking hours.

If you take more than one dose a day, take the missed dose as soon as possible. But if it's almost time for your next dose, skip the missed dose and take your next dose on schedule. Don't double dose.

What to do about side effects

Call your primary health care provider *right away* if you experience blurred vision, dry mouth, a fast pulse rate, constipation, difficulty urinating, or unusual sweating. Also call if this medication makes you feel drowsy, dizzy, or faint, especially when you get up suddenly from a sitting or lying position.

What you must know about alcohol and other drugs

Don't drink alcoholic beverages while taking doxepin unless your health care provider approves it. Also, your medication may not work well if taken with barbiturates (found in some sleeping pills and seizure medications). Taking doxepin with the ulcer medication cimetidine (Tagamet) may cause unwanted effects.

While you're taking doxepin, your primary health care provider may want you to avoid certain medications used to treat psychological disorders.

Special directions

• Tell your primary health care provider of other medical problems, especially heart disease.
• Know how this medication affects you before you drive, use machines, or perform other activities that could be dangerous if you're not fully alert.
• Before you have medical tests, tell your primary health care provider that you're taking doxepin because the medication may affect some test results.

✓ Keep in mind

• If you're pregnant or breast-feeding, check with your primary health care provider before taking doxepin.
• If you have diabetes, this medication may affect your glucose levels. If you notice a change in the results of your blood or urine glucose tests, call your health care provider.

Additional instructions

_____

_____

Taking doxycycline

Dear Patient,

Your primary health care provider has prescribed this antibiotic medication to treat your bacterial infection. The label may read Doxy Caps, Vibramycin, or Vibra-Tabs.

How to take doxycycline
This medication comes in capsule, delayed-release capsule, oral suspension, and tablet forms. Take your dose with food, milk, or a full glass (8 ounces) of water to prevent irritation of your esophagus (food tube) or stomach.

If you're taking the *oral suspension,* use a specially marked spoon to measure each dose accurately.

Continue to take your medication, even if you start to feel better after a few days. Stopping too soon may allow your infection to return. Also, try to take your doses at evenly spaced times day and night.

What to do if you miss a dose
Take it as soon as possible. But if it's almost time for your next dose, adjust your dosing schedule as follows.

If you take one dose a day, space the missed dose and the next dose 10 to 12 hours apart.

If you take two doses a day, space the missed dose and the next dose 5 to 6 hours apart.

If you take three or more doses a day, space the missed dose and the next dose 2 to 4 hours apart. Then resume your regular dosing schedule.

What to do about side effects
Call your primary health care provider *right away* if you develop any of the following symptoms of an allergic reaction to doxycycline: severe headache, vision changes, difficulty breathing, wheezing, hives, or itching.

Also check with your primary health care provider if you experience heartburn, nausea, diarrhea, rashes, or increased light sensitivity, especially if these symptoms persist or become severe.

What you must know about alcohol and other drugs
Avoid drinking alcoholic beverages because it may prevent doxycycline from working well. Other medications that may reduce the effectiveness of doxycycline are antacids, iron preparations (such as iron-containing vitamins), and some seizure medications. Also, if you use birth control pills, doxycycline may keep them from working effectively. Use another form of birth control.

Special directions
• Tell your primary health care provider if you have other medical problems, especially kidney disease. Also inform him if you're allergic to a tetracycline antibiotic.
• If your medication has changed color, tastes or looks different, has become outdated, or has been stored incorrectly (in a place too warm or too damp), don't use it; it could cause serious side effects. Discard the bottle and obtain a fresh supply.
• This medication may make your skin more sensitive to sunlight, so limit your exposure to the sun. For prolonged sun exposure, use a protecting lotion with a skin protection factor (SPF) of at least 15.

✔ Keep in mind
• If you're pregnant or breast-feeding, don't take doxycycline. It could stain your developing baby's teeth.

Additional instructions

Taking enalapril

Dear Patient,

Your primary health care provider has prescibed enalapril to lower your high blood pressure. It can also be prescribed to treat heart problems, when used with other medications. Enalapril is also called Vasotec.

How to take enalapril

Enalapril comes in tablet form. Carefully check the label on your bottle, and follow these directions exactly, unless your health care provider changes your dosage. Don't suddenly stop taking this medication without checking first with your health care provider.

What to do if you miss a dose

Take it as soon as possible. But if it's almost time for your next dose, skip the missed dose and take your next dose on schedule. Don't double dose.

What to do about side effects

Get emergency help *at once* and stop taking your medication if you have any of the following symptoms: difficulty swallowing, difficulty breathing, or swelling of your face, eyes, lips, hands, feet, or tongue. A blood problem that can cause severe infections is a rare but serious complication. Report fever, chills, weakness, or a sore throat to your health care provider *right away.*

Check with your primary health care provider as soon as possible if you feel dizzy or light-headed. Headaches and unusual tiredness also may occur, but these symptoms usually go away as your body adjusts to enalapril. However, if these symptoms persist or bother you, check with your primary health care provider.

What you must know about other drugs

Don't use salt substitutes or low-salt milk unless your primary health care provider directs you to do so. It may alter your heart rhythm or cause other problems due to a buildup of potassium in your body.

Check with your primary health care provider before taking any nonprescription medications, and be sure your he is aware of all prescription medications you're taking. If you're taking lithium (Lithane), your health care provider will closely watch your lithium level and may adjust its dosage. Your health care provider may tell you to use certain painkillers cautiously because they can prevent enalapril from working well.

Special directions

• Tell your primary health care provider about any medical conditions you have, especially kidney, liver, or collagen (immune) disease. Also tell him if you have diabetes or heart or blood vessel disease or if you've recently had a heart attack or stroke.
• Make sure you know how you react to enalapril before driving, using machines, or performing other activities that could be dangerous, in case you become dizzy.
• Your primary health care provider may prescribe a low-salt diet for you. If so, you need to limit canned soups, pickles, and other salty foods. Check with your primary health care provider first because too little salt in your body can also cause problems.

✔ Keep in mind

• If you're pregnant or think you may be, check with your primary health care provider before taking this medication.

Additional instructions

_____
_____
_____
_____

Taking ergonovine

Dear Patient,

This medication is used after delivery or miscarriage to prevent or treat excessive bleeding from your uterus. The label may read Ergotrate.

How to take ergonovine

Ergonovine comes in tablet form. Carefully check the label on your prescription bottle, which tells you how much to take at each dose. Follow these directions exactly.

Don't take more ergonovine, take it more often, or take it for a longer time than ordered because doing so could cause unwanted effects.

What to do if you miss a dose

If you miss a dose, skip it. Take your next dose on schedule. Don't double dose.

What to do about side effects

If you develop a rash or itchy skin, start to wheeze, or feel short of breath, stop the medication and call your primary health care provider *immediately.* These symptoms may be warning signs of an allergic reaction, which could be serious. If you have difficulty breathing, get emergency medical care *immediately.*

Check with your primary health care provider if you experience dizziness, headaches, chest pain, ringing in your ears, or nausea and vomiting. Also be aware that this medication can increase your blood pressure.

You may also experience menstrual-like cramps. That's because this medication causes the muscles of your uterus to tighten; this is how it controls bleeding. If your cramping becomes very uncomfortable, call your primary health care provider.

What you must know about other drugs

Tell your primary health care provider if you're taking other prescription or nonprescription medications. You may need to avoid certain medications, such as some anesthetics, because they can cause unwanted effects.

Special directions

• Tell your primary health care provider if you have other medical problems, especially chest pain or other heart problems, blood vessel disease (such as Raynaud's phenomenon), high blood pressure (now or in the past), toxemia, and kidney or liver disease. Also report any new medical problems that occur while taking this medication.
• Let your primary health care provider know if you're allergic to this medication or if you have other medication or food allergies.
• If you have an infection, check with your primary health care provider because ergonovine may have stronger effects in this case.
• Don't smoke while taking ergonovine because smoking may increase the risk of harmful side effects.
• Make sure your primary health care provider knows if you're on any special diet, such as a low-salt or low-sugar diet.
• If your bleeding doesn't slow down or if it becomes heavier, call your primary health care provider as soon as possible.

✔ Keep in mind

• If you're breast-feeding, check with your primary health care provider before taking this medication.

Additional instructions

Taking ergotamine

Dear Patient,

Ergotamine is used to relieve your headaches. The label may read Ergostat or Medihaler Ergotamine.

How to take ergotamine
Ergotamine comes in tablets to melt under your tongue, as an inhaler, or suppositories.

Place the *tablet* under your tongue so it dissolves. Don't chew or swallow it because it works faster when absorbed into the lining of your mouth.

If you have the *inhaler,* read the directions that come with it before using the medication. The inhaler gives about 300 measured sprays.

If you're using a *suppository* and it's too soft to insert, run cold water over it or chill it in the refrigerator for about 30 minutes before removing the foil wrapper. To insert it, remove the foil wrapper and moisten the suppository with cold water. Then lie on your side. With your index finger, gently push the suppository into your rectum as far as you can.

Don't exceed the prescribed amount of ergotamine without checking with your health care provider.

For best results, take ergotamine at the first sign of a headache. Also, lie down in a quiet, dark room for at least 2 hours after taking your medication.

What to do about side effects
Call your health care provider *right away* if you have any symptoms of ergotamine overdose: confusion; fast or slow heartbeat; numbness and tingling of your fingers, toes, or face; red blisters on or coldness of your hands and feet; shortness of breath; chest or stomach pains; bloating; and weakness.

If you have headaches more often than before or they are more severe or if you develop swelling in your legs or feet, check with your health care provider as soon as possible.

You may experience diarrhea, dizziness, nausea, or vomiting, but these symptoms usually stop when your body adjusts to the medication. If they continue or become bothersome, check with your primary health care provider. If you're using the inhaler and you get a cold or a sore throat or mouth, call your primary health care provider.

What you must know about alcohol and other drugs
Avoid alcoholic beverages because they can make your headaches worse. Tell your primary health care provider if you're taking other medications. Taking a beta blocker, such as propranolol (Inderal), for high blood pressure or a heart condition may cause unwanted side effects.

Special directions
• Tell your primary health care provider if you have other medical problems, especially diseases of the heart, blood vessels, kidney, liver, or thyroid. Also tell him if you have high blood pressure or a skin condition that causes severe itching.
• Tell your health care provider if you've recently had an angioplasty (to open a blocked blood vessel) or surgery on a blood vessel.

✔ Keep in mind
• If you're pregnant or breast-feeding, check with your primary health care provider before taking this medication.
• Older adults may be especially prone to side effects from ergotamine.

Additional instructions

_____

_____

Taking oral erythromycin

Dear Patient,

Your primary health care provider has prescribed erythromycin to treat your infection. The label may read E-Mycin, Erythrocin, or Wyamycin S.

How to take erythromycin

This medication is available in tablet, capsule, and oral liquid forms. Carefully check the label on your prescription bottle, and follow the directions exactly as ordered.

Take your medication with a full glass (8 ounces) of water 1 hour before or 2 hours after meals. If the tablets are coated or the medication upsets your stomach, you may take it with food. *But don't take your medication with fruit juice.*

If you're taking the *chewable tablets,* chew or crush them before swallowing. If you're taking the *delayed-release capsules,* swallow them whole.

If you're taking the *oral liquid form,* measure your dose with a special dropper or measuring spoon made especially for medications.

Continue to take your medication for the full treatment time, even if you feel better after a few days. Stopping too soon may allow your infection to return.

What to do if you miss a dose

Take the dose as soon as possible. If it's almost time for your next dose, change your schedule as follows:

If you take two doses a day, space the missed dose and the next one 5 to 6 hours apart.

If you take three or more doses a day, space the missed dose and the next one 2 to 4 hours apart.

Then resume your regular dosing schedule.

What to do about side effects

If you develop a rash or itchy skin, stop taking the medication and call your primary health care provider *immediately.* These symptoms may be warning signs of a serious allergic reaction. If you feel unusually restless or have trouble breathing, get medical care *right away.*

Tell your primary health care provider if you have stomach pain, diarrhea, nausea, or vomiting. These symptoms may go away as your body adjusts to erythromycin, but let your primary health care provider know if they bother you.

What you must know about other drugs

Tell your primary health care provider if you're taking other medications. Erythromycin may not work well if taken with certain other antibiotics. Taking erythromycin with blood thinners may increase your risk of bleeding. Because of possible unwanted effects, your health care provider may also caution you against taking erythromycin with theophylline (Theo-Dur), an asthma medication, or cisapride (Propulsid), a heartburn medication.

Special directions

● Tell your primary health care provider if you have other medical problems, especially liver disease. Inform him if you're allergic to erythromycin, another medication, or any food.
● Before you have medical tests, tell your primary health care provider that you're taking erythromycin because the medication may interfere with some test results.

Additional instructions

_____

_____

_____

Applying topical erythromycin

Dear Patient,

Your primary health care provider has prescribed erythromycin for your skin problem. The medication label may read Akne-mycin, Erycette, Eryderm, or Erygel.

How to apply erythromycin

This medication is available as an ointment, a gel, a pledget (swab), and a solution. Before applying it, wash the area with warm water and soap, rinse well, and pat dry. After washing or shaving, try to wait 30 minutes before applying the pledget, gel, or liquid forms. Otherwise, the alcohol in your medication may sting.

Keep the medication away from your eyes, nose, and mouth. If you do get some in your eyes, wash them out immediately with cool tap water.

If you're using the *ointment* or *gel,* apply a thin film of medication to cover the area lightly. If you're using the *solution,* dab the medication on with an applicator tip or a moistened pad.

What to do if you miss an application

Apply the medication as soon as possible. If it's almost time for your next application, skip the missed one and go back to your regular schedule.

What to do about side effects

Expect some mild stinging of your skin for a few minutes after you apply erythromycin. This is normal. However, check with your primary health care provider if your skin continues to itch or burn. Call your primary health care provider if your skin breaks out in a rash or becomes dry or scaly. These symptoms may go away as your body adjusts to erythromycin, but let your primary health care provider know about them, especially if they become bothersome or severe.

What you must know about other drugs

If you're using another medication on your skin along with erythromycin, wait at least 1 hour before you apply the second medication to prevent skin irritation.

Special directions

• Tell your primary health care provider if you're allergic to erythromycin, another medication, or any food.
• If you have acne, don't wash the affected area too much. Doing so could dry your skin and make your acne worse. Wash the area with a mild, bland soap two or three times a day, unless you have oily skin. Check with your primary health care provider for specific instructions.
• If you're using erythromycin for acne, you may wear cosmetics, but use only water-based products. Also, don't apply cosmetics heavily or use them too frequently because your acne could worsen.

Additional instructions

_____
_____
_____
_____
_____
_____
_____
_____
_____
_____
_____

Taking erythromycin with sulfisoxazole

Dear Patient,

Your primary health care provider has prescribed this combination medication to treat your ear infection. The label may read Eryzole or Pediazole.

How to take this medication
This medication comes as an oral liquid. Follow your primary health care provider's instructions exactly. Use a specially marked measuring spoon, not a household teaspoon, to measure your dose. Take your medication with food or extra water, if possible, to help prevent side effects.

Because this medication works best if you have a constant amount in your blood, take it in evenly spaced doses during the day and night. If you need to take four doses a day, schedule each dose 6 hours apart. Talk to your primary health care provider, nurse, or pharmacist if this schedule disrupts your sleep or other activities.

Continue to take your medication even if you start to feel better in a few days. Stopping too soon may allow your infection to return.

What to do if you miss a dose
Take the dose as soon as possible unless it's almost time for your next dose. In that case, if you take three or more doses a day, space the missed dose and the next dose 2 to 4 hours apart. Then return to your regular dosing schedule.

What to do about side effects
If you become short of breath or have difficulty breathing, stop taking this medication and get emergency medical care *at once.* You may be experiencing a serious allergic reaction.

If you have a persistent fever, a sore throat, joint pain, or start to bruise or bleed easily, don't take any more of this medica-

tion. Call your primary health care provider as soon as possible.

You may also experience some abdominal pain, nausea, vomiting, or diarrhea. Check with your primary health care provider about these symptoms, especially if they continue or become bothersome.

What you must know about other drugs
Tell your primary health care provider about other medications you're taking. Taking this medication with oral blood thinners could put you at risk for bleeding. Also, your health care provider may not want you to use theophylline (Theo-Dur), an asthma medication, with this medication or cisapride (Propulsid), a heartburn medication, because it could cause unwanted effects.

This medication can decrease the effectiveness of birth control pills. If necessary, switch to another form of birth control.

Special directions
• Tell your health care provider if you're allergic to erythromycin or sulfisoxazole.
• Drink a lot of extra water to prevent side effects, such as kidney stones, caused by the sulfa in this medication.
• Sulfisoxazole may cause an increased sensitivity to the sun. If you plan to be out in the sun for a long time, apply a sunblock with a skin protection factor (SPF) of 15 or greater.

✔ Keep in mind
• If you're pregnant or breast-feeding, don't take this medication without first checking with your primary health care provider.

Additional instructions

_____

_____

Taking estazolam

Dear Patient,

Your primary health care provider has prescribed this medication to help you sleep. The label may read ProSom.

How to take estazolam

Estazolam comes in tablet form. Follow your primary health care provider's directions exactly. Don't take more of it or take it more often or for a longer time than ordered. If you take too much estazolam, it can become habit-forming or it may not help you sleep.

Check with your primary health care provider if you think the medication isn't working well, especially if you've been taking it every night for several weeks.

What to do if you miss a dose

Skip the missed dose and go back to your regular dosing schedule. Don't double dose.

What to do about side effects

If you think you've taken an overdose, or if you experience severe side effects, such as prolonged confusion, severe drowsiness, trouble breathing, slow heartbeat, continuing slurred speech, staggering, or severe weakness, seek emergency help *at once.*

If this medication makes you drowsy in the daytime or dizzy, check with your primary health care provider, especially if these symptoms continue or bother you.

What you must know about alcohol and other drugs

Don't drink alcoholic beverages while taking this medication because the combination can cause oversedation. For the same reason, avoid other central nervous system depressants (medications that slow down the nervous system), such as tranquilizers, other sleep medications, muscle relaxers, and cold, allergy, and flu medications.

Other medications that can cause oversedation if taken with estazolam include the ulcer medication cimetidine (Tagamet); birth control pills; disulfiram (Antabuse), a medication for alcoholism; and isoniazid (Laniazid), a tuberculosis medication.

Estazolam may not work well if taken with certain medications, so be sure to tell your primary health care provider about other medications you're taking.

Special directions

• Tell your health care provider if you have other medical problems, such as a history of alcohol or medication dependence, a brain disorder, asthma or other lung diseases, kidney or liver disease, depression, myasthenia gravis, seizures, porphyria, or breathing problems while sleeping.
• Check with your primary health care provider at least every 4 months to see if you need to continue taking estazolam.
• After stopping this medication, your body may need time to adjust. Call your primary health care provider if you experience any irritability, nervousness, or trouble sleeping.
• Don't perform activities that require alertness, such as driving or operating hazardous machinery, while taking estazolam.

✔ Keep in mind

• If you're pregnant or breast-feeding, check with your primary health care provider before taking this medication.
• If you're an older adult, you may be especially prone to daytime drowsiness. So take care to prevent falls.

Additional instructions

_____

_____

_____

Taking estradiol

Dear Patient,

This estrogen-like medication is used to treat menopausal symptoms, vaginal dryness, and certain cancers. The label may read Estrace or Estraderm.

How to take estradiol

Estradiol comes in tablet, vaginal cream, and skin patch forms. Follow your primary health care provider's instructions exactly. If the tablets cause nausea, you may take them with food.

Before applying a *patch,* read the accompanying instructions. Wash and dry your hands. Apply the patch to a clean, dry, non-oily skin area, such as your abdomen or buttocks.

If you are using the *vaginal cream,* your primary health care provider may want you to use it at bedtime so it will be absorbed better. If you don't use it at bedtime, lie down for 30 minutes after use.

What to do if you miss a dose

If you forget to take a *tablet* or change a *skin patch,* do it as soon as possible. If it's almost time for your next dose, skip the missed dose. Take your next tablet or apply a new patch on schedule. Don't take double doses of tablets or use more than one patch at a time.

If you forget to apply a dose of *vaginal cream* and don't remember until the next day, skip the missed dose. Resume your regular dosing schedule.

What to do about side effects

Blood clots are a rare but serious complication. Call for emergency help *immediately* if you have one or more of these symptoms: a sudden or severe headache; sudden loss of coordination; blurred vision or other vision changes; numbness or stiffness in your legs; pain in your chest, groin, or legs; or shortness of breath.

Call your primary health care provider *right away* if you experience rapid weight gain; swelling in your feet and lower legs; breast enlargement, pain, or lumps; or unusual vaginal bleeding. Also call if you become nauseated, lose your appetite, or have stomach bloating or cramps.

If you're using the vaginal cream, call your primary health care provider if you develop swelling, redness, or itching in the vaginal area.

What you must know about other drugs

Because many medications can interfere with estradiol, tell your primary health care provider about other medications (nonprescription and prescription) you're taking.

Special directions

• Because estradiol can aggravate many medical conditions, tell your primary health care provider about other medical problems you have. Also tell him if you have female relatives who've had cancer of the breast or female organs.
• Keep all appointments for follow-up visits so your health care provider can check your progress and detect side effects early.
• Perform monthly breast self-examinations and report unusual changes.

✔ Keep in mind

• Don't take estradiol if you're pregnant or breast-feeding.
• If you have diabetes, estradiol may affect your glucose levels.

Additional instructions

_____

_____

Taking estrogen

Dear Patient,

This female hormone is used to relieve menopausal symptoms, to treat certain breast cancers, and to help prevent brittle bone disease (osteoporosis). Brand names include Premarin, Estratab, and Estinyl.

How to take estrogen

Estrogen comes in the form of tablets, capsules, and vaginal cream. Follow your primary health care provider's instructions exactly. For best results, take your medication at the same time each day.

If you take *tablets,* take them with food if you develop nausea.

If you're using the *vaginal cream,* your primary health care provider may want you to apply it at bedtime so it will be absorbed better. If you're not using it at bedtime, lie down for 30 minutes after use.

What to do if you miss a dose

If you miss a *tablet,* take it as soon as possible. If it's almost time for your next dose, skip the missed dose and take your next dose on schedule. Don't double dose.

If you forget to apply a dose of *vaginal cream* and don't remember until the next day, skip the missed dose. Go back to your regular dosing schedule.

What to do about side effects

Blood clots are a rare but serious complication. Call for emergency help *immediately* if you have any of these symptoms: sudden or severe headache; sudden loss of coordination; vision changes, such as loss of sight, blurred vision, or seeing flashing lights; numbness or stiffness in your legs; pain in your chest, groin, or legs; or shortness of breath.

Call your primary health care provider *right away* if you experience rapid weight gain; breast swelling, pain, or lumps; or unusual vaginal bleeding. If you're using the vaginal cream, call your primary health care provider if you develop swelling, redness, or itching in the vaginal area.

Check with your health care provider if you feel nauseated, lose your appetite, or your stomach becomes cramped or bloated.

What you must know about other drugs

Because many medications can interfere with estrogen therapy, make sure your primary health care provider is aware of all other medications (both nonprescription and prescription) that you're taking.

Special directions

• Tell your health care provider about other medical problems you have, especially breast disease, cancer, diabetes, high blood pressure, porphyria, gynecologic problems, or diseases of the major organs. Mention if you've ever had blood clots or a stroke. Tell him if you have female relatives who've had cancer of the breast or female organs.
• Keep all appointments for follow-up care so your health care provider can check your progress and detect side effects early.
• Perform monthly breast self-examinations and report unusual changes.

✓ Keep in mind

• If you're pregnant or breast-feeding, don't use estrogen.
• If you have diabetes, estrogen could affect your glucose level. Check with your health care provider if you notice any changes.

Additional instructions

_____

_____

_____

Taking estrogen with progestin

Dear Patient,

Your primary health care provider has prescribed estrogen with progestin. Also known as an oral contraceptive or birth control pill, this medication prevents pregnancy by changing your body's hormonal balance. This medication comes in various brand names, including Ortho-Novum, Ovcon, or Triphasil.

How to take estrogen with progestin

The medication comes in variously colored tablets. The color indicates the tablet strength. Carefully read and follow the directions. Usually, you take a certain color tablet at the same time every day in the order the tablets are arranged in the container. Don't take a tablet out of order.

To prevent nausea, take the tablet with food or just after eating.

Based on your needs, your primary health care provider will prescribe a certain dosing schedule called a *one-phase, two-phase,* or *three-phase* schedule. Here is how each works.

One-phase schedules

If you're on a 20- or 21-day schedule, take a tablet of the same strength for 20 or 21 days.

If you're on a 28-day schedule, take one tablet for 21 days and a different color tablet (containing inactive ingredients) for 7 or 8 more days.

Two-phase schedules

If you're on a 21-day schedule, take a tablet of one strength (first color) for 10 days, then a different tablet (second color) for the next 11 days.

If you are on a 24-day schedule, take a tablet of one strength (first color) for 17 days, then a different tablet (second color) for the next 7 days.

If you're on a 28-day schedule, take a tablet of one strength (first color) for 10 days

of the cycle, a different tablet (second color) for the next 11 days, then a tablet with inactive ingredients (third color) for 7 days.

Three-phase schedules

If you're on a 21-day schedule, take a tablet in the order directed by your prescription. For example, you may take the first tablet (first color) for 6 or 7 days, a different tablet (second color) for the next 5 to 9 days, and another tablet (third color) for 5 to 10 days, for a total of 21 tablets.

If you're on a 28-day schedule, follow a 21-day schedule, then take a tablet with inactive ingredients (fourth color) for the next 7 days, for a total of 28 tablets.

What to do if you miss a dose

If you forget to take your medication, consult your primary health care provider and review the following guide.

One-phase and two-phase schedules

If you're on a 20-, 21-, or 24-day one-phase or two-phase schedule and you miss one dose, take it when you remember. If you don't remember until the next day, take the missed dose and your scheduled dose; you can take two tablets on the same day. Then resume your normal schedule.

If you miss two doses in a row, take two tablets a day for the next 2 days, then resume your normal schedule. Use another birth control method to protect you for the rest of your cycle, and consult your primary health care provider.

If you miss three or more doses in a row, stop taking the tablets, and use another birth control method until you have your period or the primary health care provider tells you that you're not pregnant. Resume your normal schedule with the next cycle.

If you're on a 28-day cycle and you miss any of the first 21 tablets (which contain active ingredients), follow the instructions for

(continued)

Taking estrogen with progestin (continued)

the 21-day schedule and the number of doses you missed.

Three-phase schedules

If you're on a three-phase schedule and miss a dose during the 21-day period, take the missed tablet when you remember. If you don't remember until the next day, take the missed dose and the regular dose for that day. In this case, you can take two doses in the same day; then resume your regular schedule. Use another birth control method for the rest of your cycle, and consult your primary health care provider.

If you miss two doses in a row, take two doses for the next 2 days, then resume your normal schedule. Use another birth control method, and call your health care provider.

If you miss three doses in a row, don't take any tablets. Instead, use another birth control method until you have your period or your primary health care provider confirms that you're not pregnant. Resume your normal schedule as directed.

If you're on a 28-day cycle and you miss any of the first 21 tablets, follow the directions for the 21-day schedule, depending on how many doses you missed. Pregnancy isn't a risk if you miss any of the last seven tablets. But you must take the first tablet of the next month's cycle on your regularly scheduled day to prevent pregnancy.

What to do about side effects

Seek *emergency* care if you cough up blood or experience sudden shortness of breath, severe headache, vision changes, slurred speech, unexplained weakness in your arms or legs, or stomach, chest, groin, or leg pain.

Vaginal bleeding (spotting) may occur between your regular menstrual periods during the first 3 months of use but will lessen with continued use. Call your primary health care provider if spotting continues.

What you must know about other drugs

Certain drugs may decrease the effectiveness of this medication. Tell your primary health care provider and pharmacist what other prescription and nonprescription drugs you're taking.

Special directions

- You may need to take this medication for about 1 month before it works effectively. During this time, you may need to use an additional birth control method.
- Before having any dental work or surgery, tell the dentist or primary health care provider that you're taking this medication.

Warning: Smoking cigarettes while taking oral contraceptives greatly increases the chance of serious side effects.

Keep in mind

- If you become pregnant, stop taking this medication at once and notify your primary health care provider. Also consult your primary health care provider if you're breastfeeding.

Additional instructions

_____
_____
_____
_____
_____
_____
_____
_____
_____
_____
_____

Taking ethambutol

Dear Patient,

Your primary health care provider has prescribed ethambutol to treat your tuberculosis (TB). The medication label may read Myambutol.

How to take ethambutol

This medication comes in tablet form. Take it exactly as your primary health care provider directs. Take it at the same time each day to help you remember not to miss a dose. If the medication upsets your stomach, you can take it with food.

Keep taking ethambutol as your primary health care provider directs, even after you feel better. Otherwise, your TB may not clear up completely. Keep in mind that you may need to take it for 1 year or more.

What to do if you miss a dose

Take a missed dose as soon as you remember unless it's almost time for your next regular dose. If so, skip the missed dose and take your next dose on schedule. Don't take a double dose.

What to do about side effects

Call your primary health care provider *immediately* if you experience blurred vision; blindness; eye pain; trouble differentiating between red and green; chills or fever; pain or swelling in your joints (especially in your feet); burning, numbness, tingling, or weakness in your hands or feet; or if you cough up mucus tinged with blood.

Other possible side effects, such as an upset stomach, diarrhea, loss of appetite, severe fatigue, dizziness, itching, and rashes, may go away as your body adjusts to ethambutol. However, discuss them with your primary health care provider if they persist or become severe.

What you must know about other drugs

Don't take ethambutol within 2 hours of taking aluminum-containing antacids, such as Amphojel or AlternaGEL.

Special directions

• Before taking ethambutol, tell your primary health care provider if you have optic neuritis (eye nerve damage), cataracts, recurrent eye infections, or vision problems related to diabetes, gout, or kidney disease. Ethambutol may aggravate these conditions.
• Your primary health care provider may require you to have regular blood tests to check for certain disorders, such as gout.
• Your primary health care provider may ask you to schedule regular eye examinations while you're taking ethambutol.
• Until you know how your body responds to ethambutol, don't drive or perform activities requiring alertness and clear vision.
• Notify your primary health care provider if your symptoms don't disappear or if you feel worse after 2 to 3 weeks of ethambutol therapy.

✔ Keep in mind

• If you're breast-feeding, check with your primary health care provider before taking this medication.
• Ethambutol isn't recommended for children under age 13.

Additional instructions

_____
_____
_____
_____
_____
_____

Taking etodolac

Dear Patient,

Your primary health care provider has prescribed etodolac to treat your arthritis. This medication relieves joint swelling, pain, and stiffness. The label may read Lodine.

How to take etodolac

Etodolac comes in tablets and capsules. Follow your primary health care provider's instructions exactly. Take the medication with an 8-ounce glass of water and with food or an antacid to lessen stomach upset. Afterward, don't lie down for 15 to 30 minutes to prevent irritation to your esophagus (food tube).

If you're taking the extended release tablets, swallow them whole — don't crush, break, or chew them

It may take several weeks before you start to feel better.

What to do if you miss a dose

If you remember the missed dose within 1 or 2 hours, take it as soon as possible. Otherwise, skip the missed dose and take your next dose on schedule. Don't take two doses at the same time.

What to do about side effects

Occasionally, etodolac can cause serious bleeding from the digestive tract. Call your primary health care provider *at once* if you have any of these warning signs: black, tarry stools; severe stomach pain, severe, continuing nausea or heartburn; or vomiting of blood or material that looks like coffee grounds.

Etodolac can also cause nausea, heartburn, drowsiness, dizziness, and increased light sensitivity. Let your primary health care provider know if these symptoms continue or become bothersome.

What you must know about other drugs

Tell your primary health care provider if you're taking other medications. If you're taking lithium, cyclosporine, or phenytoin, he may need to adjust your dose of these medications. If you're taking corticosteroids, loop diuretics, or oral anticoagulants, he'll need to monitor you closely for potential problems.

The chance of serious side effects is increased if etodolac is used with aspirin or blood thinners.

Special directions

• Tell your primary health care provider if you have other medical problems, such as stomach ulcers or other digestive disorders, or diabetes, heart, kidney, or liver disease.
• Notify your primary health care provider if you've had any unusual reactions to aspirin or other medications.
• If etodolac makes you dizzy or drowsy, don't drive or perform other tasks that require alertness.

✓ Keep in mind

• If you're pregnant or breast-feeding, check with your primary health care provider before using this medication.

Additional instructions

_____

Taking eye medications

Dear Patient,

Your primary health care provider has prescribed an eyedrop or an eye ointment for you. Eyedrops and eye ointments are used for diseases such as glaucoma, for eye infections and eye inflammation, and to restore moisture to dry eyes.

How to use eyedrops and eye ointment

When putting eyedrops or ointment into your eyes, don't touch the tip of the eye dropper or ointment tube with your hands, let the dropper or tube touch any other object, or touch the tube or dropper directly to your eye. Doing so can cause germs to grow in the solution and may cause an eye infection.

Because eye ointments can caused blurred vision, it's usually better to use them at bedtime, unless your primary health care provider instructs you otherwise, or unless you need to take more than one dose per day. If so, avoid activities that require clear vision such as driving a car.

If both eyedrops and eye ointments are prescribed for you, use the eyedrop medication at least 10 minutes before you use the ointment.

Continue using eyedrops and eye ointments for the entire time of treatment, even though you may not feel any different.

Unless your primary health care provider says otherwise, don't store eyedrops or eye ointment in the refrigerator. Store them at room temperature, away from heat, light and humidity.

Using eyedrops

To put drops in your eye, follow these steps:
• Wash your hands. Tilt your head back and pull your lower eyelid away from your eye to make a pouch for the medication. Drop the medication into this pouch.

• Let go of your eyelid and close your eyes carefully. Try not to blink.
• With your eyes closed, use your finger to apply gentle pressure to the inner corner of your eye for 1 to 2 minutes. This allows the medication to be absorbed better.
• Wash your hands again. If you're also taking other eyedrop medications, wait at least 10 minutes before using them.

Using eye ointments

To put ointment in your eye, follow these steps.
• Wash your hands. Tilt your head back and pull your lower eyelid away from your eye to make a pouch for the medication.
• Move the ointment container over your eye by looking straight at it. With a slow, sweeping motion, place ¼ to ½ inch of ointment inside the lower eyelid pouch.
• Gently let go of your lower eyelid and close your eye for 1 to 2 minutes. This allows the medication to be absorbed better.
• Gently blot extra ointment from around your eye. Wash your hands again.

What to do if you miss a dose

If you miss a dose of eyedrops or ointment, use the medication as soon as you remember. If it's almost time for the next scheduled dose, skip the missed dose and go back to your regular schedule. Don't use double doses.

What to do about side effects

The side effects of eyedrops and eye ointments depend on the particular medication. Call your primary health care provider *immediately* if you have pain, itching, redness, or swelling in the eye or blurred vision that lasts for a long time.

Some common side effects include eye dryness, brief burning or stinging, increased tear production, temporary blurred vision,

(continued)

Taking eye medications (continued)

headache, and light sensitivity. These problems often go away as your body adjusts to the medicine. Contact your primary health care provider if they continue or are bothersome.

What you must know about other drugs
Check with your primary health care provider before using any other type of eye medications, either prescription or nonprescription.

Special directions
• Tell your primary health care provider about your medical history, especially if you have heart, lung, liver, or kidney problems. Although the chances are slim that eyedrops or eye ointments will cause problems within the body, some of the medication may be absorbed into your bloodstream.

✔ Keep in mind
• If you're pregnant or breast-feeding, tell your primary health care provider before taking this medication.

Additional instructions

_____
_____
_____
_____
_____
_____
_____
_____
_____
_____
_____

Taking famotidine

Dear Patient,

This medication helps treat ulcers. It's also used to treat Zollinger-Ellison disease, in which the stomach produces too much acid. The medication label may read Pepcid.

How to take famotidine

This medication comes in tablets and powder for oral suspension. Carefully follow the directions on the label.

If you're taking this medication once a day, take it at bedtime unless your primary health care provider directs otherwise. If you're taking it twice a day, take one dose in the morning and one at bedtime. If you're taking it more than twice a day, take your doses with meals and at bedtime for best results.

Keep the liquid in the refrigerator, and discard it if it's older than 30 days.

What to do if you miss a dose

Take a missed dose as soon as possible. If it's almost time for your next regular dose, skip the missed dose and take your next dose on your regular schedule. Don't take a double dose.

What to do about side effects

If you have a headache (a common side effect) that persists or becomes severe, contact your primary health care provider.

What you must know about other drugs

Warning: If you smoke, stop smoking or at least try not to smoke after taking the last dose of this medication each day. Cigarette smoking decreases famotidine's effects, especially at night.

Special directions

● Tell your primary health care provider if you have other medical problems, especial-

ly kidney or liver disease, because certain disorders may affect the way famotidine works for you.

● This medication may not begin to relieve your stomach pain for several days. Unless your primary health care provider directs otherwise, you may also take antacids to help relieve the pain. However, wait 30 minutes to 1 hour after taking the antacid before taking famotidine.

● Tell your primary health care provider that you're taking famotidine before you undergo skin tests for allergies or tests to determine how much acid your stomach produces.

● Contact your primary health care provider if your ulcer pain continues or gets worse.

✔ Keep in mind

● If you're pregnant or breast-feeding, check with your primary health care provider before taking this medication.
● Older adults may be especially sensitive to famotidine's side effects.

Additional instructions

_____
_____
_____
_____
_____
_____
_____
_____
_____
_____
_____
_____

Taking fenoprofen

Dear Patient,

Fenoprofen helps relieve the inflammation, swelling, stiffness, and joint pain of rheumatoid arthritis or osteoarthritis. The label may read Nalfon.

How to take fenoprofen

Take the medication with food or an antacid and a full glass of water. Avoid lying down for 15 to 30 minutes after taking this medication. Doing so will help prevent swallowing problems.

What to do if you miss a dose

Take a missed dose as soon as you remember if it's within 2 hours of your regular time. If it's later than that, skip the missed dose and take your next dose at the regular time. Don't take two doses at once.

What to do about side effects

Serious side effects, including ulcers or bleeding, can occur with or without warning. As a result, you should stop taking fenoprofen and call your primary health care provider *right away* if you notice any of these warning signs: severe stomach cramps, pain, or burning; severe, continuing nausea, heartburn, or indigestion; or vomit tinged with blood or material that looks like coffee grounds.

You may experience dizziness, headache, drowsiness, heartburn, nausea, vomiting, itching, and black, tarry stools while taking fenoprofen. If these symptoms persist or become severe, call your primary health care provider.

What you must know about alcohol and other drugs

Avoid alcoholic beverages; they increase your risk of stomach problems.

Also, don't take aspirin or acetaminophen (Tylenol) with fenoprofen for more than a few days (unless your primary health care provider directs otherwise) because this may increase your risk of serious side effects.

Because some other drugs interfere with fenoprofen's effects, be sure to tell your primary health care provider about other medications you're taking, particularly anticoagulants (blood thinners) and sulfonylureas (drugs for diabetes).

Special directions

• If you have other medical problems, let your primary health care provider know. They may affect the use of this medication.
• Know how you react to fenoprofen before driving or performing other activities that require alertness.
• Fenoprofen makes you more sensitive to sunlight than normal, so wear a hat and sunglasses and use a sunblock outdoors.

✔ Keep in mind

• If you're pregnant or breast-feeding, consult your primary health care provider about taking fenoprofen.
• If you're an older adult, you may be especially prone to side effects.

Additional instructions

_____
_____
_____
_____
_____
_____
_____
_____
_____

Applying a fentanyl patch

Dear Patient,

Your primary health care provider has prescribed the fentanyl transdermal patch to help relieve your pain. The label may read Duragesic-25, Duragesic-50, Duragesic-75, or Duragesic-100.

How to apply a fentanyl patch

Apply a new patch to a new site every 72 hours or as ordered by your primary health care provider. First, clip excess hair at the patch site. Don't use a razor because shaving may irritate or scratch your skin.

Wash your skin with clear water if necessary, but don't use soap, oil, lotion, alcohol, or any other substance that may irritate your skin or interfere with the patch's stickiness.

Make sure your skin is completely dry. Then put the patch on your skin and hold it in place for 10 to 20 seconds to make sure it stays on.

What to do if you miss an application

If you don't apply a new patch when scheduled, do so as soon as you can. But don't apply more than one patch at a time — this may cause serious side effects.

What to do about side effects

Seek medical care *at once* if you have trouble breathing.

Fentanyl also may make you feel drowsy and lethargic. It may lower your blood pressure, causing you to feel dizzy or light-headed. You may also experience constipation and problems with urination. If these side effects persist or become severe, contact your primary health care provider.

What you must know about alcohol and other drugs

Don't drink alcoholic beverages or take medications that affect your nervous system (such as many allergy or cold medications, narcotics, muscle relaxants, sleeping pills, and seizure medications). Combined with fentanyl, these medications may produce serious side effects.

Special directions

• Before taking fentanyl, inform your primary health care provider of other medical problems you have. They may affect the use of this medication.

! *Warning:* Don't stop taking fentanyl suddenly. Doing so may cause undesirable withdrawal effects. Consult your primary health care provider, who may reduce your dosage gradually before stopping the medication completely.

• Don't drive or perform activities requiring alertness until you know how fentanyl affects you.

• Dispose of used patches by folding them in half with the sticky sides together and flushing them down the toilet.

✓ Keep in mind

• If you're breast-feeding, consult your primary health care provider before taking fentanyl.

• Young children and older adults are especially sensitive to fentanyl.

• If you're an athlete, you should know that the U.S. Olympic Committee tests for and bans fentanyl's use.

Additional instructions

_____
_____
_____
_____
_____

Taking finasteride

Dear Patient,

Your primary health care provider has prescribed finasteride to treat your enlarged prostate and improve your urine flow. This medication blocks an enzyme that causes the prostate to grow. It's also used to treat male pattern baldness. The brand name on the label may read Proscar or Propecia.

How to take finasteride
This medication comes in tablets, which may be crushed if they're difficult to swallow. Follow your primary health care provider's orders or the directions on the label exactly. Don't stop taking this medication without first talking with your primary health care provider.

What to do if you miss a dose
Take the dose as soon as possible. However, if it's almost time for your next dose, skip the missed dose and go back to your regular dosing schedule. Don't take double doses.

What to do about side effects
Call your primary health care provider if you have a decreased interest in sex, a decreased amount of semen, the inability to have or keep an erection, or any other effects.

What you must know about alcohol and other drugs
Because finasteride improves your urine flow, avoid drinking alcohol in the evening so that your sleep won't be disturbed by having to urinate during the night.
   Tell your primary health care provider about other medications you're taking, especially theophylline. Also, don't take nonprescription medications for appetite control, asthma, colds, cough, hay fever, or si-

nus problems without first discussing it with your primary health care provider.

Special directions
• You may have to take this medication for more than 6 months before you notice an improvement in urine flow.
• Tell your primary health care provider about other medical problems you have, especially liver disease.

✔ Keep in mind
! *Warning:* Pregnant women and women of childbearing age shouldn't handle or crush the tablets because finasteride may be absorbed into the body and harm a fetus. If you're taking finasteride, wear a condom during sex to prevent semen from coming into contact with a female partner.

Additional instructions
_____
_____
_____
_____
_____
_____
_____
_____
_____
_____
_____
_____

Taking flecainide

Dear Patient,

Your primary health care provider has prescribed flecainide to help stabilize your heart rhythm. The label on your medication may read Tambocor.

How to take flecainide
This medication comes in tablet form. Take two daily doses 12 hours apart in the morning and evening unless your primary health care provider orders otherwise.

What to do if you miss a dose
Take a missed dose of flecainide as soon as you remember if it's within 6 hours of your regularly scheduled time. If it's later than that, skip the missed dose and resume your normal dosing schedule. Don't double dose.

What to do about side effects
Seek medical treatment *right away* if you experience any of these side effects: chest pain, irregular heartbeat, shortness of breath, swelling in your feet or lower legs, and trembling or shaking.

Flecainide may also cause dizziness, headache, and vision problems. If these symptoms persist or become severe, consult your primary health care provider.

What you must know about other drugs
Tell your primary health care provider if you're taking other drugs; particularly other heart medications. These may produce unpredictable effects when taken with flecainide.

Special directions
• Before taking flecainide, tell your primary health care provider about other medical problems you have, especially kidney or liver disease, a recent heart attack, or a pacemaker.

• See your primary health care provider regularly so he can check your progress and adjust your dosage as needed.
• Carry medical identification with you or wear a medical identification bracelet stating that you're taking flecainide.
• Before you undergo a dental or surgical procedure or emergency treatment, tell the dentist or primary health care provider that you're taking flecainide.
• Because flecainide may make you feel dizzy, light-headed, or sluggish, don't drive a car or perform activities requiring alertness until you know how this medication affects you.
• If you've been taking this medication regularly for several weeks, don't suddenly stop taking it. Check with your primary health care provider, who can help you reduce the dosage gradually.

✓ Keep in mind
• If you're pregnant or breast-feeding, check with your primary health care provider before taking flecainide.
• Older adults may be especially susceptible to flecainide's side effects.

Additional instructions

_____

Taking fluconazole

Dear Patient,

Your primary health care provider has prescribed fluconazole to treat your fungal infection. Your prescription label may read Diflucan.

How to take fluconazole

Take fluconazole exactly as prescribed. To help clear up your infection completely, take it for the full course of treatment even if your symptoms subside. A fungal infection may require many months of treatment even after your symptoms are no longer bothersome.

What to do if you miss a dose

Take a missed dose of medication as soon as you remember. If it's almost time for your next dose, skip the missed dose and take your next dose as scheduled. Don't double dose.

What to do about side effects

Fluconazole causes nausea in some people. If you experience persistent or severe nausea, contact your primary health care provider.

What you must know about other drugs

Combined with other medications, fluconazole may produce unwanted side effects. Be sure to tell your primary health care provider about all the medications you take, especially cisapride (Propulsid), cyclosporine (Sandimmune), phenytoin (Dilantin), isoniazid (Laniazid), rifampin (Rifadin), valproic acid (Depakene), warfarin (Coumadin), astemizole (Hismanal), oral contraceptives, and some oral medications used to lower blood glucose levels.

Special directions

- Before taking fluconazole, tell your primary health care provider about other medical problems you have, especially kidney or liver disease. They may affect the use of this medication.
- See your primary health care provider regularly so he can monitor your progress and check for unwanted effects.
- Check with your primary health care provider if your symptoms don't disappear within a few weeks or if you feel worse.

✔ Keep in mind

- If you're pregnant or breast-feeding, check with your primary health care provider before taking fluconazole.

Additional instructions

_____
_____
_____
_____
_____
_____
_____
_____
_____
_____

Applying fluocinolone

Dear Patient,

Your primary health care provider has prescribed fluocinolone cream, ointment, or solution to help relieve redness, swelling, itching, and other skin discomfort. The label may read Fluonid or Synalar.

How to apply fluocinolone

Follow your primary health care provider's directions exactly to apply fluocinolone. Use your finger to apply it to your skin. Then wash your hands. Don't bandage or wrap the area being treated unless your primary health care provider directs you to do so.

What to do if you miss a dose

If you miss a dose of this medication, apply it as soon as possible. But if it's almost time for your next dose, skip the missed dose and apply the next dose on your regular schedule.

What to do about side effects

Although side effects from using fluocinolone are uncommon, the medication may produce such skin reactions as burning, itching, dryness, changes in color or texture, or a rash and inflammation (dermatitis). Consult your primary health care provider if you have these side effects.

What you must know about other drugs

If using antifungal agents or antibiotics, stop taking fluocinolone until the infection is under control. After that time, you may resume taking this drug.

Special directions

● If you have other medical problems, be sure to let your primary health care provider know. A change in your medication may be necessary.

❗ *Warning:* Don't get fluocinolone in your eyes. If you do, flush your eyes with water.

● If your primary health care provider tells you to apply an occlusive dressing (an airtight covering, such as plastic wrap or a special patch) over fluocinolone, be sure to get complete directions for doing so.

● Don't use leftover medication for other skin problems without first consulting your primary health care provider.

● If you're applying fluocinolone to a child's diaper area, avoid using tight-fitting diapers or plastic pants, which could increase absorption of the medication through the skin and possibly cause side effects.

✔ Keep in mind

● If you become pregnant while using fluocinolone, consult your primary health care provider.

● Don't apply this medication to your breasts before breast-feeding.

● Children and adolescents using this medication should be checked closely. Fluocinolone can affect growth and cause other unwanted effects.

● Older adults may be especially susceptible to certain side effects, such as skin tearing and blood blisters.

Additional instructions

_____
_____
_____
_____
_____
_____
_____
_____

Applying fluocinonide

Dear Patient,

Your primary health care provider has prescribed fluocinonide to help relieve redness, swelling, itching, and other skin discomfort. The prescription label may read Lidex or Lidex-E.

How to apply fluocinonide

This medication comes in cream, ointment, gel, and solution forms. Apply it exactly as your primary health care provider directs. Wash your hands after using your finger to apply it. Don't bandage or wrap the skin being treated unless your primary health care provider directs you to do so.

What to do if you miss a dose

Apply a missed dose as soon as possible. If it's almost time for your next dose, skip the missed dose and apply the next dose on schedule.

What to do about side effects

Although side effects are uncommon, fluocinonide can cause such skin reactions as burning, itching, dryness, changes in color or texture, or a rash and inflammation (dermatitis). Tell your primary health care provider if such effects occur.

What you should know about other drugs

If using antifungal agents or antibiotics, stop taking fluocinonide until the infection is under control. After that time, you may resume taking this drug.

Special directions

• If you have other medical problems, be sure to let your primary health care provider know. They may affect the use of this medication.

Warning: Don't get fluocinonide in your eyes. If you do, flush your eyes with water.

• If your primary health care provider instructs you to use an occlusive dressing (an airtight covering, such as plastic wrap or a special patch) over fluocinonide, make sure you understand how to apply it.
• Don't use leftover medication for other skin problems without first consulting your primary health care provider.
• If you're applying fluocinonide to a child's diaper area, avoid using tight-fitting diapers or plastic pants. They may cause unwanted side effects.

Keep in mind

• Consult your primary health care provider if you become pregnant while using fluocinonide.
• Don't apply this medication to your breasts before breast-feeding.
• Children and adolescents who use fluocinonide should have frequent medical check-ups because this medication can affect growth and cause other unwanted effects.
• Older adults may be especially susceptible to certain side effects, such as skin tearing and blood blisters.

Additional instructions

_____
_____
_____
_____
_____
_____
_____
_____

Taking fluoxetine

Dear Patient,

This medication is prescribed to help relieve depression. The label may read Prozac.

How to take fluoxetine
Take fluoxetine exactly as prescribed. You may need to take it for 4 weeks or longer before you begin to feel better.

What to do if you miss a dose
Skip a missed dose and take your next regular dose as scheduled. Don't double dose.

What to do about side effects
If you develop a rash or hives, stop taking this medication and call your primary health care provider *immediately*— you may be having an allergic reaction.

This medication may cause nervousness, anxiety, insomnia, headache, drowsiness, shakiness, dizziness, nausea, diarrhea, dry mouth, loss of appetite, stomach upset, weight loss, itching, and weakness. If you have any of these symptoms and they persist or worsen, contact your primary health care provider.

What you must know about alcohol and other drugs
Avoid drinking alcoholic beverages while taking fluoxetine. Also avoid taking other medications that affect the nervous system (such as cough, cold, and allergy medications; narcotics; muscle relaxants; sleeping pills; and seizure medications).

Warning: Tell your primary health care provider about other medications you're taking. For example, taking fluoxetine with diazepam (Valium), warfarin (Coumadin), or monoamine oxidase (MAO) inhibitors may cause serious side effects.

Special directions
● Before taking fluoxetine, tell your primary health care provider if you have other medical problems, especially diabetes, kidney or liver disease, or a seizure disorder.
● Schedule regular checkups so your primary health care provider can monitor your progress, check for side effects, and adjust your dosage as needed.
● Because fluoxetine may cause drowsiness, don't drive or perform activities requiring alertness until you know how the medication affects you.
● If you feel dizzy, light-headed, or faint when getting up from a bed or chair, rise slowly. If the problem persists or worsens, consult your primary health care provider.
● To relieve a dry mouth, use sugarless gum, hard candy, ice chips, or a saliva substitute. Dryness that persists for longer than 2 weeks increases your chance for dental problems. Consult your primary health care provider or dentist.
● Avoid prolonged exposure to sunlight.

✓ Keep in mind
● If you have diabetes, fluoxetine may affect your glucose levels. Report changes in your home blood or urine glucose tests to your primary health care provider.
● If you're breast-feeding, check with your primary health care provider before taking fluoxetine.

Additional instructions

_____

_____

_____

_____

_____

_____

Taking fluphenazine

Dear Patient,

Fluphenazine is prescribed to treat emotional problems. The label may read Permitil or Prolixin.

How to take fluphenazine

Take fluphenazine exactly as your primary health care provider directs. You may take it with food or a full glass (8 ounces) of water or milk to minimize possible stomach upset.

If your medication comes in a dropper bottle, measure each dose with the special dropper. Dilute the medication in one-half glass (4 ounces) of orange juice, grapefruit juice, or water. Avoid spilling liquid medication on your skin because it may cause irritation and a rash.

What to do if you miss a dose

If you take one dose a day and miss the dose, take it as soon as possible. Then take your next dose at the regular time. If you don't remember the missed dose until the next day, skip it and take your next dose.

If you take more than one dose a day and miss a dose, take the missed dose as soon as you remember if it's within an hour or so of the scheduled time. If you don't remember until later, skip the missed dose and take your next dose as scheduled. Don't double dose.

What to do about side effects

Contact your primary health care provider *immediately* if you learn that your blood count is abnormal or if you develop an infection or fever, rapid heartbeat, rapid breathing, and profuse sweating.

Also call your health care provider *immediately* if you develop uncontrollable lip smacking, mouth puckering, cheek puffing, worm-like tongue movements, chewing motions, and arm or leg movements.

Fluphenazine may cause dizziness, light-headedness, or faintness when arising; blurred vision, dry mouth, constipation, urine retention, and sensitivity to sunlight. Contact your health care provider if these side effects are persistent or bothersome.

What you must know about alcohol and other drugs

Avoid alcoholic beverages and other medications that affect your nervous system. Tell your primary health care provider about all other prescription and nonprescription medications you're taking. They may interact with fluphenazine and cause problems.

Special directions

• Before taking fluphenazine, tell your primary health care provider about other medical problems you have.
• Know how you react to fluphenazine before driving or performing activities requiring alertness and clear vision.
• Relieve a dry mouth with sugarless candy or gum, ice chips, or a saliva substitute.
• Avoid exposure to direct sunlight.

✔ Keep in mind

• If you're pregnant or breast-feeding, check with your primary health care provider before taking this medication.
• Children and older adults are especially sensitive to this medication.
• If you're an athlete, be aware that the National Collegiate Athletic Association and the U.S. Olympic Committee ban the use of fluphenazine.

Additional instructions

_____

_____

Applying flurandrenolide

Dear Patient,

Your primary health care provider has prescribed flurandrenolide to help relieve redness, swelling, itching, and other skin discomfort. Your prescription label may read Cordran.

How to apply flurandrenolide

This medication is available as cream, lotion, ointment, and tape. Carefully check the medication directions. Apply flurandrenolide exactly as prescribed. Wash your hands after using your finger to apply it. Don't bandage or wrap the skin being treated unless your primary health care provider directs you to do so.

What to do if you miss a dose

Apply a missed dose as soon as possible. If it's almost time for your next dose, skip the missed dose and apply the next dose.

What to do about side effects

Although side effects are uncommon, flurandrenolide can cause such skin reactions as burning, itching, dryness, changes in color or texture, or a rash and inflammation (dermatitis). Tell your primary health care provider if these effects occur.

What you must know about other drugs

If using antifungal agents or antibiotics, stop taking flurandrenolide until the infection is under control. After that time, you may resume taking this drug.

Special directions

• If you have other medical problems, let your primary health care provider know. They may affect the use of this medication.

Warning: Don't get flurandrenolide in your eyes. If you do, flush your eyes with water.

• If your primary health care provider orders an occlusive dressing (an airtight covering, such as plastic wrap or a special patch) to be applied over this medication, make sure you understand how to apply it.
• Don't use leftover medication for other skin problems without first checking with your primary health care provider.
• If you're applying flurandrenolide to a child's diaper area, avoid using tight-fitting diapers or plastic pants. They could cause unwanted side effects.

✔ Keep in mind

• Consult your primary health care provider if you become pregnant while using flurandrenolide.
• Don't apply this medication to your breasts before breast-feeding.
• Children and adolescents using this medication should have frequent medical checkups because this medication can affect growth and cause other unwanted effects.
• If you're an older adult, you may be especially susceptible to certain side effects, such as skin tearing and blood blisters.

Additional instructions

_____
_____
_____
_____
_____
_____
_____
_____
_____
_____
_____
_____

Taking flurazepam

Dear Patient,

Your primary health care provider has prescribed flurazepam to help you sleep. Your medication label may read Dalmane.

How to take flurazepam

Take flurazepam capsules exactly as directed. Don't increase your dose because overuse may lead to mental or physical dependence.

What to do if you miss a dose

Take a missed dose as soon as you remember if it's within 1 hour of the scheduled time. If it's later than that, skip the missed dose and take your next dose as scheduled. Don't double dose.

What to do about side effects

If you think you may have taken an overdose, seek emergency help *at once*. Overdose symptoms include continuing slurred speech or confusion, severe drowsiness, and staggering.

Flurazepam may cause drowsiness, dizziness, headache, and poor coordination. If these symptoms persist or become severe, consult your primary health care provider.

What you must know about alcohol and other drugs

Avoid alcoholic beverages, cimetidine (Tagamet), and medications that depress the nervous system (such as many allergy and cold remedies, narcotics, muscle relaxants, sleeping pills, and seizure medications). The combination of flurazepam and these medications may cause excessive drowsiness.

Special directions

• Tell your primary health care provider about other medical problems you have.

They may affect the use of this medication.
• See your primary health care provider regularly to monitor your progress and check for side effects.
• Because flurazepam can affect some diagnostic test results, tell the primary health care provider that you're taking this medication before you undergo tests.
• Before you have dental work that requires an anesthetic, tell the dentist you're taking flurazepam.
• Don't drive, operate hazardous machinery, or perform activities requiring alertness until you know how the medication affects you.

Warning: Don't stop taking flurazepam suddenly; doing so may cause unpleasant withdrawal symptoms. Consult your primary health care provider about gradually reducing your dosage before stopping the medication completely.

✔ Keep in mind

• If you're pregnant or breast-feeding, consult your primary health care provider before taking this medication.
• Children and older adults are especially prone to flurazepam's side effects.
• If you're an athlete, be aware that the National Collegiate Athletic Association and the U.S. Olympic Committee ban the use of flurazepam.

Additional instructions

_____
_____
_____
_____
_____
_____
_____
_____
_____

Taking flurbiprofen

Dear Patient,

Your primary health care provider has prescribed flurbiprofen to relieve the inflammation, swelling, stiffness, and joint pain of arthritis. The label may read Ansaid.

How to take flurbiprofen
Take your medication exactly as directed. Take flurbiprofen tablets with food or an antacid and a full glass (8 ounces) of water. To prevent possible swallowing problems, don't lay down for 15 to 30 minutes after taking it.

What to do if you miss a dose
Take a missed dose as soon as you remember if it's within 1 to 2 hours of the scheduled time. If it's later than that, skip the missed dose and take your next regularly scheduled dose. Don't double dose.

What to do about side effects
Sometimes serious side effects, including ulcers and bleeding, may occur with or without warning. Stop taking flurbiprofen and seek medical attention *at once* if you experience severe abdominal cramps, pain, or burning; have severe, continuing nausea, heartburn, or indigestion; or vomit blood or material that looks like coffee grounds.

Flurbiprofen may also cause headaches, fluid retention, heartburn, nausea, diarrhea, stomach pain, burning and frequent urination, drowsiness, and dark, tarry stools. If these symptoms persist or become severe, tell your primary health care provider.

What you must know about alcohol and other drugs
Don't drink alcoholic beverages while taking flurbiprofen; stomach problems are more likely to occur. Don't take acetaminophen (Tylenol), aspirin, or another salicylate together with flurbiprofen for more than a few days because this increases your risk for unwanted effects. Aspirin may decrease flurbiprofen's effectiveness.

Taking flurbiprofen with anticoagulants (blood thinners) may increase your risk for bleeding. Diuretics (water pills) may be less effective with flurbiprofen.

Special directions
• Tell your primary health care provider about other medical problems you have. They may affect the use of this medication.
• Schedule regular medical checkups so your primary health care provider can monitor your progress and check for unwanted side effects.
• Before undergoing a dental or surgical procedure, tell the dentist or primary health care provider that you're taking flurbiprofen.
• Don't drive or perform activities requiring alertness until you know how you react to flurbiprofen.
• Protect yourself from excessive sun.

✔ Keep in mind
• Consult your primary health care provider if you're breast-feeding or become pregnant while taking flurbiprofen.
• Older adults may be especially prone to side effects from flurbiprofen.

Additional instructions
_____
_____
_____
_____
_____
_____
_____
_____

Taking flutamide

Dear Patient,

Your primary health care provider has prescribed flutamide to treat prostate cancer. The label may read Eulexin.

How to take flutamide

Take flutamide exactly as directed. Continue taking it for the full course of treatment, even after you begin to feel better. Don't stop taking the medication without first talking to your primary health care provider.

When you take flutamide, you usually take other medications also. If you do, follow your primary health care provider's instructions on their use.

What to do if you miss a dose

Take a missed dose of flutamide as soon as possible. If it's almost time for your next dose, skip the missed dose and take your next dose as scheduled. Don't double dose.

What to do about side effects

Flutamide may diminish your sexual desire and ability. It can also cause diarrhea, nausea, vomiting, and hot flashes. If these symptoms persist or become severe, call your primary health care provider.

What you must know about other drugs

Check with your primary health care provider before taking other medications.

Special directions

● If you vomit shortly after taking a dose of this medication, check with your primary health care provider. He may tell you to take the dose again or to wait until the next scheduled dose.
● Schedule regular medical checkups so your primary health care provider can monitor your progress.

✔ Keep in mind

● If you want to have children, talk to your primary health care provider because flutamide lowers your sperm count. Flutamide is used with leuprolide acetate, which also causes sterility that may be permanent.

Additional instructions

_____
_____
_____
_____
_____
_____
_____
_____
_____
_____
_____

Taking fluvastatin

Dear Patient,

Your primary health care provider has prescribed fluvastatin to lower your blood cholesterol. This medication may help prevent medical problems caused by cholesterol clogging your blood vessels. The label may read Lescol.

How to take fluvastatin
Fluvastatin comes in capsules. Take the medication at bedtime to enhance its effectiveness. Follow you primary health care provider's instructions exactly, and also follow the special diet he gives you.

What to do if you miss a dose
Take a missed dose as soon as possible. If it's almost time for your next dose, skip the missed dose and take your next dose on schedule. Don't double dose.

What to do about side effects
Report muscle aches or cramps, fever, severe stomach pain, or unusual tiredness or weakness to your primary health care provider *right away.*

Other side effects include constipation, diarrhea, gas, headache, and heartburn. Check with your primary health care provider if these become bothersome.

What you must know about alcohol and other drugs
Drinking alcohol during fluvastatin treatment can increase your risk of liver problems. Discuss your alcohol consumption with your primary health care provider.

Tell your primary health care provider and pharmacist what other medications you're taking, including those you take without a prescription or buy at a health food store.

Certain drugs, when taken with fluvastatin, can increase the risk of serious muscle side effects. These drugs include erythromycin, gemfibrozil, niacin, and cyclosporine and other drugs used to suppress the immune system. When warfarin, a blood thinner, is taken with fluvastatin, warfarin's effects may be increased. As a result, you may need frequent blood tests to monitor your blood levels.

Special directions
● Tell your primary health care provider if you have special medical problems, especially liver or kidney disease or seizures. Also report if you have received an organ transplant.

✓ Keep in mind
● If you're breast-feeding or planning on becoming pregnant, don't take fluvastatin.

Additional instructions

_____
_____
_____
_____
_____
_____
_____
_____
_____
_____
_____

Taking folic acid

Dear Patient,

Your primary health care provider has instructed you to take folic acid, a B vitamin, to help prevent or treat anemia. The label may read Folvite.

How to take folic acid
Follow your primary health care provider's instructions exactly. Don't take more than he prescribes.

What to do if you miss a dose
Although you should try to remember to take folic acid every day, don't worry if you forget to take it, even for a few days. Don't make up missed doses, and never increase your dosage.

What to do about side effects
If you experience wheezing and difficulty breathing, stop taking folic acid and call your primary health care provider *immediately.*

What you must know about other drugs
Be aware that phenytoin (Dilantin), a medication given for seizures, may decrease folic acid's effects.

Special directions
• Tell your primary health care provider about other medical problems you have, especially a blood disorder known as pernicious anemia. Taking folic acid while you have pernicious anemia may cause serious side effects.
• Eat plenty of foods high in folic acid content. Such foods include green vegetables, potatoes, fruits, grains, and organ meats. Eat fresh foods when possible; cooking may reduce a food's folic acid content.

✔ Keep in mind
• If you're pregnant or breast-feeding, ask your primary health care provider whether you should continue taking folic acid.

Additional instructions

_____

Taking fosinopril

Dear Patient,

Your primary health care provider has prescribed fosinopril to treat your high blood pressure. It may also be used to treat heart failure and kidney problems. This medication blocks production of a substance that causes blood vessels to tighten. The label may read Monopril.

How to take fosinopril

Follow your primary health care provider's directions for using fosinopril exactly. This medication comes in tablet form. Be sure to take it daily, even if you feel well. Remember that fosinopril isn't a cure for high blood pressure; it just helps control it. So you may have to take this medication for the rest of your life.

What to do if you miss a dose

Take a missed dose as soon as possible. However, if it's almost time for your next dose, skip the missed dose and go back to your regular schedule. Don't double dose.

What to do about side effects

Check with your primary health care provider *immediately* if you experience fever or chills; swelling in the face, feet or hands; trouble swallowing or breathing; yellow skin or eyes; itching skin; or stomach pain.

Check with your primary health care provider as soon as possible if you experience dizziness, light-headedness or fainting, joint pain, nausea, vomiting, or a continuing dry cough that becomes bothersome.

What you must know about alcohol and other drugs

Talk to your primary health care provider about drinking alcoholic beverages because the combined effects of alcohol and fosinopril may lower your blood pressure too much and cause drowsiness. Report other medications you're taking, especially lithium, diuretics (water pills), potassium supplements, or salt substitutes.

Take antacids 2 hours before or 2 hours after taking fosinopril.

Special directions

- Tell your primary health care provider about other medical problems you have, especially diabetes, heart disease, stroke, kidney disease, and liver disease.
- Before having medical tests done, tell your primary health care provider you're taking this medication, because it may affect the results.
- This medication can make you feel dizzy, so know how it affects your body before performing hazardous activities, such as driving or operating heavy machinery.
- To evaluate the medication's effects, your primary health care provider may order blood tests during the first few months you're taking fosinopril.

✔ Keep in mind

- If you're pregnant or breast-feeding, check with your primary health care provider before taking this medication.

Additional instructions

_____
_____
_____
_____
_____
_____
_____
_____
_____

Taking furosemide

Dear Patient,

Your primary health care provider has prescribed furosemide to help reduce the amount of water in your body. The label may read Lasix or Myrosemide.

How to take furosemide
Furosemide comes in tablet and liquid forms. Take a single dose in the morning after breakfast or, if you're taking more than one dose a day, take the last dose no later than 6 p.m., unless your primary health care provider instructs otherwise. This schedule will avoid having your sleep interrupted by the need to urinate.

If you're taking the *liquid* form, use a special measuring spoon (not a household teaspoon) to measure each dose accurately. To reduce stomach upset, take furosemide with food or milk.

What to do if you miss a dose
Take the missed dose as soon as possible. If it's almost time for your next dose, skip the missed dose and take your next dose at its scheduled time. Don't double dose.

What to do about side effects
Contact your primary health care provider *immediately* if you've been told that you have an abnormal complete blood count and you develop an infection or a fever.

Furosemide may cause dehydration and lower your body's levels of potassium, chloride, sodium, calcium, or magnesium. As a result, your primary health care provider may tell you to have your blood tested regularly.

Furosemide commonly causes dizziness, fatigue, and increased urination, particularly when you first start taking it. If these effects persist or become severe, tell your primary health care provider.

What you must know about alcohol and other drugs
Limit your intake of alcoholic beverages. Indomethacin (Indocin) can decrease furosemide's effects.

Special directions
• Tell your health care provider about other medical problems you have and if you've had a bad reaction to sulfa drugs.
• Because furosemide may lower your body's potassium level, eat plenty of foods with high potassium content, such as bananas, oranges, or other citrus fruits.
• To prevent excessive water and potassium loss, call your primary health care provider if you become ill and experience continuing vomiting or diarrhea.
• Minimize dizziness by getting up slowly after lying down or sitting. Avoid overexertion and standing for long periods.
• When exposed to sunlight, wear a hat and sunglasses and use sunblock.

✓ Keep in mind
• If you're pregnant or breast-feeding, check with your primary health care provider before taking furosemide.
• Older adults may be especially prone to side effects.
• If you have diabetes, furosemide may affect your blood glucose levels. Report any consistent change in your home test results.
• If you're an athlete, be aware that furosemide is banned by the National Collegiate Athletic Association and the U.S. Olympic Committee.

Additional instructions
_____
_____
_____

Taking gabapentin

Dear Patient,

Your primary health care provider has prescribed gabapentin to help prevent seizures. The brand name for this medication is Neurontin.

How to take gabapentin
This medication is available as a capsule. It's usually taken three times a day and can be taken either with or without food.

What to do if you miss a dose
Take the missed dose as soon as possible. If it's almost time for your next dose, skip the missed dose and take your next dose on schedule. If you're unsure what to do, call your primary health care provider or pharmacist.

What to do about side effects
You may experience sleepiness, dizziness, fatigue, blurred vision, or decreased reflexes in your muscles. Contact your primary health care provider if these symptoms persist or become severe.

What you must know about alcohol and other drugs
Check with your primary health care provider before drinking alcoholic beverages because the combined effects of alcohol and gabapentin may increase the risk of drowsiness.

Tell your primary health care provider what other medications you're taking, including those you buy without a prescription from a pharmacy, supermarket, or health food store. He needs this information to make sure that all of your medications can be taken safely together.

Cimetidine (Tagamet) may alter the time it takes for gabapentin to leave the body, so be sure to alert your primary health care provider if you're taking this medication.

Antacids such as Maalox, Mylanta, or Tums can decrease the effect of gabapentin. So take gabapentin at least 2 hours after taking antacids.

Special directions
• Before taking gabapentin, tell your primary health care provider if you've ever had an allergic reaction to this medication or any others.
• Tell your primary health care provider if you have other medical problems such as kidney or liver disease. This may affect the use of gabapentin.
• Don't drive a car, use machinery, or perform other activities that require alertness until you know how you react to this medication
• Don't stop taking gabapentin or any other medication for seizures without consulting your primary health care provider.

✓ Keep in mind
• Iif you become pregnant, plan to become pregnant, or are breast-feeding, check with your primary health care provider before taking this medication.

Additional instructions

_____
_____
_____
_____
_____
_____
_____
_____
_____

Taking gemfibrozil

Dear Patient,

Your primary health care provider has prescribed gemfibrozil to reduce cholesterol and triglyceride (fat) levels in your blood. The label may read Lopid.

How to take gemfibrozil

Gemfibrozil is available in tablets and capsules. Take the medication exactly as prescribed. Don't take more or less of it, take it more or less often, or take it for a longer or shorter time than your primary health care provider has ordered.

If your primary health care provider tells you to take two doses a day, take one dose 30 minutes before breakfast and take the second dose 30 minutes before your evening meal.

What to do if you miss a dose

Take the missed dose as soon as you remember. But if it's almost time for your next dose, skip the missed dose and take your next dose as scheduled. Never take two doses at once.

What to do about side effects

While taking gemfibrozil, you may have stomach pain, heartburn, nausea, diarrhea, and dizziness. If these symptoms persist or become severe, tell your primary health care provider.

What you must know about other drugs

Because gemfibrozil may increase the effects of blood thinners (such as Coumadin), don't take these two medications together.

Also, don't take lovastatin or simvastatin while taking gemfibrozil.

Special directions

• Carefully follow the special diet your primary health care provider has ordered for you, so that this medication can work properly.

! Warning: Don't stop taking gemfibrozil without first asking your primary health care provider. If you stop taking it, your cholesterol and triglyceride levels could rise again.

• Gemfibrozil may cause dizziness, so don't drive, operate hazardous machinery, or perform activities that require alertness until you know what effect this medication has on you.

✔ Keep in mind

• If you're pregnant or breast-feeding, check with your primary health care provider before taking this medication.

Additional instructions

_____

_____

_____

_____

_____

_____

_____

_____

_____

_____

Using gentamicin

Dear Patient,

Your primary health care provider has prescribed gentamicin to treat your eye infection. The label may read Garamycin.

How to use gentamicin
Gentamicin is available as eyedrops and as ointment. Carefully read the instructions on the medication label, which tell you how much to use for each dose.

If you're using eyedrops, follow these steps:

1 Wash your hands. Tilt your head back and pull the lower eyelid away from the eye to form a pouch.

2 Squeeze the correct number of drops into the pouch and gently close your eye. Avoid touching the tip of the eyedropper to your eye. Don't blink.

3 Keep your eye closed for 1 to 2 minutes to allow the medication to come into contact with the infection. If you think you didn't get a drop into your eye, use another drop. Repeat on the other eye, if directed.

If you're applying ointment, follow these steps:

1 Wash your hands. Pull the lower eyelid away from the eye to form a pouch.

2 Squeeze a thin strip of ointment into the pouch, and gently close your eye. Avoid touching the tip of the tube to your eye. Keep your eye closed for 1 to 2 minutes to allow the medication to come into contact with the infection. Repeat on the other eye, if directed.

What to do if you miss a dose
If you miss a dose, use the eyedrops or apply the ointment as soon as possible. If it's almost time for the next dose, skip the missed dose and take your next dose on schedule.

What to do about side effects
Your eyes may temporarily feel irritated if you're using the eyedrops.

If you're applying the ointment, expect your eyes to burn or sting; you may also have blurred vision.

If these side effects persist or become bothersome, tell your primary health care provider.

Special directions
• Tell your primary health care provider if you're allergic to this medication or to related antibiotics, such as amikacin (Amikin), kanamycin (Kantrex), neomycin (Mycifradin), streptomycin, or tobramycin (Tobrex).

Additional instructions

_____
_____
_____
_____
_____
_____
_____
_____
_____
_____

Taking glimepiride

Dear Patient,

Your primary health care provider has prescribed glimepiride along with diet and exercise to help lower the high blood glucose (sugar) levels caused by your diabetes. This medication works by stimulating insulin release from your pancreas. The label may read Amaryl.

How to take glimepiride
This medication is available as a tablet. It's usually taken once a day at breakfast, to ensure the best blood glucose control. Don't stop taking this medication without telling your primary health care provider.

What to do if you miss a dose
Take the missed dose as soon as possible. If it's almost time for your next dose, skip the missed dose and take your next dose on schedule. If you're not sure what to do, call your primary health care provider or pharmacist.

What to do about side effects
Notify your primary health care provider immediately if you develop a rash, unexplained bruising, or a sore throat.

You may also experience fatigue, excessive hunger, heavy sweating, tremors, and a fast heartbeat. Contact your primary health care provider if these symptoms persist or become severe.

What you must know about alcohol and other drugs
Alcohol, aspirin, and aspirin-containing products such as Bufferin can also lower your blood sugar levels. So don't drink alcohol or take any of these medications unless your primary health care provider gives you the okay.

Before starting glimepiride, tell your primary health care provider what other medications you're taking, including ones you buy without a prescription from a pharmacy, supermarket, or health food store. He needs this information to make sure that all of your medications can be taken safely together.

Special directions
● Before taking this medication, tell your primary health care provider if you're allergic to glimepiride or any other drugs.
● Notify your primary health care provider if you have other medical problems such as heart, kidney, liver, or thyroid disease. This may affect the use of glimepiride.
● *Warning:* Don't skip meals — your blood glucose level may fall dangerously low (a condition called hypoglycemia). Eating meals at regularly scheduled times is necessary because glimepiride causes insulin to be released into the bloodstream throughout the day. Also continue with your prescribed exercise program.
● Follow your primary health care provider's instructions for testing your blood glucose level at home.
● Wear a medical identification bracelet or necklace at all times and carry an identification card indicating that you're taking this medication.

Keep in mind
● Tell your primary health care provider if you become pregnant, plan to become pregnant, or are breast-feeding.

Additional instructions

_____

_____

_____

Taking glipizide

Dear Patient,

Your primary health care provider has prescribed glipizide, in combination with a special diet and exercise program, to control your blood glucose (sugar) level. The label may read Glucotrol.

How to take glipizide
Take glipizide exactly as prescribed. Take it at the same time each day, about 30 minutes before a meal, to ensure the best blood glucose control. If you take one dose a day, take it in the morning.

What to do if you miss a dose
Take it as soon as possible. If it's almost time for your next dose, skip the missed dose and take the next dose as scheduled.

What to do about side effects
Glipizide may cause nervousness, increased sweating, fast heartbeat, headache, and yellowing of your skin and the whites of your eyes. If these symptoms persist or worsen, tell your primary health care provider.

What you must know about alcohol and other drugs
Avoid alcoholic beverages; they can lower blood glucose levels and also cause stomach pain, nausea, vomiting, dizziness, and excessive sweating.

Glipizide can change the effects of many drugs, and other drugs can reduce glipizide's effects. Check with your primary health care provider before taking other prescription or nonprescription medications.

Special directions
• Tell your primary health care provider about other medical conditions you have, especially heart, kidney, liver, or thyroid disease. Also tell him if you develop new medical problems, especially infections.
• Test your blood glucose level as your primary health care provider instructs.
• If you experience increased sensitivity to sunlight, wear protective clothing, use sunblock, and limit sun exposure.
• Wear a medical identification bracelet or necklace at all times and carry an identification card indicating your medical problems and medications.
• Tell family members how to treat the symptoms of hyperglycemia and hypoglycemia in case you're too ill to direct them.

✔ Keep in mind
• If you're pregnant or think you may be, tell your primary health care provider, who will change your medication to insulin. If you plan to breast-feed, check with your primary health care provider first.
• Older adults may be especially sensitive to this medication.

Additional instructions
_____
_____
_____
_____
_____
_____
_____
_____
_____
_____
_____
_____
_____

Taking glyburide

Dear Patient,

Your primary health care provider has prescribed glyburide, in combination with a special diet and exercise program, to control your blood glucose level. The label may read DiaBeta, Glynase, or Micronase.

How to take glyburide
Take glyburide exactly as prescribed. Take it at the same time each day to ensure the best blood glucose control. If you take one dose a day, take it in the morning with breakfast. If you're taking more than one dose a day, you may need to take the doses before breakfast and dinner or with meals. Check with your primary health care provider.

What to do if you miss a dose
Take the dose as soon as possible. If it's almost time for your next dose, skip the missed dose and take the next dose as scheduled.

What to do about side effects
Glyburide may cause nervousness, increased sweating, fast heartbeat, headache, and yellowing of your skin and the whites of your eyes. If these symptoms persist or worsen, tell your primary health care provider.

What you must know about alcohol and other drugs
Avoid alcoholic beverages; they can lower blood glucose levels and also cause stomach pain, nausea, vomiting, dizziness, and excessive sweating.
   Glyburide can change the effects of many medications, and other medications can reduce glyburide's effects. Check with your primary health care provider before taking prescription and nonprescription medications.

Special directions
• Tell your primary health care provider about other medical conditions you have, especially heart, kidney, liver, or thyroid disease. Also tell him if you develop new medical problems, particularly infections.
• Follow your prescribed diet and exercise plan carefully.
• Test your blood glucose level as your primary health care provider instructs.
• If you experience increased sensitivity to sunlight, wear protective clothing, use sunblock, and limit sun exposure.
• Wear a medical identification bracelet or necklace at all times and carry an identification card indicating that you're taking this medication.

✔ Keep in mind
• If you're pregnant or think you may be, tell your primary health care provider, who will change your medication to insulin. If you plan to breast-feed, check with your primary health care provider.
• Older adults may be especially sensitive to this medication.

Additional instructions
_____
_____
_____
_____
_____
_____
_____
_____
_____

Taking griseofulvin

Dear Patient,

Your primary health care provider has prescribed griseofulvin to treat your fungal infection. Brand names include Fulvicin P/G, Fulvicin-U/F, Grifulvin V, and Grisactin.

How to take griseofulvin

Take griseofulvin tablets, capsules, or liquid exactly as prescribed. To help clear up your infection completely, take the medication for the full length of time ordered by your primary health care provider, even if you begin to feel better after a few days.

Take griseofulvin with or after meals, preferably with fatty foods (for example, whole milk or ice cream), which reduces stomach upset and helps your body absorb the medication.

What to do if you miss a dose

Take the missed dose as soon as possible unless it's almost time for your next dose. If so, skip the missed dose and take the next dose as scheduled. Don't double dose.

What to do about side effects

If you develop a rash or itchy skin, stop taking griseofulvin and *immediately* call your primary health care provider. Sometimes an allergic reaction such as this can be serious. If you become restless or have difficulty breathing, get emergency care *immediately.*

Griseofulvin may cause a blood problem that can increase your risk of infection. This side effect can become serious, especially when you take the medication for a long period. Promptly report fever, weakness, sore throat, or mouth sores to your primary health care provider.

Griseofulvin may cause a headache, which usually goes away as your body adjusts to the medication. If it persists or worsens, call your primary health care provider.

What you must know about alcohol and other drugs

Avoid alcoholic beverages; they could cause a fast heartbeat, sweating, and flushing of the skin.

Because griseofulvin may interfere with the action of birth control pills, consider using another birth control method while you're taking griseofulvin and for 1 month after stopping it.

Don't take barbiturates when using griseofulvin because they can decrease griseofulvin's effects.

Oral blood thinners may not work as well when taken with griseofulvin.

Taking cisapride (Propulsid) with griseofulvin has been linked to serious side effects.

Special directions

• Tell your primary health care provider about other medical conditions you have, particularly liver disease, lupus or lupus-like disease, or porphyria.
• Because griseofulvin may make you dizzy or less alert than usual, don't drive or perform other activities requiring alertness until you know how you respond to this medication.
• To protect light-sensitive skin, wear sunglasses and a wide-brimmed hat and use a sunblock when in the sun.

✔ Keep in mind

• If you're pregnant, stop the medication and check with your health care provider.

Additional instructions

_____
_____
_____
_____

Taking guaifenesin

Dear Patient,

This medication will help relieve your cough by loosening mucus or phlegm in your lungs. It's helpful for coughs due to colds but not for long-term coughs, such as those associated with asthma, emphysema, or smoking. Among the many brand names are Anti-Tuss, Glycotuss, and Robitussin.

How to take guaifenesin

Guaifenesin is available without a prescription; however, your primary health care provider may suggest the proper dosage for your specific condition. It comes in tablets, capsules, extended-release tablets and capsules, liquid, and a syrup.

Carefully read and follow the directions and precautions on the medication label. You may take a dose every 4 hours. Don't take more than the recommended total daily dosage.

Drink a full glass (8 ounces) of water with each dose to help loosen phlegm. Drink at least eight full glasses during the day unless your primary health care provider orders otherwise.

If you're taking an *extended-release tablet or capsule,* swallow it whole. Don't crush, break, or chew it.

Don't use this medication for longer than the directions recommend, unless your primary health care provider directs otherwise.

What to do if you miss a dose

If you're taking this medication regularly, take a missed dose as soon as possible. If it's almost time for the next dose, skip the missed dose and take the next dose at its regularly scheduled time. Don't double dose.

What you must know about other drugs

Check with your primary health care provider before using other medications— especially nonprescription cough or cold medications—because they may also contain guaifenesin.

Special directions

• If your cough doesn't improve within 7 days or if you develop a fever, rash, persistent headache, sore throat, nausea, vomiting, or dizziness, check with your primary health care provider.
• Because this medication may cause dizziness or drowsiness, don't drive or perform other activities requiring alertness until you know how you respond to it.
• Occasionally throughout the day, take several deep breaths and then cough to help bring up phlegm.
• Avoid fumes, smoke, and dust because they can irritate your lungs.

✔ Keep in mind

• If you're pregnant or think you may be, check with your primary health care provider before taking this medication.

Additional instructions

_____

_____

_____

_____

_____

_____

_____

_____

_____

_____

Taking haloperidol

Dear Patient,

Haloperidol is used to treat your condition. The label may read Haldol.

How to take haloperidol

Take this medication exactly as prescribed. To prevent stomach upset, take it with food or milk.

If you're taking the *liquid* form, use a specially marked dropper or measuring spoon. Avoid letting the medication come into contact with your skin.

What to do if you miss a dose

Take the missed dose as soon as possible, and space any doses remaining for that day at regular intervals. Then resume your regular dosage schedule. Don't double dose.

What to do about side effects

If you develop a fever, fast heartbeat, difficult or rapid breathing, profuse sweating, or seizures, stop taking haloperidol and get emergency care *immediately.*

Haloperidol may cause blurred vision and mouth dryness, which usually disappear as your body adjusts to the medication. If they persist or are bothersome, tell your primary health care provider. Also call if you notice fine, shaky movements of your tongue or any uncontrollable movements of your mouth, face, arms, or legs.

After you stop taking haloperidol, side effects such as trembling or uncontrolled movements, nausea, or vomiting may occur. If they do, call your primary health care provider promptly.

What you must know about alcohol and other drugs

Don't drink alcoholic beverages while taking haloperidol because the combination could cause an overdose.

Check with your primary health care provider before taking any prescription or nonprescription medications.

Special directions

• Tell your health care provider about other medical problems you have because they may affect the use of this medication.
• Don't drive or perform other activities requiring alertness until you know how you react to this medication.

! *Warning:* Don't stop taking this medication without first consulting your primary health care provider.

• Because haloperidol may make you sweat less, which raises your body temperature and increases the chance of heatstroke, be careful not to become overheated.
• Relieve mouth dryness with sugarless hard candy or gum, ice chips, mouthwash, or a saliva substitute. If this dryness continues for more than 2 weeks, tell your primary health care provider or dentist.
• Because haloperidol may make your skin more sensitive to light, wear protective clothing and sunglasses and use a sun-blocking agent when outdoors.

✔ Keep in mind

• If you're pregnant or think you may be, check with your primary health care provider before taking haloperidol. Don't breast-feed while taking this medication.
• Children and older adults are especially sensitive to haloperidol's side effects.
• If you're an athlete, be aware that haloperidol use is banned by the U.S. Olympic Committee and the National Collegiate Athletic Association.

Additional instructions

_____

_____

Taking herbal products

Dear Patient,

Your primary health care provider has ordered an herbal medication for you.

How to take an herbal product
When taking herbal medications, follow the prescription exactly. Taking too much of a medication or taking a medication inappropriately may not only diminish its effectiveness, but it may also increase the risk of dangerous side effects.

What to do if you miss a dose
Take the missed dose as soon as possible. If it's almost time for your next dose, skip the missed dose, and take your next dose on schedule. Don't double dose.

What to do about side effects
Call your primary health care provider *immediately* if you experience abdominal cramping; abnormal bleeding or bruising; changes in heart rate or rhythm; changes in vision; dizziness or fainting; hair loss; hallucinations; inability to concentrate, or other mental changes; hives, itching, rashes, or other allergic symptoms; loss of appetite; or dramatic weight loss.

What you must know about other drugs
Tell your primary health care provider about all the medications you take, including other herbal medications and vitamins.

Special directions
• Tell your primary health care provider about your medical history, including allergies.
• Purchase your herbal medication from a reputable source, such as a pharmacy.
• Never ignore symptoms you may be experiencing. Herbal medications aren't necessarily a substitute for traditional, proven

medical therapy. Never use them in place of more appropriate therapy.
• Never allow other people to take your herbal medication.
• Store herbal medications out of the reach of children and pets.
• Read the labels carefully when purchasing herbal medications. Make sure the term "standardized" is on the label. This means that the dose of the medication in each tablet or capsule in that package is the same. Also make sure that the label states specific percentages, amounts, and strengths of active ingredients.

✔ Keep in mind
• If you're a woman of childbearing age, you should use appropriate contraception and avoid taking herbal products. Little is known about the effects of herbal medications on a fetus.

Additional instructions

_____
_____
_____
_____
_____
_____
_____
_____
_____
_____
_____

Taking hormone-type medications

Dear Patient,

Your primary health care provider has prescribed a hormone-type medication. Hormones are naturally produced by the body, though the production of some hormones (such as estrogen and progesterone) decreases as we age. Hormone medications are prescribed for many different reasons. For example, they're used during menopause to replace what the body isn't making naturally. They're also used in certain diseases to limit the amount of hormones the body is making.

This sheet provides general information about hormone medications. You will also receive a sheet that gives details about the specific hormone that has been prescribed for you.

How to take hormone-type medications

Hormones may be taken by mouth, injected, placed on the skin (skin patch), or inserted vaginally.

If you're taking hormones *by mouth*, your primary health care provider may tell you to take them at a certain time each day. They can be taken either with or without food.

If you're using a *skin patch*, make sure the area where you'll place the patch is clean and dry. Clean the area with soap and water (not rubbing alcohol) and towel it dry. Then peel the protective backing off the patch to expose the adhesive. Apply the sticky side of the patch directly to your skin and press firmly. Don't puncture or cut the patch unless your primary health care provider says to. Also, don't apply the patch to your breasts.

If you're inserting a *vaginal suppository* or *cream,* wash your vaginal area with soap and water before inserting the medication. Then insert the suppository or cream high enough into the vagina to be comfortable.

Don't use tampons while using vaginal therapy. You may wish to wear a sanitary pad to protect your clothing during therapy with these medications.

What to do if you miss a dose

If you miss a dose of hormone, take it as soon as you remember. If it's almost time for your next scheduled dose, skip the missed dose and go back to your regular schedule. Don't take double doses.

What to do about side effects

You may experience side effects with hormone medications, depending on what you're taking. Call your primary health care provider *right away* if you have breast pain, increased breast size, rapid weight gain, or swelling in your legs and feet.

More common side effects include vaginal bleeding or spotting between menstrual cycles, loss of appetite, lower stomach cramps, diarrhea, nausea, and vomiting. If these side effects continue or become bothersome, call your primary health care provider.

Hormones, taken for a long time, may also increase or decrease your risk of getting certain types of cancer. Discuss these risks with your primary health care provider. He'll teach you how to do a breast self-examination and will monitor you closely for abnormal developments.

What you must know about alcohol and other drugs

Alcohol can interact with some hormone medications, so use alcohol with caution or check with your primary health care provider before using them together.

Many medications — cyclosporine (Neoral), in particular — also compete with hormones in the liver. When hormones are also

(continued)

Taking hormone-type medications *(continued)*

being taken, cyclosporine blood levels can rise and become toxic. In addition, medications called protease inhibitors for human immunodeficiency virus (HIV) can lessen the effect of some hormones. So tell your primary health care provider about all the other medications you're taking.

Special directions
• If you're of childbearing age and are taking hormones for some reason other than pregnancy prevention, be sure to use other measures to prevent pregnancy such as a diaphragm with spermicide, a condom with spermicide, or a cervical cap.

✔ Keep in mind
• If you've ever had an unusual reaction to hormone medications in the past, tell your primary health care provider.
• Be sure to perform breast self-examinations every month. Your primary health care provider or nurse will teach you how to do this.
• If you're taking hormones for menopausal symptoms, you may have withdrawal bleeding if you stop taking the hormones for a certain time period each month. This bleeding is normal and doesn't mean that you can become pregnant.
• Keep all your follow-up appointments and have an annual pelvic examination and a mammogram as directed by your primary health care provider.
• Tell your primary health care provider if you're pregnant or breast-feeding or if you become pregnant while on this medication.

Additional instructions
_____
_____
_____
_____
_____
_____
_____
_____
_____
_____
_____

Taking hydralazine

Dear Patient,

Your primary health care provider has prescribed hydralazine to lower your blood pressure or to treat your heart condition. The label may read Apresoline.

How to take hydralazine

Take hydralazine exactly as prescribed at the same time each day, preferably at mealtimes. Take it for as long as your primary health care provider orders, even after you begin to feel better. Hydralazine doesn't cure high blood pressure, it only controls it. So you must continue using it to reduce the risk of complications of high blood pressure. Don't suddenly stop taking hydralazine.

What to do if you miss a dose

Take the missed dose as soon as possible. If it's almost time for your next regular dose, skip the missed dose and resume your normal dosing schedule. Don't double dose.

What to do about side effects

A rare but possibly serious side effect of hydralazine is an irregular heartbeat. If this occurs, or if you develop chest pain, swelling of the feet or lower legs, weight gain, sore throat, fever, muscle and joint pain, or a rash, call your primary health care provider *immediately.*

Hydralazine may also cause headaches, dizziness, fast heartbeat, nausea, vomiting, diarrhea, or loss of appetite. These effects may go away as your body adjusts to the medication. Check with your primary health care provider if they continue or are bothersome.

What you must know about other drugs

Check with your primary health care provider before taking nonprescription or prescription medications because some can interfere with hydralazine's action or cause side effects.

Special directions

• Tell your primary health care provider about other medical problems you have, especially kidney, heart, or blood vessel disease, including stroke.
• Because hydralazine can cause dizziness, know how you react to this medication before driving or performing other activities requiring alertness.
• To minimize dizziness, rise slowly from a sitting or lying position.
• Follow a low-salt diet if your primary health care provider prescribes it.
• If your primary health care provider has instructed you to take your blood pressure at home, follow directions closely and notify him of any significant change.

✔ Keep in mind

• If you're pregnant or think you may be, check with your primary health care provider before taking hydralazine.
• Older adults may be especially sensitive to side effects.

Additional instructions

_____

_____

_____

_____

_____

_____

_____

_____

_____

_____

Taking hydrochlorothiazide

Dear Patient,

Your primary health care provider has prescribed this thiazide diuretic to lower your blood pressure. It works by reducing the amount of water in your body. Brand names include HydroDIURIL, Mictrin, and Oretic.

How to take hydrochlorothiazide
This medication comes in tablet and liquid forms. If you're taking one dose a day, take it in the morning after breakfast. If you're taking more than one dose a day, take the last dose before 6 p.m. so you won't wake up to urinate.

If you're taking the liquid form, use a specially marked dropper or measuring spoon.

What to do if you miss a dose
Take the missed dose as soon as you remember unless it's almost time for your next regular dose. If so, skip the missed dose and take your next dose as scheduled. Don't double dose.

What to do about side effects
If you experience persistent fever, sore throat, joint pain, or easy bruising and bleeding, stop taking this medication and call your primary health care provider *immediately.*

This medication may cause dehydration, low blood glucose level, fatigue, muscle cramps, numbness, "pins and needles" sensation, and weakness. If these side effects persist, tell your health care provider.

What you must know about other drugs
Cholestyramine (Questran), colestipol (Colestid), and nonsteroidal anti-inflammatory medications decrease hydrochlorothiazide's effects. If you're taking any of these medications along with hydrochlorothiazide, follow your dosage schedule exactly to minimize medication interactions. Avoid taking

diazoxide (Proglycem), which may worsen hydrochlorothiazide's side effects.

Special directions
● Before taking hydrochlorothiazide, tell your primary health care provider if you're allergic to sulfa medications or other medications.
● This medication may decrease your body's potassium level, so your primary health care provider may instruct you to eat foods high in potassium, such as uncooked dried fruits and fresh orange juice; take a potassium supplement; or decrease your salt intake.
● Inform your primary health care provider if you're already on a special diet, such as one for diabetes.

Warning: Contact your primary health care provider if you experience persistent or severe diarrhea or vomiting, which can cause excessive potassium and water loss and decrease blood pressure too much.
● Because hydrochlorothiazide may increase your sensitivity to sunlight, limit sun exposure, wear protective clothing and sunglasses, and use a sunblock.

✔ Keep in mind
● If you're pregnant or breast-feeding, check with your primary health care provider before taking this medication.
● If you have diabetes, this medication can interfere with blood or urine glucose tests.
● If you're an older adult, you may be especially sensitive to side effects.
● If you're an athlete, be aware that diuretics are banned and tested for by the National Collegiate Athletic Association and the U.S. Olympic Committee.

Additional instructions

Taking hydrochlorothiazide with triamterene

Dear Patient,

Your primary health care provider has prescribed this medication to control your blood pressure. It works by reducing the amount of water in your body. The label may read Dyazide or Maxzide.

How to take this medication
Take this medication exactly as prescribed. If you're taking one dose a day, take it in the morning after breakfast. If you're taking more than one dose a day, take your last dose before 6 p.m. so the need to urinate won't disturb your sleep. To prevent stomach upset, take this medication with milk or meals.

What to do if you miss a dose
Take it as soon as you remember unless it's almost time for your next dose. If so, skip the missed dose and take your next dose as scheduled. Never take two doses at once.

What to do about side effects
If you feel like your throat is closing and you have trouble breathing, stop taking this medication and get emergency care *at once.* Also stop taking this medication and call your primary health care provider if you experience persistent fever, sore throat, joint pain, or easy bleeding or bruising.

Common side effects include dehydration, low blood glucose level, chronic fatigue, anxiety, irritability, muscle cramps, numbness, pain, "pins and needles" sensation, weakness, increased urination and thirst, and weak, irregular pulse. If these symptoms persist, tell your primary health care provider.

What you must know about other drugs
Tell your primary health care provider if you're taking other prescription or nonprescription medications. For example, taking this medication with angiotensin-converting enzyme inhibitors (such as Captopril) or potassium supplements can raise blood potassium levels, possibly leading to kidney and heart problems.

Special directions
Warning: Contact your primary health care provider if you develop persistent or severe diarrhea or vomiting, which can cause excessive potassium and water loss and decrease blood pressure too much.
• This medication may make you sensitive to sunlight, so limit sun exposure, wear protective clothing and sunglasses, and use a sunblock.

✔ Keep in mind
• If you're pregnant or breast-feeding, check with your primary health care provider before taking this medication.
• Older adults are especially sensitive to this medication.
• If you're an athlete, be aware that the National Collegiate Athletic Association and the U.S. Olympic Committee ban the use of this medication.

Additional instructions
_____
_____
_____
_____
_____
_____
_____
_____
_____
_____

Applying hydrocortisone

Dear Patient,

This medication is used to help relieve the itching, redness, swelling, and discomfort of your skin problem. The label may read Cortaid, Cort-Dome, or Cortizone.

How to apply hydrocortisone

Hydrocortisone is available as an aerosol, cream, gel, lotion, ointment, or topical solution. Read and follow the instructions on the medication container. Wash your hands and skin before applying the medication. When applying the medication to hairy areas, part the hair and apply directly to the skin.

If your primary health care provider has prescribed an occlusive dressing (an airtight covering, such as plastic wrap or a special patch), apply a heavy layer of medication, cover the area with the occlusive dressing, then secure the dressing to your skin with hypoallergenic tape.

If you're using the *aerosol* form, shake the can well. Direct the spray onto the area from a distance of 6 inches. To avoid freezing the tissues, spray for no more than 3 seconds. Apply to a dry scalp after shampooing; don't rub the medication into your scalp after spraying.

Avoid breathing in the spray or getting it in your eyes. If the medication accidentally gets in your eyes, promptly flush them with water.

What to do if you miss a dose

Apply the medication as soon as you can. If it's almost time for your next regular dose, skip the missed dose and apply the next dose as scheduled.

What to do about side effects

Fever, skin tearing, painful reddened and inflamed skin with pus-filled blisters, thinning skin, reddish purple lines on the skin, or burning and itching skin with pinhead-size blisters may occur with the use of an occlusive dressing. If any of these problems occurs, remove the dressing and contact your primary health care provider.

Special directions

• Before using hydrocortisone, tell your primary health care provider if you're allergic to any medications or foods.
• For safety reasons, don't apply topical hydrocortisone near heat or an open flame or while smoking.

❗ *Warning:* Don't use topical hydrocortisone more often or for a longer time than your primary health care provider has instructed. Doing so increases the risk of side effects.
• Don't share this medication with other people.
• Don't use any remaining medication to treat other skin problems without first consulting your primary health care provider.

✔ Keep in mind

• If you're pregnant or breast-feeding, check with your primary health care provider before using this medication.
• Don't use hydrocortisone on a child under age 2 without a primary health care provider's order.
• Children, adolescents, and older adults are especially prone to side effects and should be closely monitored by a primary health care provider.

Additional instructions

_____

_____

_____

_____

_____

Using hydrocortisone with neomycin and polymyxin B

Dear Patient,

This medication helps to treat ear infections. It may also be used to relieve discomfort, irritation, and redness from other ear problems. Common brand names for this medication include Cortisporin, Otocort, and Pediotic.

How to use this medication

Insert the eardrops, following the instructions you received from the nurse or primary health care provider.

Before inserting the eardrops, warm them to body temperature (98.6° F) by holding the bottle in your hand for a few minutes. Don't heat the bottle on the stove or in the microwave; the medication won't work if it gets too warm.

To administer the drops, position the dropper above your ear and squeeze the bulb. Don't put the dropper inside your ear. Keep your ear tilted to one side for about 2 minutes, or insert a soft cotton plug just at the entrance to your ear canal, whichever is recommended by the manufacturer.

Continue using this medication as ordered even after you feel better. Complete the full treatment to make sure the infection is completely cleared up.

What to do if you miss a dose

If you miss a dose, insert the eardrops as soon as you remember. If it's almost time for your next regular dose, skip the missed dose and insert the drops when next scheduled.

What to do about side effects

If you have itching, redness, swelling, or other signs of irritation, tell your primary health care provider.

Special directions

• Before using this medication, tell your primary health care provider if you have other ear problems. Using this medication could make some problems worse.
• Inform your primary health care provider if you're allergic to this medication or others, particularly related antibiotics, such as gentamicin (Garamycin), streptomycin, or tobramycin (Nebcin).
• If your symptoms persist for more than 1 week or become worse, contact your primary health care provider.
• Don't use this medication for more than 10 days in a row unless your primary health care provider prescribes a longer course of treatment.

Additional instructions

_____
_____
_____
_____
_____
_____
_____
_____
_____
_____
_____

Taking hydromorphone

Dear Patient,

This medication is prescribed to relieve pain or cough. The label may read Dilaudid.

How to take hydromorphone

Hydromorphone comes in tablet, suppository, and injection forms. Take only as prescribed. Overuse could lead to dependency and risk of overdose.

To insert a *suppository,* follow these steps: If the suppository is too soft to insert, run cold water over it or chill it in the refrigerator for about 30 minutes before removing the foil wrapper. Then remove the wrapper and moisten the suppository with cold water. Lie down on your side. Using your index finger, gently push the suppository into your rectum as far as possible.

If you're using the *injectable* form, follow your primary health care provider's instructions for performing injections. Alternate among several injection sites to help prevent complications.

What to do if you miss a dose

Take the dose as soon as you remember. If it's almost time for your next regular dose, skip the missed dose and take the next one at the regular time. Don't take two doses at once.

What to do about side effects

If you think you've taken an overdose or develop symptoms of an overdose, get emergency medical care *immediately.* Symptoms of overdose include seizures, cold and clammy skin, confusion, severe drowsiness or dizziness, slow or troubled breathing, slow heartbeat, extreme nervousness or restlessness, severe weakness, and very small pupils.

Hydromorphone may cause drowsiness, dizziness, difficulty thinking clearly, nausea, vomiting, constipation, difficulty urinating, or a false sense of well-being. These problems may go away as your body adjusts to the medication; if they continue, tell your primary health care provider.

What you must know about alcohol and other drugs

Warning: Don't drink alcoholic beverages while taking hydromorphone; the combination can cause an overdose.

Check with your primary health care provider before taking other prescription or nonprescription medications. Some can add to hydromorphone's effects.

Special directions

• Let your primary health care provider know if you have other medical problems. They may affect the use of this medication.
• Don't drive or perform other activities requiring alertness until you know how you respond to this medication.
• To help prevent or relieve constipation, drink plenty of fluids and eat high-fiber foods.

Warning: If you've taken hydromorphone regularly for several weeks or more, don't stop without first checking with your primary health care provider. He may want to decrease your dosage gradually to minimize withdrawal side effects.

Keep in mind

• If you're pregnant or think you may be, check with your primary health care provider before taking this medication.
• Children and older adults are especially sensitive to this medication.

Additional instructions

_____

_____

Taking hydroxyzine

Dear Patient,

Hydroxyzine helps to treat many problems. For instance, it helps relieve anxiety and tension. It also treats a rash and itching. It may even be given to treat hyperactivity in children. Its brand names include Anxanil, Atarax, and Vistaril.

How to take hydroxyzine
This medication comes in tablets, capsules, a syrup, and an oral liquid. Follow your primary health care provider's instructions exactly.

Take this medication with food or a glass of water or milk to reduce stomach upset.

What to do if you miss a dose
Take the dose as soon as possible unless it's almost time for the next regular dose. If so, skip the missed dose and take the next dose at the scheduled time. Never take two doses at once.

What to do about side effects
If you think you've taken an overdose or have symptoms of an overdose — including seizures, clumsiness or unsteadiness, severe drowsiness, trouble breathing, extreme mouth dryness, and hallucinations — get emergency medical care *at once.*

Common side effects include drowsiness and dry mouth. These problems should subside as your body adjusts to the medication; if they persist or worsen, tell your primary health care provider.

What you must know about alcohol and other drugs
Don't drink alcoholic beverages while taking hydroxyzine. This combination can cause an overdose. Check with your primary health care provider before taking other prescription or nonprescription medications while you're taking hydroxyzine.

Special directions
• Tell your primary health care provider about other medical conditions you have, such as glaucoma and ulcers.
• Tell your primary health care provider if you're on a special diet, such as low-salt or low-sugar.
• Know how you react to hydroxyzine before you drive or perform other activities requiring alertness.
• Relieve mouth dryness with sugarless hard candy or gum, ice chips, mouthwash, or a saliva substitute. If dryness continues for more than 2 weeks, tell your primary health care provider or dentist as it increases your risk of tooth and gum problems.
• Avoid prolonged exposure to sunlight. Wear protective clothing and sunglasses, and use a sunblock.

✔ Keep in mind
• If you're pregnant or think you may be, check with your primary health care provider before starting this medication. Don't take this medication while breastfeeding.
• Children and older adults are especially sensitive to hydroxyzine's side effects.

Additional instructions
_____
_____
_____
_____
_____
_____
_____
_____
_____
_____

Taking ibuprofen

Dear Patient,

Ibuprofen relieves mild to moderate pain and reduces fever. It's also called Advil, Motrin, and Nuprin.

How to take ibuprofen

Ibuprofen comes in tablets, caplets, and liquid. Although its 200-mg strength is available without a prescription, only a health care provider can prescribe stronger doses.

If your primary health care provider has prescribed ibuprofen, follow his instructions. If you're taking ibuprofen without a prescription, follow the package instructions.

To reduce stomach upset, take ibuprofen with food or an antacid. However, your health care provider may instruct you to take the first few doses of ibuprofen either 30 minutes before or 2 hours after meals; taking the medication on an empty stomach helps it work faster at first.

When taking the *tablet* or *caplet*, drink a full glass (8 ounces) of water. To prevent irritation that may cause trouble swallowing, avoid lying down for 15 to 30 minutes after taking the medication.

What to do if you miss a dose

Take the dose as soon as you remember. If it's almost time for your next regular dose, skip the missed dose and take the next one at the regular time.

What to do about side effects

If your throat feels like it's closing and you have trouble breathing, get emergency medical care *immediately.*

Ibuprofen may also cause dizziness, drowsiness, headache, heartburn, and nausea. Less common effects include swelling of your ankles and feet or ringing in your ears. If these problems persist or worsen, tell your primary health care provider.

What you must know about other drugs

Furosemide (Lasix) or thiazide diuretics (water pills) may be less effective with ibuprofen. Because ibuprofen increases the effects of oral anticoagulants (blood thinners) and lithium (Lithane), don't take these medications together.

Special directions

- Don't take ibuprofen if you're allergic to aspirin. If you have other allergies, check with your primary health care provider before taking ibuprofen.
- Tell your primary health care provider if you're on a special low-salt or diabetic diet before taking ibuprofen oral liquid.
- If you're using nonprescription ibuprofen and your symptoms persist or worsen, contact your primary health care provider.
- If you're taking ibuprofen to reduce fever, call your primary health care provider if your fever lasts for more than 3 days. If you're taking it for pain, call if the injured area becomes or stays red or swollen.
- Before undergoing surgery or dental work, tell your primary health care provider or dentist that you're taking ibuprofen.
- Know how you respond to ibuprofen before driving or performing other activities requiring alertness.
- Avoid prolonged exposure to sunlight.

✔ Keep in mind

- If you're pregnant, check with your primary health care provider before taking ibuprofen.
- If you're an older adult, you may be especially susceptible to ibuprofen's side effects.

Additional instructions

_____

_____

_____

Taking imipramine

Dear Patient,

This medication is used to treat depression and to relieve severe, chronic pain. It may also be prescribed to treat childhood bed-wetting. The label may read Tofranil.

How to take imipramine

Unless your primary health care provider instructs otherwise, take imipramine with food (even at bedtime) to reduce stomach upset.

What to do if you miss a dose

If you miss a dose, and you take your medication once a day at bedtime, check with your primary health care provider.

If you take more than one dose a day, take the missed dose as soon as possible. But if it's almost time for your next dose, skip the missed dose and resume your schedule. Don't double dose.

What to do about side effects

If you experience blurred vision, trouble urinating, or constipation, call your health care provider *immediately.* If you develop symptoms of overdose (fever, seizures, confusion, severe drowsiness, difficulty breathing, muscle stiffness or weakness or fast, slow, or irregular heartbeat), stop taking imipramine and get emergency care *immediately.*

Call your health care provider if you can't sleep or have uncontrolled lip, arm, or leg movements after you stop using imipramine.

Dizziness, drowsiness, dry mouth, headache, and increased sweating may occur, but they usually go away as your body adjusts to the medication. If they persist, tell your primary health care provider.

What you must know about alcohol and other drugs

Don't drink alcoholic beverages while taking imipramine. Check with your health care provider if you're taking other prescription or nonprescription medications. They may interact with imipramine and cause problems.

Special directions

• Tell your primary health care provider about other medical conditions you have.
• Make sure you know how you react to imipramine before you drive or perform other activities requiring alertness and the ability to see clearly.
• If you feel dizzy or faint when arising from a sitting or lying position, get up slowly.
• Relieve mouth dryness with sugarless candy or gum, ice chips, or a saliva substitute. If dryness continues for more than 2 weeks, tell your primary health care provider or dentist.
• To protect light-sensitive skin, limit sun exposure; when outdoors, wear protective clothing and sunglasses and use a sunblock.
• Unless your primary health care provider instructs otherwise, drink plenty of liquids and eat a high-fiber diet to prevent constipation.

! *Warning:* Don't stop taking imipramine without first consulting your health care provider, who may decrease your dosage gradually to minimize withdrawal.

✓ Keep in mind

• If you're pregnant or breast-feeding, check with your primary health care provider before starting this medication.
• Children and older adults are at special risk for side effects.
• If you have diabetes, imipramine can affect your glucose level. If this occurs, call your primary health care provider.

Additional instructions

_____

_____

Taking indinavir

Dear Patient,

Your primary health care provider has prescribed indinavir to treat your HIV infection. This medication works by helping to slow the spread of the virus and prevent it from weakening your immune system. The brand name for this medication is Crixivan.

How to take indinavir

This medication is available as a capsule. It's usually taken three times a day on an empty stomach, 1 hour before or 2 hours after meals. Take it with a full glass (8 ounces) of water, skim milk, juice, coffee, or tea.

What to do if you miss a dose

If you miss a dose, take it as soon as possible, But if it's almost time for your next dose, skip the missed dose and take your next dose on schedule. Don't take double doses. If you're unsure what to do, call your primary health care provider.

What to do about side effects

You may experience nausea, diarrhea, stomach pain, or headache. If these persist or become severe, notify your primary health care provider.

What you must know about alcohol and other drugs

Check with your primary health care provider before drinking alcoholic beverages because the combined effects of alcohol and this medication may increase the risk of drowsiness.

Warning: Tell your primary health care provider if you're taking Hismanal (astemizole), used for allergies; Propulsid (cisapride), used for stomach problems; or Halcion (triazolam), used for anxiety or difficulty sleeping. These medications shouldn't be taken with indinavir because they can cause serious heart problems.

Tell your primary health care provider if you're taking Videx (didanosine) for HIV infection. Indinavir and Videx should be taken at least 1 hour apart and on an empty stomach. Also report if you're taking oral contraceptives or Rifadin (rifampin) for tuberculosis. The interactions between these medications and indinavir can alter how all the medications work.

Special directions

● Before taking this medication, tell your primary health care provider if you've ever had an allergic reaction to indinavir or any other medications.
● Inform your primary health care provider if you have other medical problems, such as kidney or liver disease. This may affect the use of indinavir.
● Indinavir isn't a cure for HIV infection, and you may continue to develop other infections and complications associated with HIV. This medication won't reduce the risk of transmission of HIV to other people through sexual contact or blood contamination by using the same needles.
● Store this medication in its original container. Exposure to moisture may reduce its effectiveness.

✓ Keep in mind

● Tell your primary health care provider if you're pregnant, are planning to become pregnant, or are breast-feeding.

Additional instructions

_____
_____
_____

Taking indomethacin

Dear Patient,

Indomethacin is prescribed to relieve fever, pain, swelling, or joint stiffness. The label may read Indocin or Indocid.

How to take indomethacin

Take *capsules* or *oral liquid* on a full stomach or with an antacid unless your primary health care provider instructs otherwise. Don't mix the *liquid* form with the antacid or any other liquid before taking it; take the antacid first. Take *capsules* with a full glass (8 ounces) of water, and don't lie down for 15 to 30 minutes afterward. If you're taking the *sustained-release capsule,* swallow it whole. Don't crush, break, or chew it.

To use a *suppository,* follow these steps.
• If the suppository is too soft to insert, run cold water over it or chill it in the refrigerator for about 30 minutes.
• Remove the foil wrapper and moisten the suppository with cold water.
• Lie on your side. With your index finger, gently push the suppository into your rectum as far as possible.
• Keep the suppository in place for at least 1 hour.

What to do if you miss a dose

If you're using the *regular capsules, liquid,* or *suppositories,* take a missed dose when you remember it. But if it's almost time for your next dose, skip the missed dose and take the next one as scheduled. If you're taking *sustained-release capsules* once or twice a day, take a missed dose if it's within 1 to 2 hours after the scheduled time. If it's later, skip the missed dose and take the next dose at its scheduled time.

What to do about side effects

If you develop a hive-like rash or itching, stop taking indomethacin and call your primary health care provider *immediately.* If you become restless, wheeze, and have difficulty breathing or have puffiness around your eyes, seek emergency care *immediately.*

Stop taking the medication and call your primary health care provider *at once* if you have stomach pain; pass black, tarry stools; have severe nausea, heartburn, or indigestion; or vomit coffee ground-like matter.

Tell your health care provider about other side effects, including weakness, sore throat, or swelling of your face, feet, or legs.

What you must know about alcohol and other drugs

Don't drink alcoholic beverages while taking indomethacin. Tell your primary health care provider if you're taking other medications. In particular, mention blood pressure medications, diflunisal (Dolobid), probenecid (Benemid), lithium (Eskalith), and warfarin (Coumadin).

Special directions

• Tell your primary health care provider if you have other medical problems. They may affect the use of this medication.
• Don't drive or perform other activities requiring alertness until you know how you react to this medication.

✔ Keep in mind

• If you're pregnant or think you may be, check with your primary health care provider before taking this medication. Don't breast-feed while taking indomethacin.
• If you're an older adult, you may be especially sensitive to side effects.

Additional instructions

_____

_____

Injecting insulin

Dear Patient,

Your primary health care provider has prescribed insulin injections to control your blood glucose (sugar) level.

How to inject insulin

You have been given instructions on the kind of insulin to use, the correct dose, the number of injections you need each day, and the times to perform them. Follow these instructions exactly — they're tailored especially for you.

Use the guidelines below to help you prepare and administer your insulin injection.

Drawing up insulin into the syringe

To draw up insulin into the syringe correctly, follow these steps.

1 Before you do anything else, wash your hands.

2 If your insulin is the intermediate- or long-acting kind (cloudy), mix it by slowly rolling the bottle between your hands (below) or gently tipping it over a few times. Never shake the bottle vigorously.

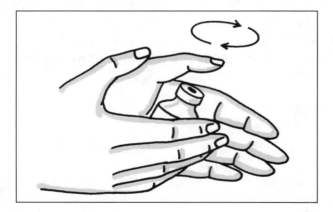

3 Inspect the insulin solution. Don't use the insulin if it looks lumpy or grainy, seems unusually thick, sticks to the bottle, or appears even a little discolored or if the bottle looks frosty. Use regular insulin (short-acting) only if it's clear and colorless.

4 Remove the colored protective cap on the bottle. Don't remove the rubber stopper.

5 Wipe the top of the bottle with an alcohol swab.

6 Remove the needle cover of the insulin syringe.

7 Draw air into the syringe by pulling back on the plunger. The amount of air that you draw into the syringe should be equal to your insulin dose.

8 Gently push the needle through the top of the rubber stopper.

9 Push the plunger in all the way to inject the air from the syringe into the bottle.

10 Turn the bottle with syringe upside down in one hand. Be sure the tip of the needle is covered by the insulin. With your other hand, pull the plunger back slowly to draw the correct dose of insulin into the syringe (below).

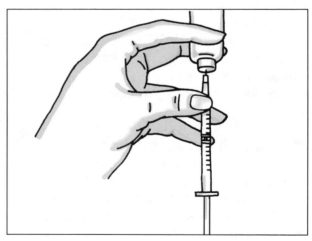

11 Check the insulin in the syringe for air bubbles. To remove air bubbles, push the insulin slowly back into the bottle and draw up your dose again.

12 Check your dose again, then remove the needle from the bottle and recover the needle.

(continued)

Injecting insulin *(continued)*

Mixing two types of insulin

If you're mixing more than one type of insulin in the same syringe, you also need to know the following.

● When mixing two types of insulin, first draw into the syringe the same amount of air as the amount of insulin you'll be withdrawing from each bottle.

● If you're mixing regular insulin with another type of insulin, *always* draw up the regular insulin into the syringe first. When mixing two types of insulin other than regular insulin, you can draw them in any order, but use the same order each time.

● Some insulin mixtures must be injected immediately. Others may be stable for a while, which means you can draw up the mixture into the syringe ahead of time. Check with your primary health care provider, nurse, or pharmacist to find out which type you have.

● If your mixture is stable and you mixed it ahead of time, gently turn the filled syringe back and forth to remix the insulins before you inject them. Don't shake the syringe.

Giving the injection

Inject the insulin into fatty tissue. Injection sites include the thighs, abdomen, upper arms, and buttocks. The abdomen is the preferred site because insulin is absorbed into the bloodstream most evenly from the abdomen. Rotate among injections sites within the same anatomic area as you've been instructed, such as moving from left to right in rows, from the top to the bottom of the area. Remember, inject each new dose at least 1 inch from the previously used site.

After you have prepared your syringe, inject the insulin, following these steps.

1 Clean the site for the injection with an alcohol swab, and let the area dry.

2 Remove the protective covering from the needle. Pinch up a large area of skin and hold it firmly. With your other hand,

push the needle straight into the pinched-up skin at a 90-degree angle (below). Be sure the needle is all the way in.

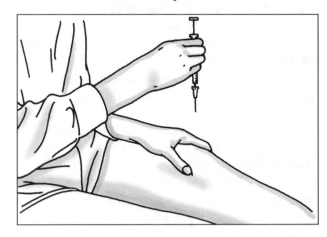

Note: If you're thin or greatly overweight, you may be given special instructions for giving yourself insulin injections.

3 Push the plunger all the way down to inject the dose quickly (in less than 5 seconds).

4 Then hold an alcohol swab near the needle, and pull the needle straight out of the skin (below).

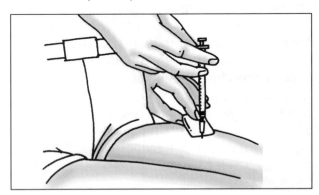

5 Press the swab against the injection site for several seconds. Don't rub.

Note: If you're using an insulin pump for continuous insulin infusion, follow your pri-

(continued)

Injecting insulin (continued)

mary health care provider's and the pump manufacturer's instructions exactly.

What to do if you miss a dose
Follow your primary health care provider's instructions. What you must do depends on the type and amount of insulin you're taking as well as how much time has elapsed since your last insulin injection.

What to do about side effects
Contact your primary health care provider *immediately* if you develop itching, hives, a rash, difficulty breathing, or wheezing after your insulin injection. You may be having an allergic reaction; your primary health care provider will need to change your type of insulin.

Insulin may cause low blood glucose, especially if you delay or miss a meal or snack, exercise much more than usual, or drink alcoholic beverages. Watch for cool pale skin, difficulty concentrating, shakiness, headache, cold sweats, or anxiety — but keep in mind that everyone has different symptoms. Learn your own early symptoms so you can take quick action.

If you have symptoms of low blood glucose, eat or drink something containing sugar, such as glucose tablets or gel or fruit juice. If possible, check your blood glucose level to confirm that it's low. If symptoms don't go away in 15 minutes, again eat or drink something containing sugar and wait another 15 minutes. If symptoms still don't go away, seek emergency medical care *immediately.*

Notify your primary health care provider if you have frequent or severe low blood glucose reactions — your insulin dosage or type may need to be changed.

Tell your primary health care provider if you note skin changes such as pitting or thickening at injection sites.

What you must know about alcohol and other drugs
Because alcohol can cause severe low blood glucose, ask your primary health care provider whether you can safely drink alcoholic beverages and, if so, how much.

Beta blockers (Inderal), clofibrate (Atromid-S), monoamine oxidase (MAO) inhibitors (medications for depression), salicylates, or tetracycline (Achromycin) can prolong a low blood glucose reaction when taken with insulin. Corticosteroids (prednisone) and thiazide diuretics (water pills) can decrease insulin's ability to lower your blood glucose level. Check with your primary health care provider before taking any of these medications.

Special directions
• Tell your primary health care provider if you have other medical problems, especially infections or kidney, liver, or thyroid disease. Other medical problems may affect the use of insulin.
• Although disposable syringes are usually used only once, you may wish to reuse a syringe until its needle becomes dull. If you reuse the syringe, check with your nurse, primary health care provider, or pharmacist for cleaning instructions. Make sure you recap the needle after each use. Throw away the syringe when the needle becomes dull or bent or comes into contact with any surface other than the cleaned and swabbed area of skin.
• Don't use insulin after the expiration date on the package, even if the bottle has never been opened. Instead, check with your pharmacist about the possibility of exchanging bottles.
• Keep unopened bottles of insulin refrigerated until needed. Never freeze insulin. Remove the insulin from the refrigerator and

(continued)

Injecting insulin (continued)

allow it to reach room temperature before injecting it.

• You may keep an insulin bottle in use at room temperature for up to 1 month. Throw away any insulin that has been kept at room temperature for longer than 1 month.

• Don't expose insulin to extremely hot temperatures or to sunlight. Extreme heat will reduce its effectiveness.

• See your primary health care provider regularly so he can check your condition and adjust your insulin therapy as needed.

• If you've been smoking for a long time and suddenly stop, tell your primary health care provider, who will probably reduce your insulin dosage.

• Follow your prescribed diet and exercise plan strictly. Don't miss or delay any meals.

• When you become sick with a cold, fever, or the flu, make sure you take your insulin, but check with the primary health care provider to determine the dose. Take your insulin even if you feel too sick to eat. This is especially true if you have nausea, vomiting, or diarrhea.

• Learn how to check your own blood glucose level and urine for ketones (an acid that may be released from your bloodstream into your urine when your blood glucose level is too high).

• You'll develop high blood glucose if you're not getting enough insulin. Contact your primary health care provider if you experience excessive thirst, hunger, and urination or if your blood glucose levels are high even without symptoms. If left untreated, high blood glucose can cause diabetic coma, an emergency condition.

• Wear a medical identification bracelet or necklace and carry an identification card indicating that you have diabetes and listing your insulin type and dosage.

• Keep a glucagon kit and a syringe and needle available, and teach your family how to prepare and use it if you develop severe low blood glucose. Keep some kind of quick-acting sugar handy to treat low blood glucose symptoms.

• Discuss travel plans with your primary health care provider, especially if you're changing time zones. You may need to make some temporary adjustments to your insulin dosage.

✔ Keep in mind

• If you become pregnant, tell your primary health care provider, who will adjust your insulin therapy.

Additional instructions

_____
_____
_____
_____
_____
_____
_____
_____
_____
_____
_____

Taking oral iron supplements

Dear Patient,

Iron supplements are used to help correct iron deficiency. Your body needs enough iron to produce the number of red blood cells that you need to stay healthy. Brand names for iron supplements may include Feosol, Feostat, Fergon, Fumerin, Mol-Iron, Niferex, Simron, or Slow FE.

How to take oral iron supplements

Iron supplements come in many forms—for example, tablets, capsules, and elixir. Carefully follow your primary health care provider's instructions. For best results, take the supplement on an empty stomach either 1 hour before or 2 hours after meals. Take the supplement with water or, even better, orange juice because vitamin C increases iron absorption into your blood.

If necessary, take iron supplements with food or immediately after meals to reduce stomach upset. However, eggs, milk, coffee, and tea can decrease the absorption of iron.

Don't crush or chew sustained relief preparations. If you're taking the elixir, sip it through a narrow straw to keep it from staining your teeth.

What to do if you miss a dose

Skip the missed dose and take your next dose as scheduled. Don't double dose.

What to do about side effects

Constipation, nausea, and black stools are common. If these problems become bothersome or severe, tell your primary health care provider.

What you must know about other drugs

Don't take iron supplements at the same time as antacids (such as Maalox or Mylanta), fluoroquinolones (such as Cipro and Floxin), tetracycline (Achromycin), cimetidine (Tagamet), levodopa (Dopar), or methyldopa (Aldomet). Ask a nurse, pharmacist, or your primary health care provider to help you schedule these medications to minimize interactions.

Special directions

● Tell your primary health care provider if you're allergic to any iron medication or to another medication, food, or chemical.

! *Warning:* Don't take high doses of iron for longer than 6 months without consulting your primary health care provider. Prolonged overuse could lead to iron poisoning. Also, unabsorbed iron could hide blood in your stool, possibly delaying discovery of a serious disorder.

● To help prevent constipation, drink plenty of fluids, exercise regularly, and eat foods high in fiber, such as fresh fruits and vegetables and foods containing bran and oats.

● Remove tooth stains caused by liquid iron supplements with baking soda or hydrogen peroxide solution (3%).

✓ Keep in mind

● If you're pregnant or breast-feeding, check with your primary health care provider before taking an iron supplement.

● Carefully follow the directions for giving an iron supplement to a child. Overdose and iron poisoning are especially dangerous in children.

● If you're an older adult, check with your primary health care provider before taking an iron supplement.

Additional instructions

_____

_____

_____

Taking isoniazid

Dear Patient,

Your primary health care provider has prescribed isoniazid to treat your tuberculosis (TB). The label may read Laniazid or Nydrazid.

How to take isoniazid

Take this medication exactly as your primary health care provider has prescribed. Take it at the same time each day to help you avoid missed doses. If the medication upsets your stomach, take it with food or an antacid.

Keep taking isoniazid as your primary health care provider directs, even after you feel better. Otherwise, your TB may not clear up completely. You may need to take this medication for 1 year or more.

What to do about side effects

Call your primary health care provider *right away* if you experience any of the following side effects:
• nausea, vomiting, diarrhea, or loss of appetite
• blurred vision, loss of vision, or eye pain
• clumsiness or unsteadiness
• burning, numbness, tingling, or weakness in your hands or feet (which may signal peripheral neuritis)
• fever, hives, itching, or rash—signs of hypersensitivity that may herald an allergic reaction to the medication
• abdominal pain, yellowing of the skin or whites of the eyes, dark urine, or light-colored stools (which may signal liver inflammation)
• behavioral changes, hallucinations, or seizures.

What you must know about alcohol and other drugs

Avoid drinking alcoholic beverages while taking isoniazid because doing so increases the risk of liver problems.

Tell your primary health care provider about prescription and nonprescription medications you're taking because some medications interact with isoniazid. For example, you should avoid taking any antacid that contains aluminum within 1 hour of the time you take isoniazid because the antacid will decrease isoniazid's effectiveness. Isoniazid may increase the potential side effects of phenytoin (Dilantin) and warfarin (Coumadin).

Special directions

• Don't drive or perform other activities requiring alertness and clear vision until you know how your body responds to this medication.

Warning: Avoid Swiss cheese and tuna. Coupled with isoniazid, these foods can cause chills, headache, lightheadedness, red and itchy skin, increased sweating, and rapid or pounding heartbeat. If these symptoms occur, call your primary health care provider *immediately.*

✔ Keep in mind

• If you're pregnant or breast-feeding, check with your primary health care provider before taking isoniazid.
• If you're an older adult, you may be especially sensitive to isoniazid's side effects.

Additional instructions

_____
_____
_____
_____
_____
_____
_____
_____

Taking isoproterenol

Dear Patient,

Isoproterenol is prescribed to relieve the wheezing and shortness of breath caused by asthma, bronchitis, or emphysema or to treat heart rhythm problems. Brand names include Aerolone, Isuprel, and Medihaler-Iso.

How to take isoproterenol

Isoproterenol comes as an aerosol inhaler, a solution used with a nebulizer inhaler, and as sublingual tablets. Follow your primary health care provider's instructions closely.

To use the *aerosol inhaler* or *nebulizer solution,* first clear your nose and throat. Then breathe out, exhaling as much air as you can. Put the mouthpiece in your mouth, release the spray, and inhale deeply. Hold your breath in for a few seconds, then remove the mouthpiece and exhale slowly.

Wait 1 to 2 minutes before using it again. You may not need another spray.

If you're also taking another inhaled medication, take isoproterenol first and wait 5 minutes before taking the other medication.

To take a *sublingual tablet,* place the tablet under your tongue and let it dissolve. Don't chew or swallow it, and don't swallow saliva until it dissolves completely.

Avoid taking isoproterenol at bedtime, if possible. It may disturb your sleep.

What to do if you miss a dose

Take the dose as soon as you can. Then evenly space your remaining doses for the day. Don't double dose.

What to do about side effects

If you think you may have taken an overdose, or if you develop symptoms of an overdose — chest pain, seizures, chills, fever, severe muscle cramps, nausea, vomiting, shortness of breath, severe trembling or weakness, and fast, slow, or fluttering heart-beat — seek emergency care *immediately.*

Also seek emergency care if your skin develops a bluish color and you experience severe dizziness, facial flushing, increased difficulty breathing, a rash, and swelling of your face or eyelids.

Isoproterenol may cause headache and rapid or pounding heartbeat. These side effects should disappear after you use the medication for a while. If they persist, call your primary health care provider.

This medication may also make your saliva a pink-red color.

What you must know about other drugs

Tell your health care provider about other prescription or nonprescription medications you're using, especially a beta blocker (such as propranolol), epinephrine (Adrenalin), or digitalis glycosides (heart medication).

Special directions

• Tell your primary health care provider about other medical problems you have. They may affect the use of this medication.
• If you don't breathe easier after taking the medication, call your primary health care provider right away.
• Avoid caffeine-containing food and drink such as coffee, tea, cola, and chocolate.

✔ Keep in mind

• If you're pregnant or think you may be, or if you're breast-feeding, ask your health care provider before taking this medication.
• If you're an athlete, be aware that isoproterenol is banned and tested for by the U.S. Olympic Committee.

Additional instructions

_____

_____

Taking isosorbide dinitrate

Dear Patient,

This medication is used to treat angina attacks and other heart conditions. The label may read Dilatrate-SR, Isordil, or Sorbitrate.

How to take isosorbide dinitrate
For best results, take isosorbide exactly as your health care provider has instructed.

Regular or extended-release tablets or capsules are used to prevent angina attacks. Take a regular or an extended-release tablet or capsule with a full glass (8 ounces) of water on an empty stomach (30 minutes before or 1 to 2 hours after meals). Swallow the extended-release tablet or capsule whole; don't crush, break, or chew it.

Sublingual or chewable tablets are used to relieve the pain of an attack that is occurring. Place a sublingual tablet under your tongue and let it dissolve. Don't chew or swallow it, and don't swallow saliva until the tablet dissolves completely. Chew a chewable tablet well and hold it in your mouth for about 2 minutes before swallowing.

If you still have chest pain after taking three sublingual or chewable tablets in 15 minutes, get emergency medical care.

What to do if you miss a dose
Take the dose as soon as possible. If it's within 2 hours of your next dose (or within 6 hours if you're taking an extended-release form), skip the missed dose and take the next one as scheduled. Don't double-dose.

What to do about side effects
If you think you may have overdosed, or if you develop bluish lips, nails, or palms; extreme dizziness or fainting; extreme head pressure; shortness of breath; severe tiredness or weakness; weak and fast heartbeat; fever; or seizures — seek emergency medical care *immediately.*

More common side effects — dizziness, rapid or pounding heartbeat, skin redness, headache, nausea, or vomiting — should go away over time. If they don't, consult your primary health care provider.

What you must know about alcohol and other drugs
Don't drink alcohol when you're taking this medication. Check with your primary health care provider if you're also taking a blood pressure medication or another heart medication. These drugs may cause your blood pressure to decrease even more.

Special directions
• Tell your primary health care provider about other medical conditions you have. They may affect the use of this medication.

Warning: Don't suddenly stop using this medication if you've been taking it regularly. This could trigger an angina attack.
• To minimize dizziness or fainting, get up slowly from a lying or sitting position.
• If you're taking extended-release tablets or capsules, call your primary health care provider if you find any partially dissolved tablets in your stool.
• Keep tablets in the original container with a tightly closed lid.

✔ Keep in mind
• If you're pregnant or think you may be, check with your primary health care provider before taking this medication.
• If you're an older adult, you may be especially susceptible to side effects.

Additional instructions
_____
_____
_____

Taking isotretinoin

Dear Patient,

Isotretinoin is prescribed to treat acne. The label may read Accutane.

How to take isotretinoin

Take isotretinoin capsules exactly as prescribed. Take each dose with a meal or shortly afterward. This will help your body absorb the medication.

What to do if you miss a dose

Take the dose as soon as you can. If it's almost time for your next dose, skip the missed dose and take the next one at the scheduled time. Don't double dose.

What to do about side effects

Call your primary health care provider if you develop a headache, nausea, vomiting, severe diarrhea, rectal bleeding, vision problems, decreased tolerance to contact lenses, or burning, redness, and itching of your eyes.

   Dry, itchy skin or pain, soreness, or stiffness in your muscles, bones, or joints should go away after you've taken this medication for a while. If they don't, check with your primary health care provider.

What you must know about alcohol and other drugs

Limit alcoholic beverages when taking isotretinoin because alcohol can increase the triglyceride (fat) level in your blood. Using drying skin preparations, medicated soaps, acne preparations that contain skin peeling agents, and alcohol preparations (such as cosmetics, after-shave lotion, and cologne) can increase skin drying and irritation. Vitamin A and tetracycline antibiotics can aggravate isotretinoin's side effects. Check with your primary health care provider before taking these medications.

Special directions

• Before taking isotretinoin, tell your primary health care provider about other medical problems you have. They may affect the use of this medication.
• When you start this medication, your acne may worsen temporarily. If it becomes severe, check with your health care provider.
• If this medication interferes with night vision, don't drive or perform other activities that could be dangerous if you can't see clearly. Notify your health care provider.
• When you start taking isotretinoin, limit sun exposure to protect light-sensitive skin.
• Relieve mouth dryness with sugarless hard candy or gum, ice chips, mouthwash, or a saliva substitute. If the dryness continues for more than 2 weeks, check with your primary health care provider or dentist.

Warning: Don't donate blood for at least 30 days after you stop taking isotretinoin, so that no pregnant woman receives blood containing this medication.
• A consent form, provided by the manufacturer, will need to be completed by you.

✔ Keep in mind

Warning: Don't take isotretinoin if you're pregnant or think you may be pregnant. Use contraceptive measures if you're a woman of childbearing age.
• Don't take this drug if you're breast-feeding.
• Children are especially susceptible to side effects.
• If you have diabetes, this medication can alter your blood glucose level. If you notice any change, tell your health care provider.

Additional instructions

_____

_____

_____

Taking oral ketoconazole

Dear Patient,

Your primary health care provider has prescribed ketoconazole to treat your fungal infection. The label may read Nizoral.

How to take oral ketoconazole
Take ketoconazole exactly as prescribed. Take it for the full time prescribed even if your symptoms disappear. If you don't, your symptoms may return.

If necessary, take the tablets with food to decrease stomach upset. If you have achlorhydria (absence of stomach acid), your primary health care provider may have you dissolve each tablet in a weak acid solution so your body can absorb it. A pharmacist will prepare the solution for you. After dissolving the tablet, add it to 1 to 2 teaspoons of water in a glass. Drink it through a straw placed far back in your mouth and away from your teeth. Then swish about half a glass (4 ounces) of water around in your mouth and swallow it.

What to do if you miss a dose
Take a missed dose as soon as possible. If it's almost time for your next dose, space the missed dose and the next dose 10 to 12 hours apart. Then resume your normal dosing schedule.

What to do about side effects
If you develop dark urine, pale stools, severe weakness, yellowing of your skin or the whites of your eyes, or loss of appetite, contact your primary health care provider *immediately.*

Nausea, vomiting, diarrhea, headache, dizziness, and drowsiness may occur when you first start taking the tablets but should disappear as your body adjusts to the medication. If these symptoms become bothersome, tell your primary health care provider.

What you must know about alcohol and other drugs
Don't drink alcoholic beverages while you're taking ketoconazole and for at least 1 day after stopping it because alcohol may aggravate liver or stomach problems.

Because many medications can interact with ketoconazole, tell your primary health care provider about other medications you're taking. Don't take antacids or cisapride (Propulsid) with this medication.

Special directions
• Tell your primary health care provider about other medical problems you have. They may affect the use of this medication.
• If your symptoms don't improve in a few weeks or if they get worse, tell your primary health care provider.
• Don't drive or perform other activities requiring alertness until you know how you react to this medication.

✔ Keep in mind
• If you're pregnant or think you may be, check with your primary health care provider before taking this medication. Don't breast-feed while you're taking ketoconazole and for 24 to 48 hours after stopping it.

Additional instructions
_____
_____
_____
_____
_____
_____
_____
_____
_____

Applying topical ketoconazole

Dear Patient,

Your primary health care provider has prescribed ketoconazole to treat your fungal infection. The label may read Nizoral.

How to apply topical ketoconazole
Apply ketoconazole exactly as prescribed. Apply it for the full time prescribed even if your symptoms disappear. If you don't, your symptoms may return.

To apply the cream, first wash your hands. Then apply enough to cover the affected area and surrounding skin. Rub it in gently. Keep the medication away from your eyes. Wash your hands again after applying the cream.

What to do if you miss a dose
Skip the missed dose and apply the cream at the next scheduled time.

What to do about side effects
Ketoconazole cream may cause skin irritation, itching, and stinging. Call your primary health care provider if these effects persist.

Special directions
• Tell your primary health care provider if you're allergic to this or another antifungal medication or to other medications, foods, dyes, or preservatives.
• If you're using this medication for a *skin infection,* keep your skin clean and dry.
• If you're using the cream to treat *ringworm of the groin (jock itch),* wear loose-fitting cotton underwear and use a bland, absorbent powder (such as talcum) on your skin between the times you apply ketoconazole.
• If you're using the cream to treat *athlete's foot,* wear clean cotton socks and change them often to keep your feet dry. Wear sandals or shoes with lots of air holes. Remember to apply talcum or another absorbent powder between your toes, on your feet, and in your socks and shoes once or twice a day, between the times you apply ketoconazole.

✔ Keep in mind
• If you're pregnant or think you may be, or if you are breast-feeding, check with your primary health care provider before using this medication.

Additional instructions
_____
_____
_____
_____
_____
_____
_____
_____
_____
_____

Taking ketoprofen

Dear Patient,

Your primary health care provider has prescribed ketoprofen to relieve fever, pain, swelling, or joint stiffness. The label may read Orudis.

How to take ketoprofen
Take ketoprofen exactly as your primary health care provider has prescribed. Overuse can aggravate side effects.

Continue taking the medication regularly for best results. You may not feel its full effects for several weeks.

Take the capsules with a full glass (8 ounces) of water either 30 minutes before or 2 hours after meals. Avoid lying down for 15 to 30 minutes after you take it. If stomach upset occurs, take the capsules with food or milk.

What to do if you miss a dose
Take the dose as soon as you remember. If it's almost time for your next dose, skip the missed dose and take the next one as scheduled.

What to do about side effects
If you develop a hive-like rash or itching, stop taking ketoprofen and call your primary health care provider *immediately*—you may be experiencing an allergic reaction. Although rare, an allergic reaction can be serious. If you become restless, wheeze, and have difficulty breathing or get puffy around your eyes, get emergency medical care *immediately.*

Ketoprofen may cause stomach ulcers and internal bleeding. Stop taking the medication and call your primary health care provider *at once* if you have stomach pain; pass black, tarry stools; have severe nausea, heartburn, or indigestion; or vomit coffee ground-like matter.

Abdominal cramps, nausea, diarrhea, constipation, gas, headache, nervousness, dizziness, and drowsiness can occur but usually disappear as your body adjusts to the medication. Tell your primary health care provider if these side effects persist or are bothersome.

What you must know about alcohol and other drugs
Don't drink alcoholic beverages while taking ketoprofen because doing so could increase stomach problems.

Tell your primary health care provider about other drugs you're taking, especially probenecid (Benemid) and blood thinners.

Special directions
• Tell your primary health care provider if you have other medical problems. They may affect the use of this medication.
• Because ketoprofen makes some people dizzy or drowsy, don't drive or perform other activities requiring alertness until you know how you react to this medication.

✔ Keep in mind
• If you're pregnant or breast-feeding, check with your primary health care provider before taking ketoprofen.
• If you're an older adult, you may be especially sensitive to side effects.

Additional instructions

_____
_____
_____
_____
_____

Taking labetalol

Dear Patient,

Your primary health care provider has prescribed labetalol to control your blood pressure. Labetalol is one of a group of medications commonly called beta blockers. The label may read Normodyne or Trandate.

How to take labetalol

Take the medication exactly as prescribed, either with food or on an empty stomach, as you prefer. Swallow the tablets whole; don't break, crush, or chew them.

What to do if you miss a dose

Take the dose as soon as you remember unless it's within 8 hours of your next dose. If so, skip the missed dose and take the next one at the scheduled time. Never take two doses at once.

What to do about side effects

Labetalol may cause dizziness and a sudden blood pressure drop when you stand up quickly. If these side effects become bothersome, tell your primary health care provider.

What you must know about alcohol and other drugs

Avoid alcoholic beverages, which in combination with labetalol may cause an excessive drop in blood pressure. Check with your primary health care provider before taking cimetidine (Tagamet), insulin, or oral antidiabetic medications with labetalol.

Special directions

• Tell your primary health care provider about other medical problems you have. They may affect the use of this medication.
• Keep in mind that labetalol controls high blood pressure but doesn't cure it. For this reason, keep taking it as prescribed even if you think you don't need it anymore.

• Make sure you always have enough labetalol on hand, even when you're away from home.

! *Warning:* Don't stop this medication suddenly. Your blood pressure might increase, making your heart problems worse.

• Carry medical identification stating that you're taking labetalol.
• Follow a low-salt diet if your primary health care provider has instructed you to.
• To minimize dizziness, get up slowly from a sitting or lying position.
• Because labetalol may make some people dizzy, don't drive or perform other activities requiring alertness until you know how you respond to this medication.

✔ Keep in mind

• If you're pregnant or breast-feeding, check with your primary health care provider before taking labetalol.
• If you're an older adult, you may be especially sensitive to side effects.

! *Warning:* If you have diabetes, be aware that labetalol may cause your blood glucose level to drop and also may mask signs of low blood glucose (hypoglycemia), such as altered pulse rate.

• If you're an athlete, be aware that the National Collegiate Athletic Association and the U.S. Olympic Committee ban beta blockers.

Additional instructions

_____
_____
_____
_____
_____

Taking lactulose

Dear Patient,

Your primary health care provider has prescribed this laxative to relieve your constipation. This medication is also used to decrease ammonia levels in the blood in patients with liver disease. Lactulose promotes bowel movements by drawing water into the bowel from surrounding body tissues. Brand names for lactulose include Cephulac, Cholac, and Chronulac.

How to take lactulose
Take each dose in or with a full glass (8 ounces) of cold water or fruit juice. For the best effect, your primary health care provider may recommend that you then drink another glass of water by itself.

What to do if you miss a dose
Take the dose as soon as you remember unless it's almost time for your next dose. If so, skip the missed dose and take the next dose at its scheduled time.

What to do about side effects
Side effects include abdominal cramps and bloating, belching, diarrhea, and flatulence (gas). Call your primary health care provider if these effects become bothersome.

What you must know about other drugs
Do not take this drug while taking antacids, antibiotics, or oral neomycin. These drugs will cause lactulose to be less effective.

Special directions
● Before taking lactulose, tell your primary health care provider if you're allergic to laxatives or to another medication or substance.
Warning: Don't use this or any other laxative if you have the following symptoms of appendicitis or an inflamed bowel—lower abdominal or stomach pain,

bloating, cramping, or soreness; nausea; or vomiting. Instead, call your primary health care provider *immediately.*
● If you notice a sudden change in your bowel habits or function that lasts longer than 2 weeks or that keeps returning on and off, contact your primary health care provider before taking lactulose.
● You may have to wait 24 to 48 hours before lactulose starts working.
● Because lactulose contains large amounts of carbohydrates, sodium, and sugar, don't take this medication if you're on a low-calorie, low-sodium, or low-sugar diet. Instead, check with your primary health care provider or pharmacist.

✔ Keep in mind
● Don't give this or any other laxative to a child under age 6 unless your primary health care provider prescribes it.

Additional instructions
_____
_____
_____
_____
_____
_____
_____
_____
_____
_____
_____
_____

Taking lamivudine

Dear Patient,

Your primary health care provider has prescribed lamivudine to treat your human immunodeficiency virus (HIV). This medication helps to slow the spread of the virus and prevent it from weakening your immune system. The brand name for this medication is Epivir.

How to take lamivudine

This medication is available as a tablet or a liquid. It's usually taken twice a day along with other medications, such as zidovudine or Retrovir, to treat your HIV infection. It can be taken either with or without food.

What to do if you miss a dose

Take the missed dose as soon as possible. If it's almost time for your next dose, skip the missed dose and take your next dose on schedule. If you're unsure what to do, call your primary health care provider or pharmacist.

What to do about side effects

You may experience headache, nausea, fatigue, or diarrhea. If these persist or become severe, notify your primary health care provider.

What you must know about alcohol and other drugs

Check with your primary health care provider before drinking alcoholic beverages because the combined effects of alcohol and this medication may increase the risk of drowsiness.

Before starting lamivudine, tell your primary health care provider what other medications you're taking, including those you buy without a prescription from a pharmacy, supermarket, or health food store. He needs this information to make sure that all of your medications can be taken together safely.

Special directions

- Before taking this medication, tell your primary health care provider if you've ever had an allergic reaction to lamivudine or any other medications.
- Tell your primary health care provider if you have other medical problems, especially pancreatic or kidney disease. They may affect the use and dose of lamivudine.
- Lamivudine isn't a cure for HIV infection, and you may continue to develop other infections and complications associated with HIV disease. This medication also won't reduce the risk of transmission of HIV to other people through sexual contact or blood contamination by using the same needles.

✔ Keep in mind

- Tell your primary health care provider if you're pregnant, are planning to become pregnant, or are breast-feeding.

Additional instructions

_____

_____

_____

_____

_____

_____

_____

_____

_____

_____

Taking laxatives

Dear Patient,

Your primary health care provider has prescribed a laxative. Laxatives help move stool through the lower bowel so it can be eliminated. They're prescribed for different reasons. For example, laxatives are taken before a procedure called a colonoscopy to clear the bowel of stool so the colon can be visualized. Laxatives are also used on a short-term basis to help a patient have regular bowel movements again and on a long-term basis to promote bowel movements in patients with certain diseases or those taking medications that cause constipation.

This sheet contains general information about laxatives. Your primary health care provider should also give you an information sheet describing the specific laxative you're taking.

How to take laxatives

Laxatives may be taken by mouth, by rectal suppositories, or by enema. If you're taking a laxative *by mouth*, your primary health care provider may tell you to take it at a certain time each day. It's best to take them on an empty stomach, especially when using bisacodyl (Dulcolax). If you're taking a bulk-forming laxative, such as psyllium (Metamucil), stir each dose into a full (8 ounce) glass of water, and drink a second full glass of water immediately after taking the dose.

If you're using a *rectal suppository*, follow the directions on the package. Unwrap the suppository, and insert the tapered end high inside the rectum. Thoroughly wash your hands before and after insertion. Because some material may leak out of the rectum as the suppository melts at body temperature, wear old undergarments or put a protective shield inside your undergarments until after you have a bowel movement.

If you're giving yourself an *enema*, follow the directions on the package for preparing and administering it. Lie on your left side, on a flat surface, with your knees bent, as shown on the package. Insert the enema tip into the rectum. Squeeze the solution bottle slowly, allowing all the solution to flow into the rectum. Remove the enema tip from the rectum, and remain in this position until you feel lower abdominal cramping and the urge to empty your bowel. Thoroughly wash your hands before and after the procedure. Because some material may leak out of the rectum, wear old undergarments or put a protective shield inside your undergarments after giving yourself an enema.

What to do if you miss a dose

If you miss a dose, take it as soon as you remember. If it's almost time for your next scheduled dose, skip the missed dose and go back to your regular schedule. Don't take double doses.

What to do about side effects

Different laxatives cause different side effects. Call your primary health care provider *right away* if you have bloody stool, black or tarry-looking stool, or severe abdominal pain.

Side effects that don't need reporting include gas, bloating, abdominal cramping for a short period of time relieved by a bowel movement, upset stomach, and a small amount of stool leakage from the rectum. Certain types of stimulant laxatives may discolor your urine reddish pink or brown. Contact your primary health care provider if any of these side effects continue or become bothersome.

What you must know about other drugs

Some medications aren't absorbed as well if they're taken with bulk forming laxatives

(continued)

Taking laxatives (continued)

such as psyllium or emollient laxative such as mineral oil. Check with your primary health care provider if you're taking other medications. He may be able to adjust the dose or timing of the medications, or to prescribe another type of laxative.

Special directions
• Different laxatives act at different times. Ask your primary health care provider or pharmacist how long your particular laxative takes to work. Then be sure to be near a bathroom at that time.
• To avoid constipation, eat 6 to11 servings of dietary fiber a day, drink plenty of fluids, and exercise regularly.

❗ *Warning:* Laxatives are for short-term use only. They should never be used as part of a weight loss or diet regimen. Continued use of laxatives beyond the time recommended by your primary health care provider can cause serious bowel problems and worse constipation.

✔ Keep in mind
• If you're of childbearing age, tell your primary health care provider if you're pregnant, if you're breast-feeding, or if you may become pregnant while on this medication.

Additional instructions

_____
_____
_____
_____
_____
_____
_____
_____
_____
_____

Taking levodopa

Dear Patient,

This medication is usually given to treat Parkinson's disease. Brand names include Dopar and Larodopa.

How to take levodopa
Levodopa comes in tablets and capsules. Check the label carefully. Take only the amount prescribed.

What to do if you miss a dose
Take the missed dose as soon as possible. However, if your next dose is within 2 hours, skip the missed one and resume your regular dosage schedule. Never double dose.

What to do about side effects
Call your health care provider *right away* if you have fatigue; headache; shortness of breath; insomnia; depression; mood, mental status, or behavior changes; or unusual and uncontrolled body movements. Also report if you feel faint, dizzy, or light-headed when rising from a lying or sitting position.

Anxiety, confusion, or nervousness may also occur. If these symptoms persist or are bothersome, call your health care provider.

This medication may turn your urine and sweat red or black. This is normal and does not require medical attention.

What you must know about other drugs
Check with your primary health care provider before taking other prescription or nonprescription medications.

Certain types of monoamine oxidase (MAO) inhibitors (medications for depression) can cause very high blood pressure when taken within 14 days of levodopa. Check with your health care provider about stopping treatment. Also check before taking iron supplements; they can increase the absorption of levodopa.

Special directions
● Tell your health care provider about your medical history before you take levodopa.
● Avoid hazardous activities such as driving until you know how the medication affects you; it may make you drowsy or less alert.
● If levodopa upsets your stomach, take it with food. Don't take it with high-protein foods, such as poultry and eggs; they can make the medication less effective.
● When getting out of bed, change positions slowly and dangle your legs for a few moments to reduce dizziness.
Warning: If your diet includes avocados, bacon, pork, peas, beans, liver, oatmeal, sweet potatoes, or tuna, ask your health care provider if you should limit these foods. They contain large amounts of vitamin B_6 (pyridoxine), which can make levodopa less effective. Don't take supplements containing vitamin B_6 unless your health care provider approves them.
● You may not notice any effects for several weeks. If you don't think it is working, don't stop taking levodopa; call your health care provider. If your symptoms persist or worsen, call your health care provider.
● Store levodopa away from light and humidity; don't use the tablets if appear brown in color.

Keep in mind
● If you're breast-feeding, check with your health care provider before taking levodopa.
● If you have diabetes, your health care provider may need to adjust your dosage of insulin or other diabetes medication. You may also need to change urine glucose tests.

Additional instructions
_____
_____

Taking levodopa with carbidopa

Dear Patient,

This medication is usually given to treat Parkinson's disease. The brand name for this medication is Sinemet.

How to take this medication
This medication is available in tablets. Your health care provider may prescribe three to six tablets daily. Carefully check the label and take only the amount prescribed.

What to do if you miss a dose
Take the missed dose as soon as possible. However, if your next dose is within 2 hours, skip the missed one and resume your regular dosage schedule. Don't double dose.

What to do about side effects
Call your primary health care provider if you experience fatigue, headache, shortness of breath, insomnia, depression, mood or behavior changes, or unusual and uncontrolled body movements.

This medication may make you dizzy, especially when you first start taking it. Tell your primary health care provider if you feel dizzy or light-headed when you get up from a lying or sitting position.

What you must know about other drugs
Check with your primary health care provider or pharmacist before taking other prescription or nonprescription medications. They can change the way levodopa works.

Certain types of monoamine oxidase (MAO) inhibitors (medications for depression) can cause very high blood pressure when taken within 14 days of levodopa. Check with your primary health care provider about stopping treatment. A MAO-B inhibitor, Selegiline, is actually used to treat Parkinson's disease.

Special directions
• Be sure your primary health care provider knows about your medical history before you take this medication.
• Avoid hazardous activities such as driving until you know how this medication affects you. It may make you drowsy or less alert.
• Your health care provider may need to change your dosage (maybe several times) to find the right amount for you to take.
• If this medication upsets your stomach, you may take it with food.
• Before getting out of bed, change position slowly and dangle your legs for a few moments to avoid dizziness.
• Contact your health care provider if you believe your behavior or mood is changing.
• Increase your physical activities gradually so your body can adjust to your changing balance, coordination, and circulation.

Warning: You may not notice this medication's effects for several weeks. If you don't think it's working, don't stop taking it; call your health care provider. Don't increase the dosage if your symptoms persist or worsen; call the health care provider.
• Never crush the tablets.

✔ Keep in mind
• If you're breast-feeding, check with your primary health care provider before taking this medication.
• If you have diabetes, your primary health care provider may need to adjust your dosage of insulin or other diabetes medication. You may also need to switch to another type of urine glucose test.

Additional instructions

_____

_____

_____

Using levonorgestrel

Dear Patient,

This contraceptive prevents pregnancy. It's commonly called Norplant.

How to use levonorgestrel
This medication is available in implant form. Your primary health care provider will make a small cut in your upper arm, put six tablets there, and close the skin over them. The tablets will start to work and won't require any action on your part. Their contraceptive effect lasts for 5 years.

What to do about side effects
Call your primary health care provider if you have pain in your stomach or muscles or discharge from your breasts or vagina.

At first, you should expect changes in your menstrual bleeding pattern. For instance, your menstrual period may stop or it may last longer than usual. You may have spotting, scanty or irregular bleeding, or frequent bleeding episodes. These changes usually go away over time. If they don't, call your primary health care provider.

What you must know about other drugs
Check with your health care provider before taking carbamazepine (Tegretol) or phenytoin (Dilantin) because these medications may make your contraceptive less effective.

Special directions
• Before you get the implants, be sure your health care provider knows your medical history, especially if you've had thrombophlebitis or problems with blood clotting; liver, kidney, or heart disease; seizures; breast cancer; or unusual genital bleeding that hasn't been diagnosed. Also report if you've ever had depression or an emotional disorder.
• Because this contraceptive can cause you to retain fluid, you may need to limit salt in your diet if you've had heart or kidney disease. Follow any specially prescribed diet.
• Don't assume you're pregnant if you miss a menstrual period. However, if your period still doesn't come after 6 or more weeks (after a pattern of regular periods), tell your primary health care provider. This could mean you're pregnant.
• Call your primary health care provider right away if one of the tablets falls out because this could reduce the contraceptive effect.
• Have a physical examination at least every year so your health care provider can check for any problems caused by levonorgestrel.

Warning: Your implants must be removed if you become pregnant, develop redness or swelling in a limb, have jaundice, or must stay in bed for a long time.
• Call your primary health care provider if you notice a change in vision; for instance, if you wear contact lenses and suddenly have vision changes or can't tolerate your lenses.
• Your primary health care provider must remove the tablets from your arm. Don't attempt to do this yourself.
• After the tablets are removed from your arm, the effects may last as long as 6 months to 1 year. But you should still use another method of contraception if you don't want to become pregnant.

✔ Keep in mind
• If you're breast-feeding, inform your health care provider before getting these implants.
• If you suspect you're pregnant—either before or after receiving the implants—make ure to tell your primary health care provider right away.

Additional instructions

_____

_____

Taking levorphanol

Dear Patient,

This medication is usually prescribed to treat moderate to severe pain. The label may read Levo-Dromoran.

How to take levorphanol
This medication is available in tablet and injection forms.

Carefully check the label on your prescription bottle, which tells you how much to take at each dose. Take only the amount prescribed by your primary health care provider.

If you're taking the *injection* form of levorphanol at home, make sure you fully understand your primary health care provider's instructions and follow them carefully.

What to do if you miss a dose
Take the missed dose as soon as you remember. If it's almost time for your next dose, skip the missed dose and resume your regular schedule. Don't double dose.

What to do about side effects
Get emergency help *immediately* if you think you may have taken an overdose. Symptoms of an overdose include slow or troubled breathing, seizures, confusion, severe drowsiness, weakness, dizziness, restlessness, and nervousness.

You may experience milder forms of dizziness or drowsiness, as well as light-headedness, fainting, an unusual feeling of well-being, nausea, vomiting, or constipation. These side effects usually go away over time as your body adjusts to the medication. Check with your health care provider if they persist or become bothersome.

What you must know about alcohol and other drugs
Avoid alcoholic beverages, sedatives (medications that relax you and make you feel sleepy), antihistamines (such as diphenhydramine [Benadryl]), and other depressant medications while taking levorphanol because of the risk of increased sedation.

Special directions
• Don't take levorphanol if you're allergic to it or to similar medications (such as codeine and morphine).
• Be sure your primary health care provider knows about your medical history, especially if you've had an abnormal heart rhythm, a head injury, liver or kidney problems, seizures, or a respiratory disorder, because this medication could cause serious problems. Also tell your primary health care provider if you've ever been addicted to any medication.
• Avoid hazardous activities, such as driving a car or using dangerous tools, because levorphanol may make you drowsy or less alert.

> *Warning:* Don't stop taking this medication suddenly without first checking with your primary health care provider. Levorphanol is a narcotic. If you use it for a long time, you may become dependent on it and have withdrawal side effects when you stop taking it.

✅ Keep in mind
• If you're pregnant or breast-feeding, tell your primary health care provider before taking this medication.
• If you're an older adult, you may be especially sensitive to side effects, particularly breathing problems, when taking levorphanol.

Additional instructions

_____

_____

_____

Applying lindane

Dear Patient,

This medication is prescribed to treat scabies and lice infestations. Other names for the medication include Kwell and Scabene.

How to apply lindane
This medication is available as a cream, lotion, and shampoo. The cream and lotion forms are used to treat scabies. The shampoo form is used to treat lice.

Don't use more than the amount your primary health care provider has ordered, and don't use the medication more often or for a longer time than ordered because this could cause poisoning.

To use the *cream* or *lotion,* apply a thin layer to your freshly washed and dried skin. Use enough medication to cover the entire skin surface from the neck down, including the soles of your feet. Rub in the cream or lotion well, then leave it on. After the prescribed number of hours (usually 8 to 12 hours), wash yourself thoroughly. If you need a second application, wait 1 week before repeating.

To use the *shampoo,* apply it undiluted to freshly washed and dried hair. Apply enough to your dry hair to thoroughly wet both the affected areas and surrounding hair-covered areas. Rub the shampoo into your hair and scalp. If you're applying it while taking a bath, make sure the shampoo doesn't drip onto other parts of your body or into the bath water. Leave it on for 4 to 5 minutes, then add enough water to create a lather. Rinse your hair thoroughly, then dry it with a clean towel. When your hair is dry, comb it with a fine-toothed comb dipped in white vinegar to remove any remaining lice eggs.

What to do about side effects
Call your primary health care provider *right away* if you have symptoms of lindane poisoning, such as seizures, dizziness, nervousness, restlessness, clumsiness, a fast heartbeat, muscle cramps, or vomiting.

If you use lindane repeatedly, your skin may become irritated and you may have toxic medication effects. Report skin irritation to your primary health care provider.

Special directions
• Don't swallow lindane. This medication is poisonous and can be fatal.

! *Warning:* Keep the medication away from your eyes, nose, mouth, and lips. If some gets in your eyes, *immediately* flush them with water and notify your primary health care provider.
• Don't use lindane on open cuts, sores, or inflamed areas of your skin.
• Don't inhale vapors from this medication.
• Your sexual partner and members of your household may need to be treated with lindane because scabies and lice spread through close contact.
• After you wash the medication off your body, change and sterilize (dry-clean or wash in very hot water) all your clothing and bed linens.
• After using lindane shampoo, clean your combs and brushes with lindane shampoo, then wash them thoroughly. Don't use as a regular shampoo.

✓ Keep in mind
• If you're pregnant or breast-feeding, tell your primary health care provider before using lindane.

Additional instructions
_____
_____
_____
_____

Taking lisinopril

Dear Patient,

This medication treats high blood pressure or other heart and kidney conditions and is also used in heart failure and in diabetics to decrease the risk of kidney damage. The label may read Prinivil or Zestril.

How to take lisinopril
Lisinopril is available in tablets. Carefully check the label on your bottle and take only the amount prescribed.

What to do if you miss a dose
Take the dose as soon as you remember. If it's almost time for your next dose, skip the missed one and resume your regular schedule. Don't double dose.

What to do about side effects
Call the primary health care provider *right away* if you suddenly have trouble breathing or swallowing or if you experience dizziness, light-headedness, nausea, vomiting, diarrhea, loss of taste, fever, chills, hoarseness, or swelling of the face, mouth, hands, or feet.

This medication may cause a dry cough. If coughing continues or becomes bothersome, call your health care provider.

What you must know about other drugs
Call your health care provider or pharmacist before using other medications, especially nonprescription remedies for asthma, colds, hay fever, cough, or appetite control. They may change how lisinopril works and cause high blood pressure or other problems.

Diuretics (water pills) or indomethacin (Indocin), an arthritis medication, may cause your blood pressure to drop too low and your potassium level to rise too high if you take them with lisinopril.

Medications and nutritional supplements that contain potassium or salt substitutes may raise your potassium level too high and cause abnormal heart beats. Your health care provider will likely order blood tests to make sure this doesn't happen.

Special directions
- Don't take lisinopril if you know you're allergic to it.
- Tell your primary health care provider about your medical history, especially if you have diabetes; heart, kidney, or liver disease; a kidney transplant; or lupus.
- *Warning:* Call your health care provider *right away* if nausea, vomiting, or diarrhea occurs after you start this medication. These symptoms may cause you to lose too much water and lead to low blood pressure.
- Avoid hazardous activities, such as driving a car or using dangerous tools, until you know how the medication makes you feel. Lisinopril makes some people feel dizzy.
- Follow any special diet the primary health care provider has prescribed.
- *Warning:* You may not notice the effects of this medication for several weeks. But don't suddenly stop taking it if you don't think it's working or if you have unpleasant side effects. Check with your primary health care provider first.
- Continue to take this medication as directed even if you feel well. You may have to take this or another blood pressure medication for the rest of your life.

✔ Keep in mind
- If you're pregnant or breast-feeding, check with your primary health care provider before taking lisinopril.

Additional instructions
_____

_____

Taking lithium

Dear Patient,

Your primary health care provider has prescribed lithium to treat your condition. This medication acts on the central nervous system to help you control your emotions and cope better with everyday problems. Other names for the medication include Eskalith, Lithane, and Lithobid.

How to take lithium

This medication is available in regular and sustained-release tablets, regular capsules, and a syrup. You may need to take up to four doses a day.

Carefully check the label on your prescription bottle, which tells you how much to take at each dose. Take only the amount prescribed by your primary health care provider.

Take doses of lithium every day at regularly spaced intervals to keep a constant amount of the medication in your blood.

If you're taking the *sustained-release tablets,* swallow the tablet whole. Don't crush, chew, or break it before swallowing.

If you're taking the *syrup,* dilute it in fruit juice or another flavored beverage.

What to do if you miss a dose

Take the missed dose as soon as you remember. However, if your next scheduled dose is within 2 hours (or 6 hours for sustained-release tablets), skip the missed dose and resume your regular dosage schedule. Don't double dose.

What to do about side effects

If you have symptoms of lithium toxicity, withhold one dose and contact your primary health care provider *immediately.* These symptoms include diarrhea, nausea, vomiting, drowsiness, muscle weakness, and clumsiness. Also contact your primary

health care provider *at once* if you feel faint or have a fast or slow heartbeat, seizures, an irregular pulse rate, trouble breathing, unusual weakness or fatigue, or weight gain.

Inform your primary health care provider if you start to lose hair, become hoarse, experience depression or unusual excitement, notice your skin getting dry, or become more sensitive to cold temperatures. Report any swelling of the neck, feet, or lower legs. These symptoms mean that lithium is affecting your thyroid function.

You may become thirstier, urinate more often, lose bladder control, and have mild nausea and slight hand trembling while taking lithium. These side effects usually go away over time as your body adjusts to the medication. You should check with your primary health care provider if they persist or become bothersome.

What you must know about other drugs

Check with your primary health care provider before taking diuretics (water pills) or nonnarcotic medications for pain or inflammation (such as indomethacin [Indocin]). These medications can increase the level of lithium in your blood and cause serious side effects.

Tell your primary health care provider if you're taking medications for psychosis (mental illness). When taken with lithium, these medications can increase your chance for side effects and may cause lethargy, tremor, and other symptoms.

Check with your health care provider before taking theophylline (TheoDur, Slo-bid), an asthma medication; sodium bicarbonate (baking soda), which is used to treat indigestion; or large amounts of sodium chloride. These medications may make lithium less effective in treating your condition.

(continued)

Taking lithium *(continued)*

Special directions
- Don't take lithium if you know you're allergic to it.
- Be sure your primary health care provider knows about your medical history, especially schizophrenia, brain or kidney disease, diabetes, difficult urination, severe infection, seizures, heart problems, psoriasis, Parkinson's disease, thyroid disease, or leukemia.
- Avoid hazardous activities, such as driving a car or using dangerous tools, until you know how the medication affects you. Lithium can make you drowsy or less alert.
- To reduce stomach upset, take lithium after meals with plenty of water.
- You probably won't get the full benefits of lithium for several weeks. However, don't stop taking it if you think you're not getting better. Instead, call your primary health care provider.
- Drink 2 to 3 quarts of water or other fluids daily and salt your food as you normally do unless your primary health care provider tells you otherwise.
- If you usually drink large amounts of caffeine-containing beverages (such as coffee, tea, or colas), you may need to cut down on these beverages to get the full benefits of lithium.
- During hot weather and activities that make you sweat heavily, take extra precautions because you could get serious side effects if you lose too much water and salt. For instance, if you start sweating too much, drink more fluids and increase your salt intake.
- **!** *Warning:* Don't switch lithium brands without your primary health care provider's approval.
- Call your primary health care provider before going on a weight-loss diet or making major changes in your diet. If you lose too much water and salt while dieting, serious side effects could occur.

- Make sure to have your lithium blood levels checked regularly because even a slightly increased level can be dangerous.
- Have regular medical checkups so your primary health care provider can make sure lithium is working properly and detect any side effects.
- Carry an identification card that tells others how to respond in case you experience lithium toxicity or another emergency.

✔ Keep in mind
- If you become pregnant while taking lithium, check with your primary health care provider.
- If you're breast-feeding, don't take lithium without your primary health care provider's approval. Lithium may be harmful to your baby.
- If you're an older adult, you may be especially sensitive to the effects of this medication.

Additional instructions

_____

_____

_____

_____

_____

_____

_____

_____

_____

_____

Taking loperamide

Dear Patient,

This medication is usually used to treat diarrhea. Brand names include Imodium and Imodium A-D.

How to take loperamide
This medication is available in tablet, capsule, and liquid forms.

If you buy this medication without a prescription and are treating yourself, carefully follow the instructions on the package. Don't take more than the recommended amount.

If you're taking loperamide by prescription, follow your primary health care provider's instructions carefully.

What to do if you miss a dose
If you're taking loperamide on a regular schedule and you miss a dose, skip the missed dose and resume your regular dosage schedule. Don't double dose.

What to do about side effects
Constipation may occur. If it's severe and occurs suddenly, check with your primary health care provider *immediately.*

What you must know about other drugs
Check with your health care provider if you're taking an antibiotic (a medication used to treat infection). Some antibiotics cause diarrhea. Taking loperamide at the same time may worsen the diarrhea.

Before taking a narcotic pain reliever, check with your health care provider. Combining a narcotic with loperamide may increase your chance for severe constipation.

Special directions
• Don't take loperamide if you're allergic to it or if you have colitis.
• Be sure your health care provider knows about your medical history. Especially mention liver disease, a severely enlarged prostate, or dependence on narcotics.
• After the initial dose, take the medication after each unformed bowel movement until your diarrhea goes away (unless your primary health care provider tells you otherwise).
• Replace the fluid your body has lost from diarrhea. For the first 24 hours, drink plenty of clear liquids that don't contain caffeine (such as caffeine-free cola and tea, ginger ale, gelatin, and broth). After that, you may eat bread, crackers, hot cereal, and other bland foods. Avoid caffeine, spicy or fried foods, vegetables, fruits, bran, candy, and alcoholic beverages.

Warning: If you lose a great deal of fluid from diarrhea, you may suffer dehydration, a serious condition. Call your primary health care provider *right away* if you have dry mouth, increased thirst, decreased urination, dizziness, light-headedness, or abnormally wrinkled skin.
• If your diarrhea doesn't go away after 2 days or if you develop a fever, stop taking loperamide and contact your primary health care provider.

✔ Keep in mind
• If you're breast-feeding or pregnant, check with your primary health care provider before using loperamide.
• Check with your primary health care provider before giving loperamide to a child.
• If you're an older adult, losing fluid from diarrhea can be especially dangerous. Call your health care provider or pharmacist for instructions on how to replace lost fluid.

Additional instructions
_____
_____
_____

Taking loracarbef

Dear Patient,

Your primary health care provider has pre-scribed loracarbef to treat your bacterial in-fection. Loracarbef eliminates bacteria that cause many kinds of infections, including bronchitis, pneumonia, sinusitis, and infec-tions of the ears, skin or urinary tract. The brand name for this medication is Lorabid.

How to take loracarbef

This medication is available in capsules and liquid. It's usually taken twice a day at least 1 hour before or 2 hours after a meal. Drink a full glass of water when taking this med-ication. Finish all of it even if you feel better. If you stop too soon, your infection may re-turn.

Liquid loracarbef may be kept at room temperature for 14 days. Discard any un-used liquid after that time.

What to do if you miss a dose

If you miss a dose, take it as soon as possi-ble. If it's almost time for your next dose, skip the missed dose and take your next dose on schedule. If you're unsure what to do, call your primary health care provider.

What to do about side effects

Contact your primary health care provider *immediately* and stop taking this medication if you develop difficulty breathing, a rash, hives, itching, or wheezing. These symp-toms may mean an allergic reaction.

Common side effects include nausea and diarrhea. If they persist or become se-vere, notify your primary health care provider.

What you must know about alcohol and other drugs

Check with your primary health care provider before drinking alcoholic beverages because the combined effects of alcohol and this medication may increase the risk of drowsiness.

Tell your primary health care provider what other medications you're taking, in-cluding medications you buy without a pre-scription from a pharmacy, supermarket, or health food store. He needs this information to make sure that all of your medications can be taken together safely.

Special directions

• Tell your primary health care provider if you're ever had an allergic reaction to lo-racarbef or any other medication or if you've ever developed a rash while taking a med-ication to treat an infection.
• Tell your primary health care provider if you have a history of kidney disease or any other medical conditions. This may affect the use of loracarbef.
• If your symptoms don't improve within a few days or if they become worse, check with your primary health care provider.
• If you develop diarrhea, don't take a diar-rhea medication without checking with your primary health care provider. It may make your diarrhea worse or make it last longer.

✔ Keep in mind

• Tell your primary health care provider if you become pregnant, plan to become pregnant, or are breast-feeding.

Additional instructions

_____
_____
_____
_____
_____
_____

Taking loratadine

Dear Patient,

Your primary health care provider has prescribed loratadine for your condition. This medication is used to treat nasal and non-nasal symptoms of seasonal allergies and to treat chronic idiopathic urticaria (hives). It's called an antihistamine because it blocks the effects of a substance produced by the body called histamine. The brand name for this medication is Claritin.

How to take loratadine

This medication is available as two kinds of tablets — regular and rapidly dissolving — and as a syrup. Both the tablets and the syrup are taken once a day on an empty stomach, 1 hour before or 2 hours after a meal. However, if loratadine upsets your stomach, it can be taken with food.

To take the rapidly dissolving tablets (Claritin Reditabs), place them on your tongue and close your mouth. The tablet will dissolve in a few seconds, and can then be swallowed with or without water.

What to do if you miss a dose

Take the missed dose as soon as possible. However, if it's almost time for your next dose, skip the missed dose and go back to your regular schedule. Don't take double doses.

What to do about side effects

If you experience a rapid heartbeat, dizziness, unusual weakness, or difficulty urinating while taking loratadine, contact your primary health care provider right away.

This medication occasionally causes headache, fatigue, drowsiness, increased thirst, blurred vision, and dry mouth or nose. These side effects usually disappear with time. Contact your primary health care provider if these symptoms persist or are severe.

What you must know about alcohol and other drugs

Check with your primary health care provider before drinking alcoholic beverages because the combined effects of alcohol and loratadine may increase the risk of drowsiness.

Certain types of medications can also increase the risk of drowsiness from loratadine. These include sleeping pills, sedative-hypnotics, muscle relaxants, narcotic pain medications, some antidepressants, certain types of over-the-counter products, erythromycin, cimetidine, and ketoconazole. Make sure your primary health care provider knows about all the medications you're taking.

Special directions

- Tell your primary health care provider if you have other medical problems, especially liver or kidney problems, because he may need to adjust the dose of loratadine.
- Know how you react to this medication before you drive, use machinery, or perform other activities that require alertness.

✔ Keep in mind

- Before taking loratadine, tell your primary health care provider if you're breast-feeding, pregnant, or trying to become pregnant.

Additional instructions

_____
_____
_____
_____
_____
_____
_____
_____

Taking lorazepam

Dear Patient,

This medication may be prescribed to treat anxiety, tension, agitation, irritability, or insomnia (difficulty sleeping). Brand names include Alzapam and Ativan.

How to take lorazepam

This medication is available in tablets. Carefully check the prescription label, and take only the amount prescribed.

What to do if you miss a dose

If you're taking this medication on a regular schedule, take the missed dose right away if you remember within an hour or so. If you remember more than 1 hour later, skip the missed dose and resume your regular dosage schedule. Don't double dose.

What to do about side effects

If you think you've taken an overdose, get emergency help *immediately.* Symptoms of an overdose include confusion, staggering, slurred speech, extreme drowsiness, and weakness.

Drowsiness, light-headedness, dizziness, and clumsiness may also occur. These side effects usually go away over time as your body adjusts to the medication. Check with your primary health care provider if they persist or become bothersome.

What you must know about alcohol and other drugs

Avoid alcoholic beverages, sedatives (medications that relax you and make you feel sleepy), antihistamines (such as diphenhydramine; [Benadryl]), and other depressants while taking this medication because of the risk of increased sedation.

Special directions

- Don't take lorazepam if you're allergic to it or if you have glaucoma.
- Tell your primary health care provider your medical history, especially psychosis (mental illness), myasthenia gravis, Parkinson's disease, respiratory problems, liver problems, drug addiction, or drug abuse.
- Avoid hazardous activities, such as driving a car or using dangerous tools, until you know how the medication affects you. Lorazepam can make you drowsy or less alert.
- Take the medication only as directed. Don't take it longer than directed because this may cause medication dependence and withdrawal symptoms.

Warning: Don't stop taking this medication without your primary health care provider's approval.

✔ Keep in mind

- If you're pregnant or breast-feeding, tell your primary health care provider before taking lorazepam.
- Older adults are especially likely to become dizzy, drowsy, light-headed, clumsy, and less alert when taking lorazepam.
- If you're an athlete, you should know that lorazepam is banned by the U.S. Olympic Committee and the National Collegiate Athletic Association for athletes participating in shooting events.

Additional instructions

_____
_____
_____
_____
_____
_____

Taking lovastatin

Dear Patient,

This medication is prescribed to lower the levels of cholesterol and other fats in the blood. Lovastatin works by blocking an enzyme that the body needs to make cholesterol. The label may read Mevacor.

How to take lovastatin

This medication is available in tablets.

Carefully check the prescription label, and take only the amount prescribed by your primary health care provider.

Taking this medication with food makes it work better. If your primary health care provider has prescribed one dose a day, take it with your evening meal. If he has prescribed several daily doses, take them with meals or snacks.

What to do if you miss a dose

Take the missed dose as soon as possible. If it's almost time for your next scheduled dose, skip the missed dose and resume your regular dosage schedule. Don't double dose.

What to do about side effects

Contact your primary health care provider *right away* if you have blurred vision, fever, unusual weakness or fatigue, or muscle aches or cramps.

What you must know about other drugs

Check with your primary health care provider if you're taking niacin, an immunosuppressive medication (such as cyclosporine; [Neoral]), or gemfibrozil [Lopid]). These medications increase the risk of side effects from lovastatin.

Special directions

• Don't take this medication if you're allergic to it or if you have liver disease.

• Tell your primary health care provider about your medical history, especially if you've had an organ transplant, if you're about to have major surgery, or if you have low blood pressure, seizures that are difficult to control, or a severe metabolic or endocrine disorder.

• Tell your primary health care provider if you drink large amounts of alcoholic beverages, which can affect your cholesterol level.

• Follow any special diet your primary health care provider has prescribed, such as a low-fat, low-cholesterol diet.

• Have regular medical checkups so your primary health care provider can make sure lovastatin is working properly and detect any side effects.

• Have regular liver function tests, if your primary health care provider orders this.

• Have regular eye examinations because this medication can cause blurred vision.

⚠ *Warning:* Don't stop taking lovastatin unless your primary health care provider approves. Stopping treatment could make your blood cholesterol level rise again.

• Before having surgery (including dental surgery), tell your primary health care provider or dentist you're taking lovastatin.

✓ Keep in mind

• If you're pregnant or breast-feeding, check with your primary health care provider. Lovastatin may cause serious problems in a fetus or breast-feeding baby.

Additional instructions

_____

_____

_____

_____

_____

Taking magnesium hydroxide (milk of magnesia)

Dear Patient,

This medication is used to relieve constipation. The label may read Phillips' Milk of Magnesia.

How to take magnesium hydroxide

This medication is available in an oral solution, an oral suspension, and granules.

You can buy magnesium hydroxide without a prescription. If you're treating yourself, carefully follow the instructions on the label. If your primary health care provider prescribed this medication or gave you special instructions on how to use it and how much to take, follow those instructions carefully.

If you're taking the *oral suspension*, shake it well and take it with a full glass (8 ounces) of fruit juice or water. Make sure that you take plenty of fluids while you're taking this medication.

What to do about side effects

Call your primary health care provider as soon as possible if you become confused, dizzy, or light-headed; if you develop an irregular heartbeat; or if you experience muscle cramps or unusual tiredness or fatigue.

Diarrhea, abdominal cramps, gas, nausea, and increased thirst may occur. These side effects usually subside as your body adjusts to the medication. But you should check with your health care provider if they persist or become bothersome.

What you must know about other drugs

Check with your primary health care provider or pharmacist if you're taking tetracycline (Achromycin) or ciprofloxacin (Cipro) because magnesium hydroxide may make them less effective.

Don't take magnesium hydroxide within 1 to 2 hours of taking another medication by mouth (such as a tablet, capsule, or liquid) because it may make the other medication less effective.

Special directions

• You shouldn't take this medication if you have kidney failure, a colostomy or an ileostomy, abdominal pain, nausea, vomiting, fecal impaction, or intestinal obstruction. Magnesium hydroxide may make these conditions worse.

• Schedule the dose so that the bowel movement it produces won't interfere with your sleep or activities. Magnesium hydroxide usually produces a watery stool in 3 to 6 hours. However, it may take longer if you take a small dose with food.

• *Warning:* Don't take laxatives regularly; they are meant only for short-term relief of constipation. Don't take a laxative if you don't need it or if you miss a bowel movement merely for 1 or 2 days.

• To help prevent the need for a laxative, eat a high-fiber diet, exercise regularly, and increase your fluid intake. Good sources of dietary fiber include bran and other cereals and fresh fruits and vegetables.

• Don't take this medication for more than 1 week unless ordered by your primary health care provider.

• If you have a sudden change in bowel habits that lasts for more than 2 weeks or returns every now and then, contact your health care provider before using this medication. You may have a serious problem.

✓ Keep in mind

• Don't give laxatives to children unless prescribed by your health care provider.

Additional instructions

_____

_____

Taking meclizine

Dear Patient,

This medication is usually prescribed to prevent and treat nausea, vomiting, and dizziness caused by motion sickness. Your primary health care provider sometimes prescribes it to treat dizziness caused by other medical problems. Brand names include Antivert, Bonine, and Ru-Vert-M.

How to take meclizine

This medication is available in regular and chewable tablets and in capsules.

Some preparations of this medication are available only by prescription. Others are available without a prescription. If you're treating yourself, carefully follow the instructions on the label, which tell you how much to take at each dose. If your primary health care provider prescribed this medication or gave you special instructions on how to use it and how much to take, follow those instructions carefully.

What to do if you miss a dose

If you're taking meclizine on a regular schedule, take the missed dose as soon as possible. If it's almost time for your next dose, skip the missed dose and resume your regular dosage schedule. Don't double dose.

What to do about side effects

Drowsiness may occur. If it persists or becomes bothersome, call your primary health care provider.

What you must know about alcohol and other drugs

Avoid alcoholic beverages, sedatives (medications that relax you and make you feel sleepy), antihistamines (such as diphenhydramine [Benadryl]), and other depressant medications while taking meclizine because of the risk of additional sedation.

Special directions

- Don't take meclizine if you're allergic to it or to similar medications, such as buclizine (Bucladin-S Softabs), cyclizine (Marezine), or dimenhydrinate (Dramamine).
- Tell your primary health care provider about other medical problems you have, especially narrow-angle glaucoma, asthma, an enlarged prostate, or a blockage of the genitourinary or GI tract. Meclizine may make these conditions worse.
- Take this medication 1 hour before starting your trip, and continue to take it regularly every travel day during the trip.
- Avoid hazardous activities, such as driving a car or using dangerous tools, until you know how the medication affects you. Meclizine may make you drowsy or less alert.
- If you've been vomiting a lot, be sure to drink plenty of fluids to prevent dehydration.
- If this medication makes your mouth dry, use sugarless gum, hard candy, or ice chips. However, if dry mouth lasts for more than 2 weeks, see your primary health care provider or dentist for further evaluation.

✔ Keep in mind

- If you're pregnant or breast-feeding, check with your primary health care provider before taking meclizine.
- If you're an athlete, you should know that meclizine is banned by the U.S. Olympic Committee and can lead to disqualification in biathlon and pentathlon events.

Additional instructions

_____
_____
_____
_____

Taking medroxyprogesterone

Dear Patient,

This medication is usually prescribed to treat abnormal bleeding of the uterus caused by hormonal imbalance, to treat amenorrhea (absence of menstruation), or to help treat cancer of the endometrium or kidney. Brand names include Amen and Provera.

How to take medroxyprogesterone
This medication is available in tablets. Carefully check the label, which tells you how much to take at each dose. Take only the prescribed amount.

What to do if you miss a dose
Take the dose as soon as you remember. However, if it's almost time for your next dose, skip the missed dose and resume your regular dosage schedule. Don't double dose.

What to do about side effects
Rarely, this medication may cause a blood clot—a life-threatening emergency. If you have any of the following symptoms, stop taking the medication and get medical help *immediately:* pain in the chest, groin, or leg; sudden shortness of breath or loss of coordination; sudden or severe headache; sudden slurring of speech; sudden vision loss or change in vision; or weakness, numbness, or pain in the arm or leg.

If this medication causes changes in your vaginal bleeding pattern, such as spotting, breakthrough bleeding, or prolonged bleeding, report these side effects to your primary health care provider *promptly.*

What you must know about other drugs
Check with your primary health care provider or pharmacist before taking rifampin (Rifadin), a tuberculosis medication, because it may make medroxyprogesterone less effective.

Special directions
• Don't take this medication if you're allergic to it or if you have a history of blood clots, severe liver disease, breast or genital cancer, or undiagnosed abnormal vaginal bleeding. Medroxyprogesterone may make these disorders worse.
• Also tell your primary health care provider about other medical problems you have, especially heart or kidney disease, fluid retention, seizures, migraine headaches, or depression.
• Contact your primary health care provider if your menstrual period doesn't start within 45 days of your last period or if vaginal bleeding lasts an unusually long time.
• Brush and floss your teeth and massage your gums carefully and regularly to help prevent your gums from bleeding. See your dentist regularly.
• Have regular medical checkups so your primary health care provider can check your progress, adjust your dosage if needed, and detect any side effects.

✓ Keep in mind
Warning: If you're pregnant, you shouldn't take this medication. If you become pregnant while taking it, stop taking it immediately because it may harm your fetus.
• If you're breast-feeding, check with your primary health care provider before taking this medication.
• If you have diabetes, report symptoms of high blood glucose (such as increased thirst and urination) to your primary health care provider.

Additional instructions
_____
_____

Taking meperidine

Dear Patient,

This medication is usually prescribed to treat moderate to severe pain. The label may read Demerol.

How to take meperidine
This medication is available in tablets and a syrup. Take only the amount prescribed.

If you're using the *syrup* form, take it with a full glass (8 ounces) of water to reduce numbness of the mouth and throat.

What to do if you miss a dose
If you're taking this medication on a regular schedule, take the missed dose as soon as possible. If it's almost time for your next regular dose, skip the missed dose and resume your regular schedule. Don't double dose.

What to do about side effects
Get emergency help *immediately* if you think you have taken an overdose of meperidine. Symptoms include cold, clammy skin; confusion; seizures; severe dizziness or drowsiness; slow heartbeat; slow or troubled breathing; and severe weakness.

This medication may cause drowsiness, dizziness, light-headedness, faintness, urine retention, nausea, vomiting, or constipation. These side effects usually subside over time; check with your health care provider if they persist or become bothersome.

What you must know about alcohol and other drugs
Don't drink alcoholic beverages or take sleeping pills, sedatives (medications that relax you), or antihistamines (such as diphenhydramine [Benadryl]) while taking meperidine because of the risk of additional sedation.

Check with your primary health care provider if you're taking other prescription or nonprescription medications. They may change the way meperidine works.

Special directions
• Don't take meperidine if you're allergic to it.
• Tell your primary health care provider about other medical problems you have, especially heart rhythm problems, a head injury, liver or kidney problems, asthma, respiratory problems, glaucoma, seizures, or drug abuse or addiction.
• To reduce nausea or vomiting from the first few doses, lie down for a while after taking the dose. If these problems persist, call your primary health care provider.
• This medication may make you feel faint, dizzy, or light-headed when rising from a lying or sitting position. To reduce this effect, get up slowly.
• Avoid hazardous activities, such as driving a car, because meperidine may make you drowsy or less alert.

Warning: If you've been taking meperidine regularly for several weeks or more, don't stop taking it suddenly; this could cause withdrawal side effects. Check with your health care provider for instructions on how to stop meperidine gradually.

✓ Keep in mind
• If you're pregnant or breast-feeding, check with your primary health care provider before taking meperidine.
• Children and older adults are especially sensitive to meperidine's effects.
• If you're an athlete, you should know that meperidine is banned by the U.S. Olympic Committee.

Additional instructions

_____

_____

Taking mesalamine

Dear Patient,

This medication is usually prescribed to treat ulcerative colitis and other inflammatory diseases of the bowel. Another name of the medication is Rowasa.

How to take mesalamine

This medication is available in a rectal suspension and rectal suppositories. Carefully check the label, which tells you how much to take at each dose. Take only the amount prescribed.

If your primary health care provider has prescribed the *suspension,* take it once a day as an enema, preferably at bedtime. You may need to take it for up to 6 weeks. Just before taking the enema, empty your bowel. Then shake the suspension well and administer the enema. Be sure to retain the medication for at least 8 hours.

What to do if you miss a dose

If you remember the same night, take the missed dose as soon as possible. If you don't remember until the next morning, skip the missed dose and resume your regular dosage schedule.

What to do about side effects

Stop taking the medication, and contact your primary health care provider *immediately* if you develop a rash, wheezing, itching, hives, severe stomach or abdominal pain or cramps, fever, bloody diarrhea, or severe headache. These symptoms may mean that you have an intolerance to the medication or a sensitivity to sulfites.

Call your primary health care provider as soon as possible if rectal irritation occurs.

You may experience a mild headache, mild stomach or abdominal pain or cramps, nausea, diarrhea, bloating, and flatulence or gas. These side effects usually go away as your body adjusts to the medication. Check with your primary health care provider if they persist or become bothersome.

Special directions

• Don't take this medication if you're allergic to it or to any of its contents (including sulfites, which are preservatives in some liquid medications).
• Tell your primary health care provider about your medical history, especially if you've had kidney disease, because this medication may further harm your kidneys. Inform your primary health care provider if you're allergic to sulfasalazine (Azulfidine), olsalazine (Dipentum), or aspirin.
• Contact your primary health care provider if you suddenly have rectal pain, bleeding, burning, itching, or other symptoms of irritation after you start using this medication.
• Continue to take this medication for the full time of treatment prescribed by your primary health care provider, even if you feel better within several days. Don't miss any doses.
• Have regular medical checkups so your primary health care provider can evaluate your progress.

Additional instructions

_____
_____
_____
_____
_____
_____
_____
_____
_____

Taking metaproterenol

Dear Patient,

This medication is usually prescribed to treat asthma. It's also used to treat bronchospasm (wheezing or difficulty breathing) associated with chronic bronchitis, emphysema, or other lung diseases or to prevent bronchospasm caused by exercise. Brand names include Alupent and Metaprel.

How to take metaproterenol

This medication is available as an inhalation aerosol, an inhalation solution, or an oral tablet or syrup. You may need to take it up to 12 times daily if you're using the inhalation aerosol, every 4 hours if you're using the inhalation solution in a nebulizer, or every 6 to 8 hours if you're taking it orally.

Carefully check the label, which tells you how much to take at each dose. Take only the amount prescribed.

To take the *aerosol,* shake the container. Then exhale through your nose completely. Inhale deeply through your mouth, then take the medication. Hold your breath for 10 seconds, then exhale slowly. Don't take more than two inhalations at a time unless prescribed. After the first inhalation, wait 1 to 2 minutes to see if you need a second inhalation.

If you're using this medication in a *nebulizer* or a *combination nebulizer and respirator,* make sure you understand how to use it. Ask your primary health care provider or pharmacist if you have any questions.

What to do if you miss a dose

If you're using this medication regularly, take the missed dose as soon as you remember. If you have more doses left that day, take them at regularly spaced intervals. Don't double dose.

What to do about side effects

Warning: If you think you may have taken an overdose, get emergency medical help *immediately.* Symptoms of an overdose include severe dizziness, lightheadedness, headache, chills, fever, nausea, vomiting, severe muscle cramps, severe weakness, blurred vision, severe shortness of breath or troubled breathing, or unusual anxiety or restlessness.

Trembling, nervousness, and restlessness may occur. These side effects usually go away over time as your body adjusts to the medication. Check with your primary health care provider if they persist or become bothersome.

If you're using an oral inhaler, you may notice an unusual or unpleasant taste. This symptom will go away when you stop using the medication.

What you must know about other drugs

Check with your primary health care provider if you're taking a beta blocker because it may prevent metaproterenol from working properly. Beta blockers are medications prescribed to treat high blood pressure or angina. Some examples are atenolol (Tenormin), labetalol (Normodyne), and propranolol (Inderal).

Notify your primary health care provider if you're taking ergoloid mesylates (Hydergine), ergotamine (Ergomar), maprotiline (Ludiomil), or a tricyclic antidepressant (a medication for depression). These medications may increase metaproterenol's effects on the heart and blood vessels.

Check with your primary health care provider if you're taking a digitalis glycoside (a medication used to treat an abnormal heart rhythm) because this medication increases the chance for an irregular heartbeat when taken with metaproterenol.

(continued)

Taking metaproterenol *(continued)*

If you're taking a monoamine oxidase (MAO) inhibitor (a medication for depression), check with your primary health care provider. Metaproterenol may increase the effects of the MAO inhibitor if the two medications are taken within 2 weeks of each other.

Special directions

• Don't take this medication if you're allergic to it. If you have tachycardia (a too-fast heart rhythm), don't take metaproterenol because it may worsen this condition.
• Be sure your primary health care provider knows your medical history, especially if you have brain damage, seizures, diabetes, an underactive thyroid, heart disease, or blood vessel disease. Metaproterenol may make these conditions worse.

Warning: Call your primary health care provider *right away* if you still have trouble breathing or if your condition gets worse after you start using this medication.
• If you're using the *aerosol* form, keep the spray away from your eyes to avoid irritation.
• If you're using the *aerosol* form and are also using an adrenocorticoid aerosol or ipratropium (Atrovent) aerosol, take metaproterenol at least 5 minutes before the other aerosol, unless your primary health care provider tells you otherwise. Adrenocorticoids available in aerosol form include beclomethasone (Beclovent), dexamethasone (Decadron Respihaler), and flunisolide (AeroBid).
• If your mouth and throat feel dry after taking this medication, try rinsing your mouth with water after each dose.
• Save the applicator because you may be able to get refills.
• Don't use more of the medication or use it more often than recommended (unless your primary health care provider tells you to)

because this could cause serious side effects.
• After using this medication for a long time, contact your primary health care provider if you find that its effects don't last as long as they did when you first started using it.

✔ Keep in mind

• If you're pregnant or breast-feeding, check with the primary health care provider before taking metaproterenol.
• If you're an older adult, you may be especially sensitive to the effects of this medication.
• If you have diabetes, your primary health care provider may need to adjust the dosage of your insulin or other diabetes medication.

Additional instructions

_____
_____
_____
_____
_____
_____
_____
_____
_____
_____
_____
_____
_____

Taking metformin

Dear Patient,

Your primary health care provider has prescribed metformin for the treatment of your type II diabetes. This medication decreases the amount of sugar made by the liver, increases the uptake of sugar by the muscle cells, and interferes with the absorption of sugar in the intestine. Unlike some diabetes medications, metformin doesn't increase the release of insulin by the pancreas.

This medication is used either alone or in combination with other diabetes medications. The brand name is Glucophage.

How to take metformin
This medication is available as a tablet. It's usually taken two or three times a day and should be taken with meals.

What to do if you miss a dose
In general, you should take the missed dose as soon as you remember it. However, if it's almost time for your next dose, skip the missed dose and go back to your regular schedule. Don't take double doses.

What to do about side effects
Rarely, this medication can cause a serious (sometimes fatal) side effect called lactic acidosis. This usually occurs in people whose kidneys aren't working properly. Signs and symptoms include weakness, fatigue, unusual muscle pain, difficulty breathing, unusual or unexpected stomach discomfort, a cold feeling, dizziness or lightheadedness, or a slow or irregular heartbeat that develops suddenly. If you notice any of these symptoms, stop taking metformin and contact you primary health care provider *immediately*.

Another rare side effect is hypoglycemia, or low blood sugar. This usually occurs when metformin is taken in combination with other blood sugar lowering medications. Symptoms include headache, sweating, shakiness, anxiety, increased heart rate, weakness, numbness or tingling of the mouth or lips, fatigue, and blurred vision. If you have any of these, drink a small glass of fruit juice or nondiet soda, or eat something with sugar, and then call your primary health care provider right away.

The most common side effects of metformin are diarrhea, nausea, upset stomach, bloating, flatulence, anorexia, and an unpleasant or metallic taste in the mouth. These side effects usually disappear with time. Contact your primary health care provider if they persist or become severe or if the stomach-related side effects go away and then come back.

What you must know about alcohol and other drugs
Avoid drinking excessive amounts of alcohol while taking metformin because it increases the risk of lactic acidosis.

Remind your primary health care provider that you're taking metformin whenever he prescribes a new medication for you or changes a dose of one of your regular medications. He may need to adjust the metformin dosage.

Special directions
● Tell your primary health care provider if you have other medical problems, especially liver or kidney disease, congestive heart failure, or a history of alcoholism. He may decide not to prescribe metformin.
● Tell your primary health care provider if you develop an illness resulting in severe vomiting, diarrhea, or fever, or if you're unable to drink your normal amount of fluids. He may need to stop your metformin temporarily.

(continued)

Taking metformin (continued)

• Tell your primary health care provider if you're having surgery or any type of X-ray procedure involving injection of contrast agents. He may need to stop your metformin temporarily.

• Don't skip or delay meals or exercise more than usual. This can cause hypoglycemia.

• Keep all appointments with your primary health care provider. He needs to monitor you closely while you're on this drug.

✔ Keep in mind

• If you're breast-feeding, pregnant, or trying to become pregnant, let your primary health care provider know. He'll need to monitor your blood and kidney and liver function periodically while you're on metformin.

Additional instructions

_____

_____

_____

_____

_____

_____

_____

_____

_____

_____

Taking methimazole

Dear Patient,

Methimazole is used to treat an overactive thyroid gland. Another name is Tapazole.

How to take methimazole
This medication is available in tablets. Carefully check the label and take only the amount prescribed.

If your health care provider has prescribed more than one daily dose, take the doses at evenly spaced intervals throughout the day and night. If you need help in planning the best times to take the doses, call your health care provider or pharmacist.

Take this medication at a consistent time in relation to meals. Either take all doses on an empty stomach or take all doses with meals. If this medication upsets your stomach, you may want to take it with meals.

What to do if you miss a dose
Take the missed dose as soon as possible. If it's almost time for your next regular dose, take both doses together, then resume your regular schedule. If you miss two or more doses, check with your health care provider.

What to do about side effects
Call your primary health care provider *immediately* if you experience nausea, vomiting, fever, chills, a sore throat, malaise, unusual bleeding, or yellowing of the eyes.

What you must know about other drugs
Tell your health care provider if you are taking potassium iodide (Pima), lithium (Lithane), or iodinated glycerol (Iophen). These drugs may reduce thyroid function too much and increase the risk for goiter (swollen thyroid gland) when taken with methimazole.

Avoid nonprescription cough remedies because they may contain iodine, which may make methimazole less effective.

Tell your health care provider if you're taking digoxin (Lanoxin) for your heart. Methimazole can increase digoxin blood levels.

Special directions
• Avoid this medication if you're allergic to it.
• Tell your primary health care provider about other medical problems you have, especially an infection or liver disease.
• To maintain the proper amount of this medication in your blood, don't skip any doses.
• When your thyroid function becomes normal, your primary health care provider may reduce your dosage.
• Ask your primary health care provider whether you can eat shellfish or use iodized salt. The iodine in these substances may make methimazole less effective.
• If you're injured or get sick, you may need to stop taking this medication or take a different dosage for a while. Call your primary health care provider for instructions.

! *Warning:* Contact your health care provider if you have symptoms of an underactive thyroid (mental depression, intolerance to cold, or swelling); your dosage may need to be changed.
• This medication may take several weeks to work. Don't stop taking it without consulting your primary health care provider.
• Tell your health care provider or dentist before having surgery (including dental surgery).

✓ Keep in mind
• If you're pregnant, make sure your health care provider monitors you during therapy.
• If you're breast-feeding, ask your health care provider before using methimazole.

Additional instructions

_____

_____

Taking methocarbamol

Dear Patient,

This medication is usually prescribed to relax muscles and to relieve pain and discomfort caused by muscle injury (such as sprains and strains). Brand names include Delaxin and Robaxin.

How to take methocarbamol

This medication is available in tablets. Carefully check the prescription label. Take only the amount prescribed. If you have trouble swallowing tablets, you may crush the tablets and mix them with food or liquid.

What to do if you miss a dose

Take the dose right away if you remember within an hour or so. Otherwise, skip the missed dose and resume your regular dosage schedule. Don't double dose.

What to do about side effects

Call your primary health care provider *right away* if you develop a fever, a fast heartbeat, skin rash or redness, itching, hives, shortness of breath, troubled breathing, wheezing, tightness in the chest, stinging or burning of the eyes, red or bloodshot eyes, or a stuffy nose.

You may experience vision changes (including blurring or double vision), dizziness, light-headedness, or drowsiness. These effects usually go away as your body adjusts to the medication. But check with your primary health care provider if they persist or become bothersome.

This medication may discolor your urine. This effect goes away once you stop taking the medication.

You may notice a metallic taste. If it becomes bothersome, try eating sugarless hard candy.

What you must know about alcohol and other drugs

Avoid alcoholic beverages, sedatives, antihistamines (such as diphenhydramine [Benadryl]), and other depressant medications while taking methocarbamol because of the risk of oversedation.

Special directions

• Don't take this medication if you're allergic to it.
• Tell your health care provider about other medical problems you have, especially allergies, kidney disease, seizures, or a blood disease caused by an allergy to another medication.
• Tell your primary health care provider if you've ever abused or been dependent on drugs.
• To prevent stomach upset, take this medication with meals or milk.
• Avoid hazardous activities, such as driving a car or using dangerous tools. Methocarbamol may make you drowsy or less alert and may affect your vision.
• If you're taking this medication for more than a few weeks, have regular medical checkups so your primary health care provider can evaluate your progress and detect any unwanted side effects.

✔ Keep in mind

• If you're breast-feeding, ask your health care provider before taking methocarbamol.
• If you're an athlete, you should know that methocarbamol use is banned and tested for by the U.S. Olympic Committee and the National Collegiate Athletic Association.

Additional instructions

_____

_____

Taking methotrexate

Dear Patient,

This medication is often prescribed to treat psoriasis or rheumatoid arthritis. (In higher doses, it's also used to treat cancer. However, this instruction sheet doesn't apply to that use.) Brand names include Folex and Rheumatrex.

How to take methotrexate

This medication is available in tablets. Carefully check the prescription label, and take only the prescribed amount.

What to do if you miss a dose

If you miss a dose, skip it and resume your regular schedule. Then call your primary health care provider. Don't take double doses.

What to do about side effects

Call your primary health care provider *immediately* if you have diarrhea; reddened skin; red spots on the skin; stomach pain; mouth or lip sores; black, tarry stools; bloody urine or stools; blurred vision; seizures; cough; hoarseness; fever; chills; lower back or side pain; painful urination; shortness of breath; or unusual bleeding or bruising.

Check with your primary health care provider *promptly* if you have dark urine, dizziness, drowsiness, headache, unusual fatigue or weakness, or yellow eyes or skin.

Hair loss may occur. However, after you finish methotrexate treatment, your hair should grow back.

If nausea and vomiting occur, check with your primary health care provider. If you vomit shortly after taking a dose, ask your primary health care provider whether you should take the dose again or wait until the next scheduled dose.

What you must know about alcohol and other drugs

Avoid drinking alcoholic beverages, which may increase unwanted effects on the liver.

Check with your health care provider before taking other drugs, including nonprescription medications. Especially avoid taking aspirin and other medications used for pain and inflammation because they may increase the risk of serious side effects.

Special directions

• Tell your primary health care provider about other medical problems you have, especially a stomach ulcer, colitis, an immune system disease, liver or kidney disease, or a blood disorder.

❗ *Warning:* Don't get immunizations during treatment except with your health care provider's approval. Also, avoid people who've recently taken the oral polio vaccine.

✅ **Keep in mind**

• If you're breast-feeding, check with your primary health care provider before taking methotrexate because it may cause serious side effects in your baby.

❗ *Warning:* Don't take this medication if you're pregnant, and practice birth control during treatment and at least 3 months after it ends. Methotrexate may cause birth defects if either the mother or father takes it at the time of conception or if the mother takes it during pregnancy. Call your primary health care provider immediately if you think you're pregnant.

• If you're an older adult, you may be especially sensitive to the effects of methotrexate.

Additional instructions

_____

_____

Taking methyldopa

Dear Patient,

This medication is usually prescribed to treat high blood pressure. It controls impulses along certain nerve pathways, which relaxes blood vessels. The prescription label may read Aldomet.

How to take methyldopa

This medication is available in tablets and an oral suspension. Carefully check the label, and take only the prescribed amount.

What to do if you miss a dose

Take it right away. If it's almost time for your next dose, skip the missed dose and resume your regular schedule. Don't double dose.

What to do about side effects

Call your primary health care provider *immediately* if you develop a fever shortly after you start taking this medication.

Contact your primary health care provider *as soon as possible* if you experience swelling of the feet or lower legs, depression, anxiety, nightmares, stomach pain or cramps, pale stools, diarrhea, nausea, vomiting, fever, chills, joint pain, troubled breathing, fast heartbeat, weakness, a rash, itching, dark or amber urine, or yellow eyes or skin.

Drowsiness, dry mouth, and headache may occur. You may feel dizzy or light-headed when getting up from a lying or sitting position. Check with your primary health care provider if these side effects persist or become bothersome.

What you must know about other drugs

Check with your primary health care provider before taking levodopa. When combined with methyldopa, this medication may lower your blood pressure too much and cause other problems.

Contact your primary health care provider before taking a tricyclic antidepressant or a monoamine oxidase (MAO) inhibitor (medications for depression) or a phenothiazine (used for anxiety, nausea and vomiting, or psychosis). Combining one of these medications with methyldopa may cause high blood pressure.

Don't take any nonprescription remedies (such as for colds, hay fever, or cough) without first checking with your primary health care provider or pharmacist. These medications may increase your blood pressure.

Special directions

• Tell your primary health care provider your medical history, especially if you're taking diuretics (water pills) or other medications to reduce your blood pressure. Also report if you have Parkinson's disease, kidney or liver problems, or mental depression or if you've ever had liver problems when taking methyldopa in the past.
• Avoid hazardous activities, such as driving a car or using dangerous tools, until you know how the medication affects you. Methyldopa can make you drowsy or less alert.
• Follow any special diet the health care provider prescribed, such as a low-salt diet.
• *Warning:* Don't suddenly stop taking this medication if you don't think it's working or if unpleasant side effects occur. Instead, contact your health care provider.

✔ Keep in mind

• If you're an older adult, you may be especially sensitive to methyldopa's side effects.

Additional instructions

_____

_____

_____

Taking or giving methylphenidate

Dear Patient or Caregiver,

Your primary health care provider has prescribed methylphenidate to treat attention deficit hyperactivity disorder (ADHD) or narcolepsy. This medication activates various places in the brain causing a stimulant effect. The brand names include Ritalin and Ritalin-SR.

In children with ADHD, this medication has a calming effect, increasing attention span and decreasing restlessness. In narcolepsy, it reduces the number of daytime sleep attacks so the patient can lead a more normal life.

How to take or give methylphenidate
This medication is available as a regular-release and a sustained-release tablet. If you're an adult, you'll probably be instructed to take the regular-release tablet two or three times a day, 30 to 45 minutes before meals. Take the last dose several hours before bedtime to avoid sleeplessness.

If the patient is a child, you'll probably be instructed to give methylphenidate twice a day before breakfast and lunch. The sustained-release tablet is usually given every 8 hours and should be swallowed whole; don't crush it or let your child chew it.

What to do if you or your child miss a dose
Take or give the missed dose as soon as possible; then divide remaining doses for that day at evenly spaced intervals. Avoid taking or giving the medication late in the day or near bedtime. If you remember a missed dose and it's almost time for the next dose, skip the missed dose and go back to the regular schedule. Don't take or give double doses.

What to do about side effects
If you or your child experience dizziness, drowsiness, heart palpitations, loss of appetite, skin rash, fever, sore throat, or unusual bleeding or bruising, call your primary health care provider *right away*. Also report nervousness or difficulty sleeping if these symptoms are bothersome or severe.

What you must know about other drugs
Tell your primary health care provider about all the other medications you or your child are taking, especially warfarin (Coumadin), guanethidine (Ismelin), monoamine oxidase (MAO) inhibitors, and medications for seizures.

Special directions
• Tell your primary health care provider if you or your child have other medical problems, especially anxiety, glaucoma, seizures, hypertension, drug dependence, alcoholism, motor tics, or a family history or diagnosis of Tourette syndrome.

✔ Keep in mind
• Loss of appetite, stomach pain, weight loss with long-term use, insomnia, and increased heart rate occur more commonly in children.
• If you're pregnant or breast-feeding, inform your primary health care provider before taking this medication.

Additional instructions
_____
_____
_____
_____
_____
_____

Taking methylprednisolone

Dear Patient,

This medication is usually given to treat severe inflammation caused by allergies, asthma, skin problems, or arthritis. Brand names for this medication include Depo-Medrol and Medrol.

How to take methylprednisolone

This medication is available in tablets and as an enema. Carefully check the prescription label, and take only the prescribed amount. This medication can also be given as an injection by the nurse or the primary health care provider.

If you're taking the *enema,* use the entire contents of the bottle unless your primary health care provider tells you otherwise. Insert the rectal applicator tip gently. If your primary health care provider has instructed you to take the enema slowly, shake the bottle every so often during administration.

What to do if you miss a dose

If you're taking one dose every other day, take the missed dose as soon as possible if you remember it the same morning. Then resume your regular schedule. If you don't remember until later, take the missed dose the next morning, then skip a day and start your regular schedule again.

If you're taking one dose a day, take the missed dose as soon as you remember, then resume your regular schedule. If you don't remember until the next day, skip the missed dose. Don't double the next dose.

If you're taking several doses a day, take the missed dose as soon as possible, then resume your regular schedule. If you don't remember until it's time for your next regular dose, double the next dose.

What to do about side effects

Call your primary health care provider *as soon as possible* if you have decreased or blurred vision, frequent urination, increased thirst, confusion, excitement, hallucinations, depression, mood swings, a false sense of well-being, unusual feelings of self-importance or of being mistreated, or restlessness.

If you've been taking this medication for a long time, report any of the following side effects to your primary health care provider: nausea; vomiting; stomach pain or burning; skin problems; bloody or black, tarry stools; filling out of the face; irregular heartbeat; menstrual problems; muscle cramps, pain, or weakness; pain in the back, hips, arms, shoulders, ribs, or legs; pitting, scarring, or skin depression (at the place of injection); reddish purple lines on the arms, legs, face, trunk, or groin; swelling of the feet or lower legs; thin, shiny skin; unusual bruising; unusual weakness or fatigue; rapid weight gain; or wounds that won't heal.

This medication may also cause increased appetite, indigestion, nervousness, or trouble sleeping. Call your primary health care provider if these side effects persist or become bothersome.

If you're taking the *enema,* call your primary health care provider if you experience rectal pain, bleeding, burning, blistering, itching, or other irritation that wasn't present before you started using this medication.

If you take the medication for a long time, you may experience side effects when you stop taking it. For instance, you may have an upset stomach, loss of appetite, fatigue, weakness, joint pain, fever, dizziness or light-headedness (especially when rising from a sitting or lying position), lethargy, depression, or fainting.

(continued)

Taking methylprednisolone *(continued)*

What you must know about alcohol and other drugs

Avoid drinking alcohol while taking this medication. Combining alcohol with this medication increases the chance for stomach problems.

Check with your primary health care provider or pharmacist if you're taking other medications. They may change the way methylprednisolone works, methylprednisolone may change the way other medications work, or serious problems could occur. For instance, barbiturates (such as phenobarbital), phenytoin (Dilantin), and rifampin (Rifadin) may make methylprednisolone less effective. Aspirin and indomethacin (Indocin) may increase the risk of stomach upset and bleeding.

Special directions

• Tell your primary health care provider about other medical problems you have, especially bone, heart, liver, or kidney disease; colitis; diverticulitis; a stomach or an intestinal disorder; diabetes; infection; glaucoma; high blood pressure; kidney stones; high cholesterol levels; an overactive or underactive thyroid; myasthenia gravis; or lupus. Also tell him if you've ever had tuberculosis or if you've recently had surgery or a serious injury.
• Take this medication in the morning unless your primary health care provider tells you otherwise.
• You may take the tablets with food if they cause stomach upset.
• Follow any special diet your primary health care provider has prescribed, such as a low-salt, high-potassium diet. He also may want you to add protein to your diet and take potassium supplements.
• Have regular medical examinations so your primary health care provider can check your progress.

❗ *Warning:* Don't get immunizations when taking this medication unless your primary health care provider approves. Avoid close contact with people who have recently taken oral polio vaccine.
• Don't suddenly stop taking this medication after long-term use (greater than 2 weeks) because this can be fatal. Check with your primary health care provider for instructions on reducing the dosage gradually before stopping treatment.
• If this medication is injected into one of your joints, don't put too much strain or stress on that joint at first. While the joint is healing, don't move it more than your primary health care provider permits. Call him if you have persistent redness or swelling at the place of injection.

✔ Keep in mind

• If you're pregnant or breast-feeding, tell your primary health care provider before taking methylprednisolone.
• Older adults are especially likely to develop high blood pressure or bone disease when taking this medication.
• If you have diabetes, you may need to change the dosage of your diabetes medication. Call your primary health care provider for instructions.
• If you're an athlete, you should know that the U.S. Olympic Committee and the National Collegiate Athletic Association restrict athletes' use of this medication.

Additional instructions

_____
_____
_____
_____
_____

Taking metoclopramide

Dear Patient,

This medication may be prescribed to prevent nausea and vomiting after treatment with anticancer medications, to help diagnose stomach or intestinal problems, or to treat stomach reflux disease. It also may be used to treat certain GI disorders or to help relieve nausea, vomiting, and bloating after meals. The label may read Reglan.

How to take metoclopramide
This medication is available in tablets and as a syrup. Carefully check the label and take only the amount prescribed. Take this medication 30 minutes before meals and at bedtime unless otherwise directed.

What to do if you miss a dose
Take the dose as soon as you remember. If it's almost time for your next dose, skip the missed dose and resume your regular schedule. Don't double dose.

What to do about side effects
Warning: Call your primary health care provider *promptly* if you experience a fever, chills, sore throat, loss of balance, odd tongue movements, arm or leg stiffness, shuffling walk, or difficulty swallowing or speaking.

If you're taking high doses, a panic-like sensation, lower leg discomfort, or unusual restlessness, nervousness, or irritability may occur within minutes. Report these effects to the primary health care provider *as soon as possible.*

Drowsiness usually goes away over time. If it persists or becomes bothersome, check with your primary health care provider.

What you must know about other drugs
Avoid sedatives (medications that relax you and make you feel sleepy), antihistamines (such as diphenhydramine [Benadryl]), and other depressants while taking this medication because of the risk of oversedation.

Check with your primary health care provider before taking a narcotic pain reliever or an anticholinergic medication (used to treat spastic disorders of the stomach or intestine). These medications can prevent metoclopramide from working properly.

Special directions
• Don't take this medication if you're allergic to it or to a sulfonamide.
• Tell your primary health care provider about other medical problems you have, especially stomach bleeding, breast cancer, intestinal blockage, Parkinson's disease, seizures, or severe kidney or liver disease.
• Avoid hazardous activities, such as driving a car or using dangerous tools, until you know how this medication affects you. Metoclopramide can make you drowsy or less alert.
• Don't take this medication for more than 12 weeks unless instructed to by your primary health care provider.

✔ Keep in mind
• If you're an older adult, you may become sensitive to metoclopramide if you take it for a long time. Children are more sensitive than adults to the effects of this drug.
• If you're an athlete, you should know that metoclopramide use is banned by the U.S. Olympic Committee and the National Collegiate Athletic Association.

Additional instructions
_____
_____
_____
_____
_____

Taking metolazone

Dear Patient,

This medication is usually prescribed to treat high blood pressure. Your primary health care provider also may prescribe it to treat heart failure or kidney disease. Brand names include Mykrox and Zaroxolyn.

How to take metolazone
This medication is available in tablets. Carefully check the prescription label. Take only the prescribed amount.

What to do if you miss a dose
Take it right away. If it's almost time for your next dose, skip the missed dose and resume your schedule. Don't double dose.

What to do about side effects
Call your primary health care provider *right away* if you have fever; chills; lower back, side, or joint pain; severe stomach pain; a rash; hives; red spots on the skin; unusual bleeding or bruising; yellow skin or eyes; bloody urine or stools; or black, tarry stools.

Call your primary health care provider if you experience increased thirst, irregular heartbeat, muscle pain or cramps, nausea or vomiting, unusual fatigue or weakness, or mood or mental changes.

You may notice appetite loss, diarrhea, decreased sexual performance, stomach upset, and increased sensitivity to sunlight. You may feel dizzy or light-headed when getting up from a sitting or lying position. Check with your primary health care provider if these side effects persist or become bothersome.

What you must know about other drugs
Check with your primary health care provider before taking another medication, especially nonprescription medications for colds, cough, hay fever, asthma, or appetite control.

Cholestyramine (Questran) and colestipol (Colestid), medications used to lower cholesterol levels, may prevent metolazone from working properly. Digitalis (a heart medication) may increase the risk for digitalis side effects. Nonsteroidal anti-inflammatory medications (such as ibuprofen, naproxen [Naprosyn], and indomethacin [Indocin]) may decrease the effects of metolazone.

Special directions
• Don't take this medication if you're allergic to it.
• Tell your primary health care provider about other medical problems you have, especially diabetes, gout, lupus, inflammation of the pancreas, or heart, blood vessel, liver, or kidney disease.
• Follow any special diet your primary health care provider has prescribed, such as a low-salt, high-potassium diet.
• Keep taking this medication exactly as directed, even if you feel well.

✔ Keep in mind
• If you're breast-feeding or you become pregnant while taking this medication, check with your primary health care provider.
• If you're an older adult, you may feel dizzy and light-headed. Get up slowly when moving from a lying to a standing position.
• If you have diabetes, this medication may increase your blood glucose level. Be sure to test your blood or urine for glucose regularly.
• If you're an athlete, you should know that metolazone use is banned by the U.S. Olympic Committee and the National Collegiate Athletic Association.

Additional instructions

_____

_____

Taking metoprolol

Dear Patient,

Metoprolol is prescribed to treat high blood pressure and is sometimes used after a heart attack. The label may read Lopressor.

How to take metoprolol

This medication is available in regular and sustained-release tablets. Take only the amount prescribed. To help the medication work better, take the tablets with meals.

What to do if you miss a dose

Take the missed dose as soon as possible. If it's within 4 hours of your next regular dose, skip the missed dose and resume your regular schedule. Don't double dose.

What to do about side effects

Call your primary health care provider *right away* if you experience wheezing or difficulty breathing, confusion, hallucinations, slow or irregular heartbeat, cold feet or hands, or swelling of the feet or ankles.

You may experience trouble sleeping, drowsiness, dizziness, light-headedness, reduced sexual ability, or unusual fatigue or weakness. Call your primary health care provider if these effects persist.

What you must know about other drugs

Ask your health care provider before taking other drugs, including nonprescription ones. They may alter the way metoprolol works.

Barbiturates and rifampin (Rifadin) may decrease the effects of metoprolol.

Chlorpromazine (Thorazine), cimetidine (Tagamet), and verapamil (Calan) may cause your blood pressure to drop too much when taken with metoprolol.

Monoamine oxidase (MAO) inhibitors (medications for depression) may cause severe high blood pressure if taken within 14 days of metoprolol.

Special directions

• Tell your health care provider if you have heart or blood vessel disease, diabetes, kidney or liver disease, depression, asthma, bronchitis, emphysema, hay fever, hives, an unusually slow heartbeat, or an overactive thyroid.

Warning: Ask your health care provider about checking your pulse rate regularly while taking metoprolol. If it's slower than your usual rate (or below 50 beats per minute), don't take metoprolol; call your health care provider. Don't stop taking metoprolol even if you feel well or if side effects occur. Check with your health care provider.

• If metoprolol makes you urinate frequently, take it early to prevent sleep disruption.

• Avoid hazardous activities, such as driving a car, until you know metoprolol's effects.

• Follow any diet your primary health care provider prescribes.

✔ Keep in mind

• If you're pregnant or breast-feeding, check with your primary health care provider before taking metoprolol.

• If you're an older adult, you may be sensitive to the effects of this medication.

• If you have diabetes, tell your health care provider. Metoprolol may decrease your blood glucose level and may mask signs of low blood glucose (such as a change in your pulse rate). The dosage of your diabetes medication may need to be changed.

• If you're an athlete, you should know that metoprolol use is banned by the U.S. Olympic Committee and National Collegiate Athletic Association.

Additional instructions

_____

_____

Taking metronidazole

Dear Patient,

This medication is usually prescribed to treat trichomoniasis (an infection of the sex organs) or amebiasis (an infection of the intestine). Brand names include Flagyl, Metizol, and Protostat.

How to take metronidazole
This medication is available in tablets and as an oral suspension. Carefully check the label and take only the amount prescribed.

To keep a constant amount of this medication in your blood, space doses evenly.

You may crush the tablets before swallowing, if necessary. If this medication causes stomach upset, take it with meals.

What to do if you miss a dose
Take the dose as soon as you remember. If it's almost time for your next dose, skip the missed dose and resume your regular schedule. Don't double dose.

What to do about side effects
Call your primary health care provider *immediately* if you have seizures or if you experience pain, tingling, numbness, or weakness in your hands or feet.

This medication may cause a metallic taste. You can use sugarless hard candy if this is bothersome.

Metronidazole may turn your urine reddish brown.

Headache, dizziness, light-headedness, diarrhea, nausea, vomiting, stomach pain, and appetite loss may occur. Call your primary health care provider if these side effects persist or become bothersome.

What you must know about alcohol and other drugs
Don't drink alcoholic beverages or take medications that contain alcohol (such as cough syrup) during treatment and for at least 48 hours afterward.

Check with your primary health care provider before taking an anticoagulant (blood thinner). Combining metronidazole with an anticoagulant may increase your chance for bleeding.

Special directions
● Tell your primary health care provider about your medical history, especially if you have heart or liver disease, blood problems, central nervous system problems (such as seizures), or edema (swelling).
● Avoid hazardous activities, such as driving a car or using dangerous tools, until you know how this medication affects you. Metronidazole may make you dizzy.
● If you're taking this medication to treat amebiasis, see your primary health care provider for follow-up visits. You may need to provide stool specimens for 3 months after treatment ends to make sure your infection is gone. To prevent reinfection, wash your hands after bowel movements and before handling and eating food. Avoid eating raw foods.

Warning: If you're taking this medication to treat trichomoniasis, avoid intercourse or use a condom. Your primary health care provider may want to treat your sexual partner while you're being treated.

Keep in mind
● If you're in the first 3 months of pregnancy or if you're breast-feeding, check with your primary health care provider before taking this medication.

Additional instructions
_____
_____
_____

Using miconazole

Dear Patient,

This medication is usually prescribed to treat fungus infections, such as athlete's foot, jock itch, and vaginal yeast infections. Brand names include Micatin, Monistat-Derm, and Monistat.

How to use miconazole
This medication is available in cream, lotion, powder, spray, vaginal cream, and vaginal suppositories.

You can buy some preparations of this medication without a prescription. If you're treating yourself, carefully follow the instructions on the package.

If your health care provider prescribed this medication or gave you instructions on how to use a nonprescription preparation, follow those instructions carefully.

If you're using the *spray,* shake it well before applying. Spray it on the affected area from a distance of 4 to 6 inches. If you're using the spray on your feet, spray it between your toes, on your feet, and in your socks and shoes. Don't inhale the spray.

If you're using the *powder* on your feet, sprinkle it between your toes, on your feet, and in your socks and shoes.

If you're using the *vaginal cream* or *suppositories,* insert the applicator or suppository high into your vagina at bedtime for the number of days specified on the package or prescribed by your health care provider.

What to do if you miss a dose
Administer the dose as soon as you remember. If it's almost time for your next dose, skip the missed dose and resume your regular schedule.

What to do about side effects
Call your health care provider *as soon as* you notice a rash, burning, redness, blister-ing, or other type of skin irritation that wasn't there before you started using miconazole.

Special directions
• Don't take miconazole if you're allergic to it. If you have liver disease, ask your health care provider before using miconazole.
• Don't apply an airtight cover (such as plastic wrap) over the treated area unless your primary health care provider tells you to because this may irritate your skin.
• If you plan to use a vaginal form and are using any other vaginal medication, check with your primary health care provider before starting treatment.
• If you're using the vaginal cream or suppositories, wear a sanitary pad to prevent clothing stains. To help clear up your infection, wear only freshly washed, cotton underwear and avoid using tampons during treatment. If you have intercourse during treatment, don't stop using this medication.

! *Warning:* Avoid using latex contraceptive diaphragms or latex condoms because the latex could cause an interaction with the medication. Your sexual partner may also need to be treated.
• Take this medication for the full time of treatment, even if your condition improves. If your condition doesn't improve within 4 weeks or if it gets worse, call your primary health care provider.

✔ **Keep in mind**
• If you're pregnant, check with your primary health care provider before using the vaginal form of this medication.

Additional instructions

_____

_____

_____

Applying minoxidil

Dear Patient,

This medication is prescribed to stimulate hair growth. The label may read Rogaine.

How to apply minoxidil

This medication is available as a topical solution.

Carefully check the label on your prescription applicator, which tells you how much to use at each dose. Use only the amount prescribed. Using more won't speed hair growth or cause more hair to grow. In fact, using too much might cause unwanted side effects.

Apply the medication once in the morning and again at bedtime, using the applicator provided. Before applying the morning dose, shampoo your hair and towel-dry it thoroughly. Then use the applicator to spread the medication. Start at the center of the bald area.

After applying your bedtime dose, let the medication dry for at least 30 minutes. This allows more to be absorbed by your scalp and less by your pillowcase.

What to do if you miss a dose

Apply the missed dose as soon as possible, then resume your regular dosage schedule. If it's almost time for your next dose, skip the missed dose and go back to your regular schedule. Don't apply the medication twice or try to make up for a missed dose some other way.

What to do about side effects

Call your health care provider *at once* if you have difficulty breathing, chest pain, a fast or irregular heartbeat, flushing, headache, dizziness, faintness, rapid weight gain, swelling of the feet or lower legs, or numbness or tingling in your hands, feet, or face.

Check with your primary health care provider if your scalp starts burning or itching, if your face swells, or if you notice a rash.

Your skin may become reddened or dry and flake, and you may have increased hair growth on your face, arms, and back. These side effects usually go away over time as your body adjusts to the medication. But you should check with your primary health care provider if they persist or become bothersome.

What you must know about other drugs

Don't apply other medications to your scalp while using minoxidil. Other medications may prevent minoxidil from working properly or cause unwanted side effects.

Special directions

• Tell your primary health care provider about your medical history, especially if you have heart disease or high blood pressure or if you've had other skin problems, irritation, or sunburn on your scalp.
• If you apply minoxidil by hand, wash your hands thoroughly when you're finished.
• Don't use a hair dryer during treatment because this might make the medication less effective.
• Stop using the medication temporarily if your scalp gets irritated or sunburned; but check with your primary health care provider first.
• You may have to use minoxidil for 4 or more months before you see results, and you must use it every day. If you stop using it, hair growth stops and you can expect to lose any new hair within a few months.

Additional instructions

_____

_____

Taking mirtazapine

Dear Patient,

Your primary health care provider has prescribed mirtazapine for the treatment of depression. Antidepressants are thought to increase the amount of certain chemicals in the brain, helping to improve your mood, appetite, and sleep problems. The brand name for this medication is Remeron.

How to take mirtazapine
This medication is available as a tablet. Take it exactly as your primary health care provider orders—usually, once a day at bedtime. You may not notice the full benefits for several weeks. Don't stop taking the medication without checking with your primary health care provider.

What to do if you miss a dose
Take the missed dose as soon as you remember it. However, if you don't remember until the next morning, skip the missed dose, and then go back to your regular schedule. Don't take double doses.

What to do about side effects
Contact your primary health care provider *right away* if you have a sore throat, fever, chills, mouth sores, flulike symptoms, or other signs of infection. Also report dry mouth, constipation, abnormal dreams, abnormal thinking, and confusion. These side effects may disappear with time.

The most common side effects are drowsiness, dizziness, light-headedness, increased appetite, and weight gain. Call your primary health care provider if these problems persist or become severe.

What you must know about alcohol and other drugs
Don't drink alcohol while taking mirtazapine.

This medication also shouldn't be taken in combination with diazepam (Valium), a monoamine oxidase (MAO) inhibitor (such as Nardil or Parnate), or within 14 days of stopping an MAO inhibitor. Check with your primary health care provider before taking any nonprescription medications or herbal products.

Special directions
- Tell your primary health care provider if you have other medical problems, especially liver, kidney, or heart disease; drug dependency; high cholesterol; high blood pressure; seizures; or a history of stroke or transient ischemic attacks.
- Know how you react to this medication before you drive, use machinery, or perform other activities that require alertness.

✔ Keep in mind
- Before taking mirtazapine, tell your primary health care provider if you're pregnant, trying to get pregnant, or breast-feeding.
- Older adults are especially sensitive to the effects of mirtazapine.

Additional instructions

_____
_____
_____
_____
_____
_____
_____
_____
_____

Taking misoprostol

Dear Patient,

This medication is usually prescribed to prevent stomach ulcers in patients who are taking anti-inflammatory medications (such as aspirin). A brand name of this medication is Cytotec.

How to take misoprostol
This medication is available in tablets. You may need to take it four times a day.

Carefully check the prescription label. Take only the amount prescribed.

To make the medication work better, take it with or after meals and at bedtime.

What to do if you miss a dose
Take the missed dose as soon as possible. If it's almost time for your next regular dose, skip the missed dose and resume your regular dosage schedule. Don't double dose.

What to do about side effects
Diarrhea and abdominal or stomach pain may occur. These side effects usually go away over time as your body adjusts to the medication. Check with your primary health care provider if diarrhea lasts more than 1 week or if abdominal or stomach pain persists or becomes bothersome.

Special directions
• Tell your primary health care provider about your medical history, especially if you have blood vessel disease or have had uncontrolled seizures. Misoprostol may worsen blood vessel disease and may trigger seizures.
• Avoid smoking cigarettes because this increases stomach acid secretion and may make your ulcer worse.
• If your primary health care provider has prescribed this medication to treat a duodenal ulcer, you may take an antacid to help

relieve stomach pain (unless he tells you not to). However, avoid antacids that contain magnesium because they may worsen diarrhea caused by misoprostol.
• Keep taking this medication for the full time of treatment, even if you start to feel better. Don't take it for more than 4 weeks, unless your primary health care provider wants you to continue treatment for another 4 weeks to make sure your ulcer heals completely.

✓ Keep in mind
• If you're breast-feeding, check with your primary health care provider before using misoprostol.
• If you're a woman of childbearing age, you must have had a negative pregnancy test within 2 weeks before starting misoprostol. You must begin taking this medication on the second or third day of your next normal menstrual period and must use an effective birth control method during treatment.

Warning: If you become pregnant or even suspect you're pregnant while taking this medication, stop taking it immediately and call your primary health care provider. This medication may cause miscarriage, uterine contractions, and uterine bleeding.

Additional instructions
_____
_____
_____
_____
_____
_____
_____
_____

Taking morphine

Dear Patient,

Morphine is usually prescribed to relieve pain. Brand names include Astramorph, Duramorph, and MSIR.

How to take morphine
Take only the amount prescribed. If you're taking the *extended-release tablets,* be sure to swallow them whole. Don't break, crush, or chew them.

If you're taking the *liquid* form, use a measuring spoon to measure your dose. Mix it with juice to improve its taste.

If you're using *suppositories,* remove the wrapper and moisten the suppository with cold water. Lie on your side. Using your finger, push the suppository well up into your rectum.

If you're taking the *injection* form, your primary health care provider or nurse will teach you how to administer it.

What to do if you miss a dose
If you're taking morphine on a regular schedule, take the missed dose as soon as you remember. If it's almost time for your next regular dose, skip the missed dose and resume your schedule. Don't double dose.

What to do about side effects
Get emergency help *immediately* if your heartbeat seems unusually fast, slow, or pounding; if you start wheezing or have trouble breathing; if your hands and face swell; or if you start sweating a lot.

Call your primary health care provider *right away* if your breathing rate drops to 8 to 10 breaths a minute, if you have hallucinations, or if you feel confused, dizzy, or unusually weak or tired.

If itching or a rash develops, you may have an allergic reaction. Stop the medication and contact your health care provider.

Nausea, vomiting, or constipation may occur, especially at first. If these side effects continue, call your health care provider.

What you must know about alcohol and other drugs
Avoid alcohol and sleeping pills or antihistamines during morphine treatment.

Check with your health care provider or pharmacist if you're taking other prescription or nonprescription medications. They may change the way morphine works.

Special directions
• Take morphine at regular times. Don't wait until your pain is severe.
• Get up slowly from a lying or sitting position to avoid feeling faint or dizzy.
• Avoid hazardous activities such as driving because morphine may make you drowsy.
• If nausea is severe or if you vomit, ask your health care provider for medication to prevent this.
• To help prevent constipation, eat a well-balanced, high-fiber diet.

! *Warning:* If you've been taking morphine regularly, don't stop taking it suddenly. Ask your primary health care provider how to discontinue it gradually.

✓ **Keep in mind**
• If you're pregnant or breast-feeding, check with your primary health care provider before taking morphine.
• Children and older adults are especially sensitive to the effects of morphine.
• If you're an athlete, know that morphine is banned by the U.S. Olympic Committee.

Additional instructions

_____

_____

Applying mupirocin

Dear Patient,

This medication is usually prescribed to treat bacterial infections of the skin (such as impetigo). The label may read Bactroban.

How to apply mupirocin

This medication is available in an ointment.

In Canada, you can buy this medication without a prescription. If you're treating yourself, carefully follow the instructions on the package, which tell you how much to take at each dose.

If your primary health care provider prescribed this medication or gave you special instructions on how to use it, follow those instructions carefully. Apply only the amount prescribed by your primary health care provider.

Your primary health care provider will probably instruct you to apply mupirocin to affected skin areas two or three times daily. Before applying it, clean the affected area with soap and water and dry it thoroughly. Then apply a small amount of the ointment, rubbing it in gently.

What to do if you miss an dose

Apply the missed dose as soon as possible. If it's almost time for your next regular dose, skip the missed dose and resume your regular dosage schedule.

What to do about side effects

This medication may cause a rash, redness, or dryness. Also, you may notice itching, burning, pain, tenderness, or swelling at the place where you apply it. These side effects usually go away over time as your body adjusts to the medication. Check with your primary health care provider if they persist or become bothersome or if you have other side effects.

Special directions

- Don't use mupirocin if you're allergic to it.
- If desired, you may cover the treated area with a gauze dressing.
- Keep this medication out of your eyes.
- Don't apply mupirocin on burns.

! *Warning:* To make sure your infection heals completely, continue to use this medication for the full time of treatment prescribed by your primary health care provider, even if your symptoms disappear. Don't skip any doses.

- Don't use this medication for a longer period than your primary health care provider prescribes or the package instructions specify.
- Call your primary health care provider or pharmacist if your condition doesn't improve within 3 to 5 days or if it gets worse.

Additional instructions

_____
_____
_____
_____
_____
_____
_____
_____
_____
_____
_____

Taking nabumetone

Dear Patient,

Nabumetone is usually prescribed to reduce joint pain, swelling, and stiffness caused by arthritis. The label may read Relafen.

How to take nabumetone
This medication is available in tablets.

Carefully check the prescription label. Take only the prescribed amount.

If nabumetone gives you heartburn, you may take it with food or an antacid. However, you should check with your primary health care provider first.

What to do if you miss a dose
Take the missed dose as soon as you remember. However, if it's almost time for your next regular dose, skip the missed dose and resume your regular dosage schedule. Never take a double dose.

What to do about side effects
Call your primary health care provider *right away* if you see blood in your urine, if you start urinating less often, or if you have diarrhea, black stools, sore throat, wheezing, dizziness, drowsiness, light-headedness, ringing in your ears, vision changes, swollen ankles, or a rash.

You may experience stomach or abdominal cramps or pain, headache, heartburn, indigestion, nausea, or vomiting. These side effects usually go away over time as your body adjusts to the medication. But you should check with your primary health care provider if they persist or become bothersome.

What you must know about alcohol and other drugs
Don't drink alcoholic beverages while you're taking this medication. The combination may make you overly drowsy.

Check with your primary health care provider or pharmacist before taking other medications. Many medications increase the chance for serious side effects when taken with nabumetone. Especially avoid taking aspirin or steroids because these medications increase the risk of stomach or intestinal side effects.

Special directions
Warning: Don't take this medication if you're allergic to it or to aspirin.
• Tell your health care provider about your medical history, especially if you have intestinal disease, stomach ulcers, kidney disease, or heart or blood vessel disease.
• Take all doses at the prescribed times. Don't postpone taking a dose to make the medication last longer than intended.
• Avoid driving or performing any activities that require alertness until you know the effects of nabumetone.
• Keep taking this medication even if your symptoms don't get better right away. Nabumetone may take about 1 month to achieve its full effect.
• If you're taking this medication for a long time, be sure to get regular medical checkups so your primary health care provider can evaluate your progress.

Keep in mind
• If you're pregnant or breast-feeding, check with your primary health care provider before taking this medication.
• If you're an older adult, you may be especially sensitive to the medication's side effects.

Additional instructions

_____

_____

Taking nadolol

Dear Patient,

This medication is usually prescribed to treat angina (chest pain) or high blood pressure. The label may read Corgard.

How to take nadolol
Carefully check the prescription label. Take only the amount prescribed.

What to do if you miss a dose
Take the dose right away if you remember within an hour or so. However, if it's within 8 hours of your next dose, skip the missed dose and resume your regular schedule. Don't double dose.

What to do about side effects
Call your primary health care provider at once if you start wheezing, have difficulty breathing, or experience confusion, hallucinations, a slow or irregular heartbeat, cold feet or hands, or swelling of the feet or ankles.

You may have trouble sleeping, drowsiness, dizziness, light-headedness, reduced sexual ability, or unusual fatigue or weakness. These usually go away over time. Check with your health care provider if they persist or become bothersome.

What you must know about other drugs
Check with your primary health care provider before taking other medications, including nonprescription medications. Some medications may prevent nadolol from working properly. Prescription medications used to reduce blood pressure may increase the effects of nadolol on the heart.

Digitalis (a heart medication) may cause a too-slow heart rate when combined with nadolol.

Other medications used to treat angina may cause increased effects on your blood pressure when taken with nadolol.

Epinephrine may constrict your blood vessels and slow your heart rate when taken with nadolol.

Special directions
• Don't take nadolol if you're allergic to it.
• Tell your primary health care provider about your medical history, especially if you have heart or blood vessel disease, diabetes, kidney disease, liver disease, mental depression, asthma, hay fever, hives, bronchitis, emphysema, an unusually slow heartbeat, or an overactive thyroid.
• While taking nadolol, check your pulse rate regularly. If it's slower than your usual rate, don't take the dose, and call your primary health care provider.
• Avoid hazardous activities such as driving a car; nadolol may make you drowsy.
• Your health care provider may need to increase your dosage gradually to find the amount that causes the best response.

✔ Keep in mind
• If you have diabetes, check with your primary health care provider. This medication may cause your blood glucose level to drop and may mask signs of low blood glucose (such as a change in your pulse rate). Also, the dosage of your diabetes medication may need to be changed.
• If you're pregnant or breast-feeding, check with your health care provider before taking nadolol.
• Older adults may be especially sensitive to the side effects of this medication.
• Athletes should be aware that nadolol is banned by the U.S. Olympic Committee and the National Collegiate Athletic Association.

Additional instructions

_____

_____

Taking naproxen

Dear Patient,

Naproxen is usually prescribed to reduce joint pain, swelling, and stiffness caused by arthritis. The label may read Naprosyn.

How to take naproxen
Naproxen comes in regular and extended-release tablets and an oral suspension. Check the label. Take only as prescribed.

Take each dose with a full glass (8 ounces) of water. Stay upright for about 30 minutes afterward.

Be sure to swallow the *extended-release tablets* whole. Don't crush or break them.

Take *regular tablets* with food or an antacid if naproxen causes heartburn. Check with your primary health care provider first.

Shake the *oral suspension* well before measuring a dose; don't mix it with an antacid.

What to do if you miss a dose
Take the dose as soon as you remember. However, if it's almost time for the next dose, skip the missed dose and resume your regular schedule. Don't double dose.

What to do about side effects
Call your primary health care provider *at once* if you see blood in your urine or start urinating less often, or if you have diarrhea, black stools, sore throat, wheezing, dizziness, drowsiness, light-headedness, ringing in your ears, vision changes, swollen ankles, or a rash.

Headache, heartburn, indigestion, nausea, vomiting, or stomach or abdominal cramps or pain may occur. Call your health care provider if these side effects persist or become bothersome.

What you must know about alcohol and other drugs
Avoid alcohol while taking this medication. The combination may make you drowsy.

Check with your health care provider before taking other medications. Many medications increase the chance for serious side effects when taken with naproxen. Avoid aspirin and steroids because these medications increase the risk of stomach or intestinal (GI) side effects.

Special directions
Warning: Don't take this medication if you're allergic to it or to aspirin.
• Tell your health care provider of your medical history, especially if you've had stomach or intestinal disease, ulcers, kidney disease, or heart or blood vessel disease.
• Avoid hazardous activities, such as driving a car, until you know how you react to naproxen because it may make you drowsy.
• Take all doses at the prescribed times. Don't postpone a dose to make the medication last longer than intended.
• Keep taking naproxen even if your symptoms don't get better right away. Naproxen may take 1 month to achieve its effect.
• If you're taking this medication for a long time, your primary health care provider should evaluate your progress regularly.

Keep in mind
• If you're pregnant, check with your health care provider before taking this medication.
• If you're an older adult, you may be especially likely to have GI side effects.

Additional instructions

_____

_____

_____

Taking a narcotic pain medication

Dear Patient,

Your primary health care provider has prescribed a narcotic pain medication (analgesic) to relieve your pain. This medication works on the brain and spinal cord to relieve pain.

This information sheet contains general information about narcotic pain medications. It's not meant to replace a sheet describing the particular medication you're taking.

How to take a narcotic pain medication

This medication comes in tablet, capsule, liquid, injection, or rectal suppository form. Take it exactly as directed by your primary health care provider.

If you're taking a long-acting *tablet,* swallow it whole. Don't break, crush, or chew it.

If you're taking the *liquid* form, check with your primary health care provider to see if you can mix it with water or another liquid to improve the taste.

If you're using the *suppository* form, remove the foil wrapper and moisten the suppository with cold water. Then lie down on your side and insert the suppository well up into the rectum.

If you're using the *injection* form of this medication at home, make sure you clearly understand your primary health care provider's instructions.

What to do if you miss a dose

If you're taking the medication on a regular schedule and you miss a dose, take it as soon as possible. However, if it's almost time for your next dose, skip the missed dose and resume your regular schedule. Don't take double doses.

What to do about side effects

Stop taking the medication and get emergency help *immediately* if you have clammy skin, confusion, convulsions, severe drowsiness, slow heart beat, slow or troubled breathing, severe nervousness, a rash, or facial swelling.

If you develop pale stools, ringing ears, nausea, decreased urine output, constipation, severe dry mouth, unusual dreams, or a general feeling of illness, notify your health care provider as soon as possible.

What you must know about alcohol and other drugs

Don't drink alcohol while on this medication. This combination may make you dangerously drowsy and slow your breathing.

Tell your health care provider about other medications you're taking, especially other analgesics; allergy, cold, or flu medications; sleeping pills; muscle relaxants; antidepressants; and medications for seizures.

Special directions

• Inform your health care provider about other medical problems you have, especially alcohol abuse; head injury; enlarged prostate; heart, kidney, lung, or liver disease; colitis; or convulsions.
• This medication may make you drowsy. Know how it affects you before you drive or perform activities that require alertness.
• If you're taking this medication on a regular basis, don't stop taking it without first checking with your health care provider.

✔ Keep in mind

• If you're pregnant or breast feeding, check with your primary health care provider before taking this medication.
• Children or older adults are more sensitive to the effects of this medication.

Additional instructions

_____

_____

Taking nefazodone

Dear Patient,

Nefazodone is used for the treatment of mood disorders and depression. The brand name is Serzone.

How to take nefazodone
Take this medication exactly as your primary health care provider instructs. The usual dosage is twice a day in equal doses. You can take it either with or without food.

What to do if you miss a dose
Take the dose as soon as you remember it. However, if it's close to the time for your next dose, skip the missed dose and resume your regular schedule. Don't take double doses.

What to do about side effects
Tell your primary health care provider *immediately* if you develop an irregular heartbeat, a skin rash, hives, vision changes, confusion, agitation, or dizziness while taking this medication.

   After starting this medication, some patients may develop sleepiness, nausea, diarrhea, constipation, dry mouth, shortness of breath, or eye pain. Notify your primary health care provider if these continue or bother you.

What you must know about alcohol and other drugs
Don't drink alcohol while on this medication. It may increase stomach irritation.

Warning: Before starting this medication, notify your primary health care provider if you've taken a monoamine oxidase (MAO) inhibitor during the past 2 weeks. These medications include isocarboxazid (Marplan), phenelzine (Nardil), or tranylcypromine sulfate (Parnate). Combining nefazodone and MAO inhibitors can cause serious side effects.

Special directions
• People respond to medications differently. Your primary health care provider may begin this medication at a low dose and ask you to increase the dose after he evaluates you. Don't stop taking this medication or change the dose without instructions from your primary health care provider.
• Several weeks of medication may be necessary before you notice an improvement in your condition. Often 6 months to 1 year of total therapy may be necessary depending on your condition.
• Don't drive or perform any activities that require alertness until you know the effects of the medication.

✓ Keep in mind
• Notify your primary health care provider if you're pregnant, think you're pregnant, or wish to breast-feed.

Additional instructions

_____
_____
_____
_____
_____
_____
_____
_____
_____
_____
_____

Applying neomycin

Dear Patient,

This medication is usually prescribed to treat skin infections, minor burns, or minor wounds. The label may read Myciguent.

How to apply neomycin

This medication is available in a cream and an ointment.

You can buy this medication without a prescription. If you're treating yourself, carefully follow the package instructions. If your primary health care provider prescribed this medication or gave you special instructions on how to use it, follow those instructions carefully.

To apply neomycin, wash the affected area with soap and water, then dry it thoroughly. Apply a generous amount of medication to the affected area and rub it in gently. If you're using the *cream* form of neomycin, rub it in until it disappears. You may cover the area with a gauze dressing.

What to do if you miss a dose

Apply the missed dose to the affected area as soon as possible. However, if it's almost time for your next regular dose, skip the missed dose and resume your regular dosage schedule.

What to do about side effects

Call your primary health care provider *immediately* if you have breathing problems, dizziness, fainting, or a fever or if you notice a rash, itching, redness, or other symptoms of skin irritation that weren't there before you started using this medication.

Report any hearing changes to your primary health care provider.

What you must know about other drugs

Check with your primary health care provider or pharmacist before applying another medication to the same skin area where you're using neomycin.

Special directions

• Check with your primary health care provider before using this medication if you have a kidney problem or if you've ever had an allergic or unusual reaction to this medication or to another antibiotic, including the oral form of neomycin (Mycifradin), amikacin (Amikin), gentamicin (Garamycin), kanamycin (Kantrex), netilmicin (Netromycin), streptomycin, and tobramycin (Nebcin).

• If you're using this medication without a prescription, don't apply it on a puncture wound, deep wound, serious burn, or raw area unless your primary health care provider approves this.

• Keep this medication away from your eyes.

• Continue to use this medication for the full time of treatment, even if your symptoms go away. This will help eliminate your infection completely.

• If your skin condition doesn't improve within 1 week or if it gets worse, call your primary health care provider or pharmacist.

• Don't use this medication for a long time without your primary health care provider's approval.

Additional instructions

_____

_____

_____

_____

_____

_____

_____

_____

Taking niacin

Dear Patient,

This medication is used to treat niacin deficiency or to help lower blood cholesterol and fat levels. Brand names include Nia-Bid, Niacor, and Nicotinex.

How to take niacin
Niacin is available as regular and extended-release tablets and capsules and an oral suspension. Take niacin with milk or meals if it causes diarrhea or stomach upset.

If you're taking the *extended-release tablets,* swallow them whole. If they're scored, you may break them before swallowing, but don't crush or chew them.

If you're taking the *extended-release capsules,* swallow them whole. Don't chew, crush, or break them. If they're too large to swallow, mix the contents with jelly or jam and swallow without chewing.

What to do if you miss a dose
If you're taking niacin without your primary health care provider's recommendation, missing 1 or 2 days is harmless. If niacin is prescribed to treat high cholesterol levels, take the missed dose as soon as possible. However, if it's almost time for your next dose, skip the missed dose and resume your regular schedule. Don't double dose.

What to do about side effects
If you're taking extended-release niacin, call your health care provider *at once* if you have dark urine, light gray stools, appetite loss, severe stomach pain, or yellow skin or eyes.

You may feel dizzy, especially when getting up quickly. This effect should decrease after 1 or 2 weeks.

If you're taking high doses of niacin, you may have stomach pain, diarrhea, vomiting, dizziness, fever, frequent urination, itching, joint pain, muscle or back pain, unusual weakness, or a fast, slow, or irregular heartbeat. A feeling of warmth, skin flushing, and headache may occur. Call your health care provider if these persist or worsen.

What you must know about other drugs
If you're taking niacin with lovastatin, you may experience serious muscle problems. Tell your primary health care provider about any other medications you're taking.

When taken with high blood pressure medications, niacin may cause sudden episodes of very low blood pressure and fainting or dizziness when standing.

Niacin may reduce the effectiveness of sulfinpyrazone, a drug used for gouty arthritis.

Special directions
• Before using niacin, check with your primary health care provider if your medical history includes diabetes, bleeding problems, glaucoma, gout, liver disease, low blood pressure, or a stomach ulcer.
• Avoid taking large doses of niacin except under your health care provider's direction.
• If you're taking niacin to lower your cholesterol level, follow the prescribed diet.
• Take niacin as directed. Call your health care provider before stopping treatment.
• If you're taking niacin as a vitamin supplement, know that this isn't meant to replace a varied, well-balanced diet. Meat, eggs, and dairy foods contain niacin.

✓ Keep in mind
• If you're pregnant or breast-feeding, check with your primary health care provider before taking niacin.

Additional instructions

_____

_____

Applying a nicotine patch

Dear Patient,

This medication helps you stop smoking. Use it only as part of a comprehensive stop-smoking program. Brand names for this medication include Habitrol, Nicoderm, and ProStep.

How to apply a patch

This medication is available by prescription only. It comes in a stick-on patch.

Carefully follow the instructions on the package, which tell you when and how often to apply a new patch and how long to leave it on. You should apply a new patch daily, preferably at the same time each day.

To apply the patch, choose a hairless part of your body, such as the outer part of your upper arm or your stomach or back above the waist. This site should be free from cuts and irritation. Press the patch firmly to your skin. Then wash your hands with water only.

What to do if you miss an application

If you miss an application, apply a new patch as soon as you remember. Then change the patch at the regular time.

What to do about side effects

Call your primary health care provider *immediately* if you have symptoms of nicotine overdose: severe headache, vomiting, diarrhea, dizziness, weakness, or confusion.

The first patch you apply may cause mild itching, tingling, and burning. These problems should go away within 1 hour. If the skin under the patch becomes red or swollen or a rash appears, remove the patch and call your primary health care provider; you could be allergic to it.

What you must know about other drugs

Check with your primary health care provider or pharmacist to find out if the dosages of any medications you're taking need to be changed.

Special directions

● Don't use this medication if you're allergic to nicotine or to any component in the patch.
● Tell your primary health care provider about your medical history, especially if you have high blood pressure, ulcers, kidney or liver disease, heart rhythm problems, or angina (chest pain), or if you've recently had a heart attack.
● Be sure to stop smoking completely before starting this medication to prevent nicotine overdose.
● To avoid skin irritation, apply each new patch to a different site. Wait at least 1 week before reusing a site.
● Discard patches properly — and always where children and animals can't reach them. Used patches contain enough nicotine to poison children and pets.
● If the patch falls off, apply a new one, then change it at your usual time.
● Continue to use this medication for the full time prescribed by your primary health care provider. Don't stop using it suddenly.
● Follow the other parts of your stop-smoking program.

✔ Keep in mind

● If you're pregnant, don't use this patch. If you become pregnant while using it, remove it until you've talked to your primary health care provider.
● If you're breast-feeding, check with your primary health care provider before using the patch.

Additional instructions

_____

_____

Taking nifedipine

Dear Patient,

Nifedipine is usually given to treat angina (chest pain), high blood pressure, and Raynaud's disease (episodes of reduced blood supply to the fingers or toes). Brand names include Adalat and Procardia.

How to take nifedipine
This medication comes in capsules and sustained-release tablets. Check the label, and take only the prescribed amount.

Take nifedipine exactly as your primary health care provider has ordered. Swallow capsules and tablets whole. Don't break, crush, or chew them. Don't take medication with grapefruit juice.

What to do if you miss a dose
Take the dose as soon as you remember. But if it's almost time for your next dose, skip the missed dose and resume your regular schedule. Don't double dose.

What to do about side effects
Chest pain may occur when you first start taking nifedipine. Although such pain is usually temporary, report it to your primary health care provider *immediately.*

Call *at once* if you have ankle swelling, a very fast or very slow heartbeat, shortness of breath, severe headache, or fainting.

Constipation, dizziness, flushing, headache, and nausea may also occur. These side effects usually go away over time as your body adjusts to the medication. Call your health care provider if they persist or become bothersome.

What you must know about other drugs
Check with your health care provider before taking other drugs, including nonprescription medications. Heart failure or very low blood pressure may occur if you take nifedipine with other angina medication or with medications used to treat blood pressure or heart rhythm problems.

Special directions
• Don't take nifedipine if you're allergic to it.
• Tell your health care provider if you've had heart failure or constriction of the aorta.
• Call your health care provider if this medication doesn't relieve your chest pain.
• Avoid hazardous activities such as driving a car; you may feel dizzy or light-headed.
• Avoid eating excessive amounts of calcium-rich foods, such as cheese.
• Check with your health care provider before taking calcium supplements.
• If swelling occurs, your health care provider may want you to drink less fluid and limit your salt intake.
• Schedule your activities so you can get enough rest.
• Get up slowly from a sitting or lying position to help prevent dizziness.
• If constipation occurs, drink more fluids and add more bulk to your diet. Ask your health care provider about taking a bulk laxative if needed.
• Keep taking this medication as prescribed, even if you feel better.
Warning: Don't stop taking this medication suddenly. Your health care provider may need to reduce your dosage gradually.

Keep in mind
• If you're pregnant, check with your health care provider before taking nifedipine.
• If you're an older adult, you may be especially sensitive to the effects of nifedipine.

Additional instructions

_____

_____

Taking nitrofurantoin

Dear Patient,

This medication is usually prescribed to treat urinary tract infections. Brand names include Furadantin, Macrodantin, and Nitrofuracot.

How to take nitrofurantoin
This medication is available in tablets, capsules, and an oral suspension.

Carefully check the prescription label, and take only the prescribed amount.

If you're taking the *oral suspension,* shake it forcefully before each dose. Use a specially marked measuring spoon (not a household teaspoon) to measure doses accurately.

What to do if you miss a dose
Take the missed dose as soon as you remember. However, if it's almost time for your next regular dose and your primary health care provider has prescribed three or more daily doses, space the missed dose and the next dose 2 to 4 hours apart. Then resume your regular dosage schedule.

What to do about side effects
Contact your primary health care provider *immediately* if you have chest pain, fever, chills, sore throat, cough, troubled breathing, dizziness, drowsiness, headache, numbness or tingling of the face or mouth, joint pain, itching, a rash, yellow skin or eyes, or unusual tiredness or weakness.

This medication may cause stomach or abdominal pain or upset, diarrhea, nausea, vomiting, and appetite loss. These side effects usually go away over time as your body adjusts to the medication. Check with your primary health care provider if they persist or become bothersome.

This medication may turn your urine a brown or darker color.

What you must know about other drugs
Check with your primary health care provider or pharmacist before taking other medications. Taken at the same time, many medications can worsen the side effects of nitrofurantoin.

Antacids that contain magnesium may make nitrofurantoin less effective. If you must take such an antacid, take it at least 1 hour before or after nitrofurantoin.

Special directions
• Don't take this medication if you're allergic to it.
• Tell your primary health care provider about your medical history, especially if you have glucose-6-phosphate dehydrogenase deficiency, kidney or lung disease, diabetes, asthma, anemia, vitamin B deficiency, electrolyte imbalance, or nerve damage.
• To reduce stomach upset, take this medication with milk or meals.
• Store this medication in its original container, and keep it away from all metals except aluminum and stainless steel.

✓ Keep in mind
• If you're pregnant or breast-feeding, check with your primary health care provider before using nitrofurantoin.
• If you have diabetes, don't use the copper sulfate test (Clinitest) to test your urine glucose because nitrofurantoin may cause a false-positive result.
• Check with your primary health care provider about which test to use.

Additional instructions
_____
_____
_____
_____

Applying nitroglycerin ointment

Dear Patient,

This ointment is prescribed to prevent or reduce the number of angina (chest pain) attacks. It's also called by the brand names Nitro-Bid, Nitrol, Nitrong, and Nitrostat.

How to apply nitroglycerin ointment
Carefully check the label on your prescription tube, and apply only the amount prescribed at each dose.

Measure the prescribed amount of ointment onto the special paper. Spread it lightly over the area specified by your primary health care provider—usually your upper arm or chest. *Don't rub it into your skin.* For best results, spread the ointment to cover an area about the size of the application paper (roughly 3½ inches by 2¼ inches). Cover the ointment with paper and tape it in place.

You may want to cover the paper (including the side edges) with plastic wrap to protect your clothes from stains. However, check with your primary health care provider first. This covering will make your skin absorb more medication and may increase the chance for side effects.

What to do if you miss an application
Apply the missed application as soon as you remember. However, if your next scheduled application is within 2 hours, skip the missed one and resume your regular schedule. Don't increase the amount you apply.

What to do about side effects
Call your primary health care provider *right away* if you get a severe or prolonged headache, dry mouth, or blurred vision.

This ointment may cause a headache, fast pulse rate, flushing of the face and neck, nausea, vomiting, and restlessness. Also, you may feel dizzy or light-headed when rising from a sitting or lying position. These side effects usually go away over time as your body gets used to the medication. Check with your primary health care provider if these side effects persist or become bothersome.

What you must know about alcohol and other drugs
Drink alcoholic beverages in moderation, if at all. Alcohol will increase the chance for feeling dizzy or light-headed when you get up quickly from a lying or sitting position.

Check with your primary health care provider before taking other heart or blood pressure medications. When taken with your ointment, these medications may lower your blood pressure too much.

Special directions
• Tell your health care provider of your medical history, especially if you have glaucoma, kidney or liver disease, an overactive thyroid, or severe anemia, or if you've recently had a heart attack, stroke, or head injury.
• To prevent skin irritation and other problems, apply each dose to a different skin site.

! *Warning:* If you're using this medication for several weeks or more, don't suddenly stop using it because this may bring on angina attacks. Your primary health care provider may tell you to gradually reduce your dosage before stopping completely.

✔ Keep in mind
• If you're an older adult, you may be especially sensitive to the effects of nitroglycerin.

Additional instructions
_____

_____

Taking nitroglycerin tablets

Dear Patient,

This medication is prescribed to prevent or relieve angina (chest pain) attacks. It's also called by the brand names Nitrogard and Nitrostat.

How to take nitroglycerin tablets

Place one tablet under your tongue, between your lip and gum, or between your cheek and gum. Let it dissolve there. Don't chew, crush, or swallow the tablet.

To *prevent* an angina attack, take a tablet 5 to 10 minutes before expected physical exertion or emotional distress that has caused an attack in the past.

To *relieve* an angina attack, place one tablet in your mouth when you start to feel an attack coming on. If your pain doesn't go away within 5 minutes, take a second tablet. If you still have pain after another 5 minutes, take a third tablet. If three tablets don't provide relief, call your primary health care provider and have someone take you to the nearest hospital. Never take more than three tablets.

What to do about side effects

Call your primary health care provider *right away* if you get a severe or prolonged headache, dry mouth, or blurred vision.

This medication may cause a fast pulse rate, flushing of your face and neck, headache, nausea, vomiting, and restlessness. Also, it may make you feel dizzy or light-headed when you get up from a sitting or lying position. These side effects usually go away over time as your body gets used to the medication. Check with your primary health care provider or pharmacist if these effects persist or become bothersome.

What you must know about alcohol and other drugs

Drink alcoholic beverages in moderation, if at all. Alcohol increases the chance for feeling dizzy or light-headed when you get up quickly from a lying or sitting position.

Check with your health care provider or pharmacist before taking other heart or blood pressure medications. When taken together with nitroglycerin, your blood pressure may become very low.

Special directions

• Tell your primary health care provider about your medical history, especially if you have kidney or liver disease or an overactive thyroid, or if you've recently had a heart attack.
• This medication works best when you're sitting or standing. Sitting is safer than standing because you may become dizzy or light-headed soon after taking a tablet. If you get dizzy or light-headed while sitting, take a few deep breaths and bend forward with your head between your knees.
• Don't eat, drink, smoke, or use chewing tobacco while the tablet is in your mouth.
• Get new tablets after 3 months, even if you have some left in the container.

❗ *Warning:* If you've been on nitroglycerin regularly for several weeks, don't suddenly stop using it because this may bring on angina attacks. Your health care provider may tell you to gradually reduce the dosage before stopping completely.

✅ **Keep in mind**
• If you're an older adult, you may be especially sensitive to the effects of nitroglycerin.

Additional instructions

_____

_____

Applying a nitroglycerin patch

Dear Patient,

This medication is prescribed to treat attacks of angina (chest pain). It's also called by the brand names Deponit, Nitro-Dur, Transderm-Nitro, Minitran, and Nitrodisc.

How to apply a patch
This medication comes in a stick-on patch.

Carefully check the label on the prescription package, which tells you how often to apply a new patch. Apply a patch only as often as prescribed by your primary health care provider.

To apply the patch, choose a clean, dry skin area with little or no hair. The area should be free from cuts, scars, or irritation. Don't choose the lower part of your arm or leg because the medication won't work as well at these sites.

What to do if you miss an application
Apply a new patch as soon as you remember. Then resume your regular schedule.

What to do about side effects
Call your primary health care provider *right away* if you get a severe or prolonged headache, dry mouth, or blurred vision.

This medication may cause a fast pulse rate, flushing of your face and neck, headache, nausea, vomiting, and restlessness. Also, it may make you feel dizzy or light-headed when you get up from a sitting or lying position. These side effects usually subside as your body gets used to the medication. Check with your primary health care provider if these effects persist or become bothersome.

What you must know about alcohol and other drugs
Drink alcoholic beverages in moderation, if at all. Alcohol will increase the chance for feeling dizzy or light-headed when you get up quickly from a lying or sitting position.

Check with your primary health care provider or pharmacist before taking other heart or blood pressure medications. Taken with nitroglycerin, these medications may lower your blood pressure too much.

Special directions
• Tell your primary health care provider about your medical history, especially if you have glaucoma, kidney or liver disease, an overactive thyroid, or severe anemia, or if you've recently had a heart attack, stroke, or head injury.
• Always remove the previous patch before applying a new one.
• To prevent skin irritation or other problems, apply each new patch to a different skin area.
• If you think this medication isn't working properly, don't trim or cut the patch to adjust the dosage. Instead, check with your primary health care provider.

Warning: If you've been using this medication for several weeks or more, don't suddenly stop using it because this may bring on angina attacks. Your primary health care provider may instruct you to gradually reduce your dosage before stopping treatment completely.

Keep in mind
• If you're an older adult, you may be especially sensitive to the effects of nitroglycerin.

Additional instructions
_____
_____
_____
_____

Taking nizatidine

Dear Patient,

Your primary health care provider has prescribed nizatidine to treat your duodenal ulcers or prevent their return. The label may read Axid.

How to take nizatidine
Nizatidine comes in capsules. Follow the directions on the prescription label exactly. If you're taking one capsule daily, take it at bedtime unless your primary health care provider gives you other instructions. If you're taking two capsules, take one in the morning and one at bedtime.

Continue to take this medication even after you begin to feel better. Stopping too soon may prevent your ulcer from healing completely.

What to do if you miss a dose
Take the dose as soon as possible. However, if it's almost time for your next dose, skip the missed capsule and take your next dose as scheduled. Don't double dose.

What to do about side effects
Call your primary health care provider *at once* if you start to bleed or bruise easily or you become unusually tired. Also tell him right away if you develop rashes or other skin problems.

This medication may make you sleepy or sweaty or, rarely, may cause an irregular heartbeat. Check with your primary health care provider if these symptoms persist or are troublesome.

What you must know about other drugs
Tell your primary health care provider if you're taking other medications and check with him before taking new medications. In particular, reveal if you regularly take aspirin

in high doses because nizatidine may increase aspirin's side effects.

If you take antacids to relieve stomach pain, wait 30 minutes to 1 hour between taking the antacid and nizatidine.

Special directions
• Nizatidine may aggravate certain medical conditions. For this reason, tell your primary health care provider if you have other medical problems, especially kidney or liver disease.
• Before you have skin tests for allergies or tests to measure how much acid is in your stomach, tell your primary health care provider you're taking nizatidine. This medication may affect the test results.
• Avoid foods and other substances that irritate your stomach, such as alcohol, carbonated soft drinks, and citrus products.
Warning: Don't smoke while taking this medication because cigarette smoking reduces nizatidine's effectiveness. If you can't stop smoking completely, at least wait until after you've taken your last dose for the day.
• Keep appointments for follow-up examinations, so your primary health care provider can check your progress.

Keep in mind
• If you're pregnant or breast-feeding, check with your primary health care provider about using nizatidine.
• If you're an older adult, you may be especially prone to nizatidine's side effects, particularly dizziness and confusion.

Additional instructions
_____
_____
_____

Taking a nonsteroidal anti-inflammatory medication

Dear Patient,

Your primary health care provider has prescribed a nonsteroidal anti-inflammatory medication for your condition. These medications are used to relieve symptoms of arthritis; to treat painful conditions, such as muscle sprains or strains, menstrual cramps, gout attacks, or eye inflammation; or to reduce fevers.

This information sheet contains general information about nonsteroidal anti-inflammatory medications. It's not meant to replace a sheet describing the particular medication you're taking.

How to take a nonsteroidal anti-inflammatory medication

This medication is available as a tablet, capsule, liquid, rectal suppository, or as eyedrops. Take it exactly as directed by your primary health care provider.

Take the *tablet or capsule* with a full glass (8 ounces) of water. To reduce stomach irritation, take the tablet or capsule with a full glass (8 ounces) of milk or with food or an antacid to reduce stomach irritation (unless your primary health care provider says otherwise).

Take the *liquid form* of these drugs with a full glass (8 ounces) of milk, food, or with an antacid to reduce stomach irritation.

To insert the *suppository*, remove the foil wrapper and moisten the suppository with cold water. Lie on your side and use your finger to insert the suppository well up into the rectum.

To use the *eyedrops*, first wash your hands. Next tilt your head back and pull the lower eyelid away from the eye to form a pouch. Squeeze the drops into the pouch and gently close your eye. Wash your hands again.

What to do if you miss a dose

If you're taking the medication on a regular schedule and you miss a dose, take it as soon as possible. But if it's almost time for your next dose, skip the missed dose and resume your regular schedule.

If you're taking a long-acting tablet or capsule, take the missed dose only if you remember it within 1 to 2 hours after the regularly scheduled time. Otherwise, skip the missed dose and go back to your regular schedule. Don't double dose.

What to do about side effects

Stop taking this medication and get emergency help *immediately* if you faint or have an irregular heartbeat, swelling of the face, shortness of breath, or tightness in your chest. Also call your primary health care provider *immediately* if you have a rash; stomach pain; bloody or black, tarry stools; fever; heartburn; unexplained nosebleeds; or if you spit up blood or material that looks like coffee grounds.

What you must know about alcohol and other drugs

Avoid alcohol while taking this medication because alcoholic beverages may increase stomach irritation.

Tell your primary health care provider about other medications you're taking, especially blood thinners, aspirin, other anti-inflammatory agents, oral diabetic medications, phenytoin (Dilantin), water pills, medications for high blood pressure, digoxin (Lanoxin), lithium (Lithane), methotrexate (Folex), or nonprescription pain relievers.

Special directions

● Tell your primary health care provider about other medical problems you have, especially alcohol abuse; bleeding problems;

(continued)

Taking a nonsteroidal anti-inflammatory medication *(continued)*

stomach ulcers; diabetes; liver, heart, or kidney disease; high blood pressure; heart disease; or an allergy to aspirin or another nonsteroidal anti-inflammatory medication.
- It may take several weeks to reach the medication's peak effectiveness.
- This medication may make you drowsy. Don't drive or perform activities that require alertness until you know its effect on you.

✔ Keep in mind
- If you're pregnant or breast-feeding, check with your primary health care provider before taking this medication.
- If you're an older adult, you may be especially sensitive to the effects of this medication.

Additional instructions

_____

_____

_____

_____

_____

_____

_____

_____

_____

_____

Taking norfloxacin

Dear Patient,

Your primary health care provider has prescribed norfloxacin to treat your bacterial infection. This medication usually is prescribed to treat urinary tract infections. The label may read Noroxin.

How to take norfloxacin

Norfloxacin comes in tablets. Follow your primary health care provider's instructions exactly. Take your tablet with a full glass (8 ounces) of water on an empty stomach, either 1 hour before or 2 hours after meals. Also, try to drink several extra glasses of water every day.

For best results, take your tablets at evenly spaced times during the day and night. For example, if you take two doses daily, you might take one dose at 8 a.m. and the other at 8 p.m.

Continue to take your medication, even after you begin to feel better. Stopping too soon might allow your infection to return.

What to do if you miss a dose

Take the dose as soon as possible. But if it's almost time for your next dose, skip the missed tablet and go back to your regular dosing schedule. Don't double dose.

Try not to forget a dose because norfloxacin works best with a constant amount in your blood or urine.

What to do about side effects

Call your primary health care provider *right away* if you start to wheeze, have difficulty breathing, or break out in hives or a rash.

Check with your primary health care provider if you become dizzy, drowsy, or unusually tired. Also tell him if you develop constipation, heartburn, nausea, a dry mouth, headache, or trouble sleeping.

What you must know about other drugs

Tell your primary health care provider about other medications you're taking. If you use antacids, zinc supplements, iron supplements, or sucralfate (Carafate), an ulcer medication, don't take these medications with norfloxacin. Instead, take antacids, zinc, iron or sucralfate at least 2 hours after you take norfloxacin.

Your primary health care provider also needs to know if you're taking nitrofurantoin (Macrodantin), another medication for urinary tract infections, or probenicid (Benemid), a gout medication.

Special directions

• Tell your primary health care provider if you have other medical problems, especially kidney disease or a history of seizures.
• Because norfloxacin may increase your sensitivity to light, wear sunglasses and use a sunscreen while outdoors on bright days. Call your primary health care provider if you have a severe reaction from the sun.
• Norfloxacin can make you drowsy, so make sure you know how you react to it before you drive or perform other activities that might be dangerous if you're not fully alert.

✓ Keep in mind

• If you're pregnant or breast-feeding, don't use norfloxacin unless your primary health care provider instructs you to do so.

Warning: Don't give this medication to infants, children, or adolescents because it may cause bone problems.

Additional instructions

_____

_____

_____

Taking nortriptyline

Dear Patient,

Your primary health care provider has prescribed nortriptyline to treat your depression. Brand names include Aventyl and Pamelor.

How to take nortriptyline

This medication comes in capsules and an oral solution. Follow the directions for using nortriptyline exactly.

To lessen stomach upset, take nortriptyline with food unless your primary health care provider has told you to take it on an empty stomach.

If you're taking the *oral solution,* use the dropper provided to measure each dose. Dilute each dose with about one-half cup (4 ounces) of water, milk, or orange juice. Then drink the liquid.

Check with your primary health care provider before you stop taking this medication.

What to do if you miss a dose

Adjust your dosage schedule as follows.

If you take one dose a day at bedtime, don't take the missed dose the next morning because it may cause side effects during the waking hours. Check with your primary health care provider instead.

If you take more than one dose a day, take the missed dose as soon as possible. If it's almost time for your next dose, skip the missed dose and take your next dose as scheduled. Don't double dose.

What to do about side effects

Check with your primary health care provider if you have blurred vision, a dry mouth, increased sweating, constipation, dizziness, drowsiness, rapid or irregular heartbeat, or difficulty urinating.

What you must know about alcohol and other drugs

Don't drink alcoholic beverages while taking nortriptyline because the combination may cause you to be overly drowsy. For the same reason, don't use other medications that slow the nervous system, such as sleeping pills, sedatives, tranquilizers, and cold, flu, and allergy medications.

Tell your primary health care provider about other medications you're taking. In particular, he needs to know if you take barbiturates (for seizures or sedation); cimetidine, or Tagamet (for ulcers); epinephrine, or Sus-Phrine (for asthma or severe allergic reactions); or medications for depression or other emotional problems.

Special directions

● Tell your primary health care provider if you have other medical problems. They may affect the use of this medication.
● Because this medication may make you drowsy, avoid driving or performing other activities requiring alertness until you know how it affects you.
● If nortriptyline makes your mouth feel dry, use sugarless gum or hard candy, ice chips, or a saliva substitute.

✓ Keep in mind

● If you're pregnant or breast-feeding, don't use nortriptyline, unless you've discussed the risks and benefits with your primary health care provider.
● Children and older adults are especially prone to nortriptyline's side effects.

Additional instructions

_____

_____

_____

Taking oral nystatin

Dear Patient,

Your primary health care provider has prescribed nystatin by mouth to treat your fungal infection. Brand names include Mycostatin, Nilstat, and Nystex.

How to take nystatin

This medication comes in tablets, lozenges, an oral solution, and a dry powder that's mixed with water. Follow your primary health care provider's directions for taking nystatin exactly.

If you're taking the *lozenges,* hold the lozenge in your mouth to allow it to dissolve slowly. Don't chew or swallow lozenges whole.

If you're taking the *oral solution,* place half of the dose in each side of your mouth. Then swish the dose in your mouth, gargle, and swallow.

If you're using the *dry powder,* follow these steps:
• Read the prescription label to find out what proportions of water and powder to use for each dose.
• Thoroughly mix the powder and water. Then take the medication by dividing the whole amount into several portions.
• Swish each portion in your mouth for as long as possible, gargle, then swallow.

Continue to take nystatin, as directed, even if your symptoms disappear. Stopping too soon might allow your infection to return.

What to do if you miss a dose

If you miss a dose, take it as soon as possible. However, if it's almost time for your next dose, skip the missed dose and go back to your regular dosing schedule.

What to do about side effects

Check with your primary health care provider if you have a digestive upset, such as diarrhea, nausea, vomiting, or stomach pain.

Special directions

• To prevent fungal infections of your mouth, take good care of your teeth and mouth. Don't overuse mouthwash or wear poorly fitting dentures because doing so may lead to a mouth infection.
• Check with your primary health care provider or pharmacist about how to store the form of nystatin you're using. Keep nystatin lozenges in the refrigerator. Don't allow the oral solution to freeze.

✔ Keep in mind

• Don't give the lozenges to a child under age 5 because he might choke.

Additional instructions

_____

_____

_____

_____

_____

_____

_____

_____

_____

_____

_____

Applying topical nystatin

Dear Patient,

Topical nystatin is prescribed to treat a fungal infection of the skin or vagina. Brand names include Mycostatin, Nilstat, and Nystex.

How to apply nystatin

For a skin infection, this medication comes in cream, ointment, and powder forms. For a vaginal infection, it's available as vaginal tablets. Follow your primary health care provider's directions for applying nystatin.

If you have a *skin infection,* apply just enough cream or ointment to cover the affected area. If you're using the powder on your feet, sprinkle it between your toes, on your feet, and in socks and shoes.

Don't cover the treated skin with a bandage, wrap, or other tight dressing unless directed to do so by your primary health care provider.

If you have a *vaginal infection,* you'll probably insert the tablets with an applicator. Check with your primary health care provider about how to use the applicator. Keep using this medication even if you begin to menstruate during the time of treatment.

Continue to use nystatin for as long as your primary health care provider directs, even if your symptoms disappear. Stopping too soon might allow your infection to return.

What to do if you miss a dose

If you miss a dose of cream, powder or ointment, apply it as soon as possible, than resume your regular dosing schedule. Insert vaginal tablets as soon as possible. However, if it's almost time for the next regular dose, skip the missed dose and go back to your normal schedule.

What to do about side effects

Check with your primary health care provider if you have skin or vaginal irritation that wasn't present before you began using nystatin.

If you're using vaginal tablets, expect some vaginal drainage. Wear a sanitary napkin to protect your clothing.

Special directions

• Tell your primary health care provider if you're allergic to nystatin. Also reveal if you have other allergies, especially to foods, other medications, or preservatives.
• If you have a vaginal infection, practice good health habits to prevent reinfection. Wear cotton panties (or panties or pantyhose with cotton crotches) instead of synthetic underclothes. Also wear only freshly washed underwear.
• Check with your primary health care provider or pharmacist about how to store the form of nystatin you're using.

✔ Keep in mind

• If you're pregnant and have a vaginal infection, check with your primary health care provider before using the applicator to insert the vaginal tablets.

Additional instructions

_____
_____
_____
_____
_____
_____
_____
_____
_____

Applying nystatin with triamcinolone

Dear Patient,

Your primary health care provider has prescribed nystatin with triamcinolone to treat your fungal infection and relieve the discomfort it's causing. Brand names include Dermacomb, Myco II, or Tri-Statin II.

How to apply this medication
This combination medication comes in cream and ointment forms. Follow your primary health care provider's directions for using this medication exactly. Don't use it more often or for a longer time than prescribed.

To apply the cream or ointment, rub a small amount into the affected area gently and thoroughly. Take care to keep it away from your eyes.

Don't put a bandage, wrap, or other tight dressing over the treated skin unless your primary health care provider directs you to do so. Wear loose-fitting clothing when using this medication on your groin area.

Use the medication for the full time of treatment, even if your symptoms go away. Stopping too soon might allow your infection to return.

What to do if you miss a dose
Apply the medication as soon as possible. But if it's almost time for your next dose, skip the missed dose and take your next dose on schedule.

What to do about side effects
Call your primary health care provider *right away* if you start to have skin irritation, such as blistering, burning, dryness, itching, or peeling.

If you use this medication for a long time, you may experience other side effects. Let your primary health care provider know if you start to have acne or oily skin; in-creased hair growth or loss of hair; reddish purple lines on your arms, face, legs, trunk, or groin; thin skin with easy bruising;

Special directions
• Tell your primary health care provider about other medical problems you have or have had in the past, especially herpes, chickenpox, tuberculosis, or viral infections of the skin. Certain medical conditions may prevent your using this medication.
• Don't use this medication for other skin problems without checking first with your primary health care provider.
• If your skin problem isn't better within 2 to 3 weeks, check with your primary health care provider.
• If you're using this medication to treat a child's diaper rash, avoid tight-fitting diapers and plastic pants.

✔️ Keep in mind
• If you're pregnant or breast-feeding, check with your primary health care provider before using this medication.
• If you have severe diabetes, also talk to your primary health care provider before using this medication. In rare instances, it can raise blood and urine glucose levels.

Additional instructions

_____
_____
_____
_____
_____
_____
_____
_____

Taking ofloxacin

Dear Patient,

Ofloxacin has been prescribed to treat your bacterial infection. This antibiotic is used to kill the bacteria that cause gonorrhea, urinary tract infections, and other infections. The label may read Floxin.

How to take ofloxacin

This medication comes in tablets. Take them exactly as ordered. For best results, take each dose with a full glass (8 ounces) of water on an otherwise empty stomach. Drink several extra glasses of water daily unless your primary health care provider tells you otherwise.

Take the tablets at evenly spaced times day and night. Don't take antacids, iron, or zinc within 2 hours before or 2 hours after taking ofloxacin.

Continue to take ofloxacin, even after you begin to feel better. Stopping too soon may allow your infection to return.

What to do if you miss a dose

Take the dose as soon as possible. However, if it's almost time for your next dose, skip the missed dose and take your next dose as scheduled. Don't double dose.

What to do about side effects

Call your primary health care provider *right away* if you start to wheeze, feel short of breath, have difficulty breathing, or break out in a rash or hives.

Check with your primary health care provider if you have abdominal pain, diarrhea, dizziness, drowsiness, headache, light-headedness, nausea, vomiting, nervousness, or trouble sleeping.

What you must know about other drugs

Tell your primary health care provider about other medications you're taking because many of them can interfere with the absorption of ofloxacin. These medications include aluminum- or magnesium-containing antacids; iron supplements; sucralfate (Carafate), an ulcer medication; and products that contain zinc.

If you take blood thinners, you should know that combined use with ofloxacin may increase the risk of bleeding. If you take theophylline (Theo-Dur), a medication for asthma or bronchitis, ofloxacin may worsen the side effects from this medication.

Special directions

- Tell your primary health care provider about your medical history, especially if you have brain or spinal cord disease or a kidney problem.
- Ofloxacin may make you drowsy. So know how you react to it before you drive or perform other activities that might be dangerous if you're not fully alert.
- This medication may make you unusually sensitive to sunlight, so limit your exposure to direct sun.

✔ Keep in mind

- If you're pregnant or breast-feeding, don't use ofloxacin unless you and your primary health care provider have discussed the possible risks.

- *Warning:* Don't give this medication to infants, children, or teenagers unless instructed by your primary health care provider. It may cause bone problems.

Additional instructions

_____
_____
_____
_____
_____

Taking omeprazole

Dear Patient,

This medication is used to treat duodenal ulcers, severe or chronic heartburn, and other problems in which the stomach has too much acid. The label may read Prilosec.

How to take omeprazole

Omeprazole comes in delayed-release capsules. Carefully check the label, and follow the directions exactly as ordered. Don't break, chew, or crush the capsule—swallow it whole.

Keep taking omeprazole for the full treatment period even after you feel better.

What to do if you miss a dose

Take the dose as soon as possible. However, if it's almost time for your next dose, skip the missed dose and take your next scheduled dose. Don't double dose.

What to do about side effects

Call your primary health care provider *immediately* if you have bloody or cloudy urine; difficult, frequent, or painful urination; easy bruising or bleeding; fever; persistent sores or ulcers in your mouth; sore throat; unusual tiredness.

Check with your primary health care provider if you get a cough, a headache, back or chest pain, or a rash. Also let him know if you have digestive troubles, such as abdominal or stomach pain, constipation, diarrhea, gas, heartburn, nausea, or vomiting.

What you must know about other drugs

Tell your primary health care provider about other medications you're taking. Some of them are more likely to cause side effects if taken with omeprazole. These medications include blood thinners, the muscle relaxant diazepam (Valium), and the seizure medication phenytoin (Dilantin).

Special directions

- Tell your primary health care provider about other medical problems you have, especially liver disease. Also mention if you're allergic to omeprazole or to other substances, such as foods or dyes.
- Keep appointments for follow-up examinations, so your primary health care provider knows when you can stop taking this medication.
- After you start therapy, several days may pass before you experience pain relief. Until then, you may take antacids with omeprazole unless your primary health care provider gives you other instructions.

✔ Keep in mind

- If you're pregnant or breast-feeding, check with your primary health care provider before taking this medication.

Additional instructions

_____
_____
_____
_____
_____
_____
_____
_____
_____
_____
_____

Taking oxacillin

Dear Patient,

Your primary health care provider has prescribed oxacillin to treat your bacterial infection. The label may read Bactocill or Prostaphlin.

How to take oxacillin

This antibiotic, a form of penicillin, comes in capsules and an oral solution. Follow the medication instructions exactly. For best results, take your medication 1 hour before or 2 hours after meals.

Try to take the doses at evenly spaced times to keep a constant amount of oxacillin in your blood or urine.

Keep taking this medication for the full treatment period even after you feel better. Stopping too soon may allow your infection to return.

What to do if you miss a dose

Take the dose as soon as possible. However, if it's almost time for your next dose, adjust your dose as follows.

If you take two doses daily, space the missed dose and the next dose about 5 hours apart.

If you take three or more doses daily, space the missed dose and the next dose 2 to 4 hours apart.

Then resume your regular dosing schedule.

What to do about side effects

Stop taking oxacillin *at once* and call for emergency medical help if you have symptoms of an allergic reaction. These symptoms include difficulty breathing, light-headedness, fever, chills, a rash, hives, itching, and wheezing. Rarely, this medication may cause seizures. If you experience a seizure, a friend or family member must call for medical help *at once*.

Also check with your primary health care provider if you have diarrhea or other digestive troubles, especially if these side effects persist or become bothersome.

What you must know about other drugs

Tell your primary health care provider if you're taking any other medications including probenecid (Benemid), a medication for gout, because this medication can increase blood levels of oxacillin.

Special directions

- Tell your primary health care provider about your medical history, especially if you have allergies, bleeding problems, kidney disease, mononucleosis, or stomach or intestinal disease.
- If you're allergic to oxacillin or another form of penicillin, don't use this medication, and carry a medical identification card or wear a medical identification bracelet stating that you're allergic.
- Before you have medical tests, tell your primary health care provider that you're taking oxacillin because it may affect the results.

✔ Keep in mind

- If you're breast-feeding, check with your primary health care provider before using this medication.

Additional instructions

_____
_____
_____
_____
_____
_____
_____

Taking oxycodone

Dear Patient,

Your primary health care provider has prescribed oxycodone to help relieve your pain. The label may read Roxicodone.

How to take oxycodone
This narcotic medication is available in tablets and an oral solution. Follow the directions exactly as ordered. Don't take more oxycodone than directed because it may become habit-forming or cause an overdose.

Check with your primary health care provider before you stop taking this medication.

What to do if you miss a dose
If your primary health care provider has ordered you to take this medication on a scheduled basis and you miss a dose, take it as soon as possible. However, if it's almost time for your next dose, skip the missed dose and take your next dose on schedule. Don't double dose.

What to do about side effects
Confusion, seizures, difficulty breathing, severe dizziness or drowsiness, slow heartbeat, and weakness are possible signs of overdose. If you have any of these side effects, call for emergency medical help *right away.*

This medication can cause drowsiness, a false sense of well-being, nausea, vomiting, constipation, or difficult urination. Check with your primary health care provider if you develop any of these symptoms, especially if they continue or become severe.

What you must know about alcohol and other drugs
Don't drink alcoholic beverages while taking oxycodone because the combination can make you dangerously drowsy.

For the same reason, avoid taking medications that slow the nervous system unless your primary health care provider gives you other directions. These depressant medications include many allergy and cold medications, sleeping pills, and muscle relaxants.

If you regularly take blood thinners, aspirin, or products containing aspirin, check with your primary health care provider before using oxycodone. Combined use may lead to easy bleeding.

Special directions
• Tell your primary health care provider if you have other medical problems. They may affect the use of this medication.
• Oxycodone may make you drowsy. So know how it affects you before you perform hazardous activities, such as driving or operating machinery.
• Oxycodone may make you feel faint, dizzy, or light-headed, especially when you get up suddenly from a lying or sitting position. To prevent falls, get up slowly from these positions.
• Tell your primary health care provider or dentist that you're taking this medication before you have surgery.

✔ Keep in mind
• If you're pregnant or breast-feeding, check with your primary health care provider before using this medication.
• If you're an athlete, you should know that oxycodone is banned and tested for by the U.S. Olympic Committee.

Additional instructions

_____

_____

Taking oxycodone with acetaminophen

Dear Patient,

This medication contains two kinds of pain relievers: a narcotic analgesic (oxycodone) and acetaminophen. Brand names include Endocet, Percocet, Roxicet, Roxilox, and Tylox.

How to take this medication

This medication is available in capsules, tablets, and an oral solution. Follow the instructions exactly. Don't take more than the prescribed amount of this medication because it may become habit-forming or lead to overdose. If you think this medication isn't helping you, call your primary health care provider.

What to do if you miss a dose

If your primary health care provider has ordered you to take this medication on a scheduled basis and you miss a dose, take it as soon as you remember it. However, if it's almost time for your next dose, skip the missed dose and take your next dose on schedule. Don't double dose.

What to do about side effects

Call for emergency help *immediately* if you think you may have taken an overdose. Symptoms include cold, clammy skin; confusion; seizures; difficulty breathing; severe dizziness or drowsiness; increased sweating; slow heartbeat; stomach cramps; and weakness.

Call your primary health care provider *at once* if you have black, tarry stools; bloody or dark urine; easy bruising or bleeding; facial swelling; irregular heartbeat or breathing; mental depression; skin problems; sore throat or fever.

Also check with your primary health care provider if this medication makes you feel dizzy or faint or causes nausea or vomiting.

What you must know about alcohol and other drugs

Don't drink alcohol while taking this medication; the combination may make you dangerously drowsy. Avoid medications that depress the nervous system, including many cold and flu remedies, muscle relaxants, sleeping pills, and seizure medications.

Check with your health care provider before taking aspirin or aspirin-containing products; nonsteroidal anti-inflammatory medications, such as Motrin and Naprosyn; acetaminophen-containing products; or zidovudine (AZT).

Special directions

• Tell your primary health care provider if you have other medical problems, especially alcohol or drug abuse, emotional problems, brain disease or head injury, or diseases of any of the major organs.
• This medication can make you dizzy or drowsy. So know how it affects you before you drive or perform any activities that require alertness.
• Tell your primary health care provider or dentist that you're taking this medication before you have surgery.

✔ Keep in mind

• If you're pregnant or breast-feeding, check with your primary health care provider before using this medication.
• Children and older adults may be especially sensitive to the medication's effects.
• If you're an athlete, you should know that oxycodone is banned and tested for by the U.S. Olympic Committee.

Additional instructions

_____

_____

Taking oxycodone with aspirin

Dear Patient,

This medication contains two kinds of pain relievers: a narcotic analgesic (oxycodone) and aspirin. Brand names include Percodan, Percodan-Demi, and Roxiprin.

How to take oxycodone with aspirin

This medication comes in tablets. Take it exactly as directed. Don't take more than the prescribed amount because it may become habit-forming or lead to overdose. If this medication isn't relieving your pain, check with your primary health care provider.

What to do if you miss a dose

If your primary health care provider has ordered you to take this medication on a scheduled basis and you miss a dose, take it as soon as you remember it. However, if it's almost time for your next dose, skip the missed dose and take your next dose on schedule. Don't double dose.

What to do about side effects

Call for emergency help *immediately* if you think you may have taken an overdose. Symptoms include cold, clammy skin; confusion; seizures; severe dizziness or drowsiness; increased sweating or thirst; slow heartbeat; severe stomach pain; vision problems; and weakness.

Call your primary health care provider *right away* if you have black, tarry stools; confusion; dark urine; facial swelling; irregular heartbeat or breathing; mental depression; rashes or other skin problems; unusual tiredness or weakness; vomiting that looks like coffee grounds.

Check with your primary health care provider if you feel faint or dizzy or have an upset stomach.

What you must know about alcohol and other drugs

Don't drink alcoholic beverages while taking this medication because the combination may make you dangerously drowsy. For the same reason, avoid taking other medications that depress the nervous system, including many cold and flu remedies, muscle relaxants, and sleeping pills.

Check with your primary health care provider before you take other medications, especially blood thinners, acetaminophen (Tylenol), aspirin or aspirin-containing products, diabetes medications, probenecid (Benemid) for gout, and zidovudine (AZT).

Special directions

• Tell your primary health care provider if you have other medical problems. They may affect the use of this medication. Also mention if you're allergic to any medication.
• This medication may make you drowsy. So know how it affects you before you drive or perform other activities that require full alertness.

✔ Keep in mind

• If you're pregnant or breast-feeding, check with your primary health care provider before using this medication.
• If you're an older adult, you may be especially prone to this medication's side effects.
• If you're an athlete, you should know that the oxycodone in this medication is banned and tested for by the U.S. Olympic Committee.

Additional instructions

_____

_____

_____

Taking penicillin G

Dear Patient,

Your primary health care provider has prescribed penicillin G to treat your bacterial infection.

How to take penicillin G
Penicillin G comes in tablet and oral liquid forms. Take this medication exactly as your primary health care provider directs.

If you're taking the *oral liquid,* use a specially marked measuring spoon (not a household teaspoon) or dropper to measure each dose.

If you're taking the *tablets,* don't drink acidic beverages, such as fruit juices, within 1 hour of taking penicillin G.

Try to take your medication at evenly spaced times day and night. Continue to take penicillin G as directed, even if you start to feel better. Stopping too soon may allow your infection to return.

What to do if you miss a dose
Take the dose as soon as possible. But if it's almost time for your next dose, follow these guidelines.

If you take two doses a day, space the missed dose and the next dose 5 to 6 hours apart.

If you take three or more doses a day, space the missed dose and the next dose 2 to 4 hours apart.

Then resume your regular schedule.

What to do about side effects
Call for emergency help *at once* if you have an allergic reaction to penicillin G. Symptoms include difficulty breathing, light-headedness, rash, hives, itching, or wheezing.

Call your primary health care provider *right away* if you have severe abdominal or stomach cramps, bloody or decreased urine, seizures, severe diarrhea, fever, joint pain, sore throat, or unusual bleeding or bruising.

Check with your primary health care provider if this medication causes mild diarrhea, nausea, vomiting, or sore mouth or tongue.

What you must know about other drugs
Tell your primary health care provider about other medications you're taking. Probenicid (Benemid), a gout medication, may increase blood levels of penicillin G.

Don't take diarrhea medication without first checking with your primary health care provider. Severe diarrhea may be a sign of a serious side effect.

Special directions
• Tell your primary health care provider if you have other medical problems, especially asthma, bleeding disorders, mononucleosis, or kidney, stomach, or intestinal disease. Also mention if you're allergic to any penicillin or another medication.
• Before you have medical tests, tell your primary health care provider you're taking penicillin G because it may affect the test results.
• If you're allergic to penicillin, your primary health care provider may want you to carry a medical identification card or wear a medical identification bracelet stating this.

✔ Keep in mind
• If you're breast-feeding, check with your primary health care provider before using this medication.

Additional instructions
_____
_____
_____

Taking pentamidine

Dear Patient,

Pentamidine is prescribed to prevent or treat pneumocystis pneumonia. If you're receiving the *injection* form of this medication, the label may read Pentam 300. The *inhalant* form may read NebuPent.

How to take pentamidine

Take pentamidine exactly as directed by your primary health care provider.

If you're using the *inhalant* form, use the aerosol device until the chamber is empty. This may take as long as 45 minutes.

If you're receiving the *injection* form, lie down during the injection. That's because the medication may cause your blood pressure to drop suddenly, making you feel light-headed or dizzy.

Continue to take pentamidine as directed, even after you begin to feel better. Stopping too soon may allow your infection to return.

What to do if you miss a dose

If you're using the *inhalant* device and you miss a dose, use your medication as soon as possible. If you miss an *injection,* check with your primary health care provider about when to receive the next dose.

What to do about side effects

Call your primary health care provider *right away* if you have:
• decreased urination
• sore throat and fever
• easy bleeding or bruising
• symptoms of high blood glucose: increased urination, loss of appetite, increased thirst, fruit-like breath odor
• symptoms of low blood glucose: anxiety; chills; cold sweats; cool, pale skin; headache; increased hunger; nervousness; shakiness
• symptoms of low blood pressure: blurred vision, confusion, dizziness, fainting or light-headedness, and unusual tiredness or weakness.

Also check with your primary health care provider if you develop diarrhea, loss of appetite, nausea, or vomiting.

If you're receiving the injections, tell your health care provider if you have pain, redness, or swelling at the injection site.

What you must know about other drugs

Tell your primary health care provider of other medications you're taking. You may be at risk for kidney damage if you take pentamidine with certain antibiotics; amphotericin B (Fungizone), a medication for fungal infections; cisplatin (Platinol), a cancer medication; or zidovudine (AZT), an AIDS medication.

Special directions

• Tell your health care provider if you have other medical problems, especially anemia, asthma, diabetes, bleeding disorders, low blood pressure, and kidney, heart, or liver disease; also if you're allergic to pentamidine.
• If you're receiving the injections, apply warm compresses to the injection site if the area hurts.
• If you're using the inhalant, don't smoke because it can cause coughing and difficulty breathing.

✓ Keep in mind

• If you're pregnant or breast-feeding, check with your primary health care provider before using this medication.

Additional instructions

_____

_____

_____

_____

Taking pentazocine

Dear Patient,

Pentazocine is prescribed to relieve your pain. If you're taking the *tablet* form of this narcotic pain reliever, the label may read Talwin NX. If you're using the *injection* form, the label may read Talwin.

How to take pentazocine

If you're taking the *tablets,* carefully follow the prescription directions. If you're *injecting* yourself with pentazocine at home, make sure you understand and follow your primary health care provider's instructions exactly.

Don't take more pentazocine or use it for a longer time than directed because it may become habit-forming. If you think this medication isn't helping your pain, check with your primary health care provider.

What to do if you miss a dose

If your primary health care provider has ordered you to take this medication on a regular basis and you miss a dose, take it as soon as you remember. However, if it's almost time for your next dose, skip the missed dose and take your next dose at the scheduled time. Don't double dose.

What to do about side effects

Get emergency help *at once* if you think you may have taken an overdose. Symptoms include seizures; confusion; severe nervousness, restlessness, dizziness, weakness, or drowsiness; and slow or troubled breathing.

Let your primary health care provider know if you feel dizzy, light-headed, faint, or drowsy. Also tell him if you have difficulty urinating or nausea and vomiting.

What you must know about alcohol and other drugs

Don't drink alcoholic beverages while taking pentazocine. Combined use increases the chance of oversedation. For the same reason, don't take other medications that slow the nervous system, such as sleeping pills, tranquilizers, and cold and flu medications unless your primary health care provider tells you otherwise. Likewise, avoid other narcotic pain relievers, such as Darvon.

Special directions

• Tell your primary health care provider if you have other medical problems, especially lung disease, colitis, or a history of seizures, emotional problems, or alcohol or drug abuse. Also reveal if you have any disease that affects a major organ, such as the heart, kidneys, and liver.
• Because this medication may make you drowsy or light-headed, don't drive or perform activities requiring alertness until you know how you respond.

Warning: Don't stop taking pentazocine suddenly without checking first with your primary health care provider. He may want you to reduce your dosage gradually to lessen the chance of withdrawal effects.

✓ Keep in mind

• If you're pregnant or breast-feeding, check with your primary health care provider before using this medication. If you're an older adult, you may be especially prone to pentazocine's side effects.
• If you're an athlete, you should know that pentazocine is banned and tested for by the U.S. Olympic Committee.

Additional instructions

_____
_____
_____
_____
_____

Taking pentobarbital

Dear Patient,

Pentobarbital is prescribed to relax you. It belongs to a group of medications called barbiturates, which act by slowing down the nervous system. Brand names may include Nembutal and Nembutal Sodium.

How to take pentobarbital

This medication comes in capsule, elixir, and suppository forms. Take it exactly as your primary health care provider directs. Because it can become habit-forming, don't take it for a longer time than recommended.

To use the suppository, first remove the foil wrapper. Then moisten the suppository with cold water. Next, lie down on your side and use your finger to push the suppository well up into your rectum. Wash your hands afterward.

What to do if you miss a dose

If you're taking this medication regularly, take a missed dose as soon as possible. However, if it's almost time for your next dose, skip the missed dose and go back to your regular schedule. Don't double dose.

What to do about side effects

Get emergency help *immediately* if you think you may have taken an overdose. Symptoms include severe drowsiness, confusion, or weakness; shortness of breath; slow heartbeat; slow or troubled breathing; slurred speech; and staggering.

Check with your primary health care provider if you become drowsy or lethargic or feel as if you have a hangover.

What you must know about alcohol and other drugs

Don't drink alcoholic beverages while you're taking pentobarbital because the combination may cause oversedation. Likewise,
don't take other medications that slow down the nervous system, such as many allergy and cold medications, narcotic pain relievers, and sleeping pills, without checking first with your primary health care provider.

Tell your primary health care provider about other medications you're taking. In particular, he needs to know if you're using adrenocorticoids (cortisone-like medications); blood thinners (aspirin or warfarin); griseofulvin (Grisactin), an antifungal medication; or birth control pills.

Special directions

• Tell your primary health care provider if you have other medical problems. They may affect the use of this medication.
• Because pentobarbital may make you drowsy or light-headed, don't drive or perform activities requiring alertness until you know how it affects you.

! *Warning:* After prolonged use, don't suddenly stop taking this medication.

✓ Keep in mind

• If you're pregnant or breast-feeding, check with your primary health care provider before using this medication.
• If you're an older adult, you may be especially prone to pentobarbital's side effects.
• If you're an athlete, you should know that pentobarbital is banned and, in some cases, tested for by the U.S. Olympic Committee and the National Collegiate Athletic Association.

Additional instructions

_____

_____

_____

_____

Taking pentoxifylline

Dear Patient,

Your primary health care provider has prescribed pentoxifylline to improve your blood circulation. This medication is used to relieve leg pain and cramps caused by poor circulation. The label may read Trental.

How to take pentoxifylline

Pentoxifylline comes in extended-release tablets. Take your medication with meals to lessen the chance of stomach upset. You may also take the tablets with an antacid unless your primary health care provider tells you otherwise.

Swallow the tablet whole—don't chew, crush, or break it.

Don't stop taking this medication suddenly without first checking with your primary health care provider. It may take several weeks before you feel that pentoxifylline is working.

What to do if you miss a dose

Take the dose as soon as possible. But if it's almost time for your next dose, skip the missed dose and take your next dose on schedule. Don't double dose.

What to do about side effects

Rarely, this medication causes chest pain or an irregular heartbeat. If you have these symptoms, call your primary health care provider *as soon as possible.*

Pentoxifylline can also cause headache, dizziness, heartburn, nausea, or vomiting. Check with your primary health care provider if these symptoms continue or bother you.

What you must know about other drugs

Tell your primary health care provider about other medications you're taking. Taking pentoxifylline with blood thinners may increase your risk of bleeding. If you take medications for high blood pressure, your primary health care provider may need to adjust your dosage of these medications because pentoxifylline can increase their effect.

Special directions

• Tell your primary health care provider if you have other medical problems, especially stomach ulcers, strokes, and kidney or liver disease. Also mention if you've ever had an unusual or allergic reaction to caffeine or any foods or medications.

! *Warning:* Because nicotine can narrow your blood vessels, cigarette smoking may worsen your condition. So if you smoke, make an effort to quit, perhaps by joining a smoking-cessation program.

✓ Keep in mind

• If you're pregnant or breast-feeding, check with your primary health care provider before you take pentoxifylline.
• If you're an older adult, you may be especially prone to side effects from pentoxifylline.

Additional instructions

_____
_____
_____
_____
_____
_____
_____
_____
_____
_____
_____
_____

Taking perphenazine

Dear Patient,

Perphenazine is used to treat psychological disorders and to relieve severe nausea, vomiting, or hiccups. The label may read Trilafon.

How to take perphenazine
Perphenazine comes in tablets, syrup, and an oral solution. Take your medication exactly as your primary health care provider directs. Take your dose with food, water, or milk to prevent stomach irritation.

To use the *concentrated oral solution*, dilute your dose in fruit juice, ginger ale, or semisolid food, such as applesauce. Don't mix your medication with colas, black coffee, grape or apple juice, or tea.

Don't stop taking perphenazine without first checking with your primary health care provider.

What to do if you miss a dose
If you take one dose a day, take the missed dose as soon as possible. If you don't remember until the next day, skip it and go back to your regular schedule.

If you take more than one dose a day, take the missed dose within 1 hour if you remember it. If not, skip the missed dose and go back to your regular dosing schedule. Don't double dose.

What to do about side effects
Call your primary health care provider *at once* if you develop a fever, fast heartbeat, difficulty breathing, and increased sweating. or if you start to feel extremely tired or unwell.

Tell your health care provider if this medication causes uncontrolled movements of your mouth, tongue, or other body parts. Also tell him if you have blurred vision, a dry mouth, difficulty urinating, constipation, or dizziness or faintness, especially when you get up from a sitting or lying position.

What you must know about alcohol and other drugs
Don't drink alcoholic beverages while taking this medication because it could cause excessive drowsiness. Also avoid other medications that depress the nervous system, including tranquilizers and sleeping pills.

To avoid harmful medication interactions, check with your primary health care provider before you use other medications. If you take antacids, take them at least 2 hours before or after taking perphenazine.

Special directions
• Tell your health care provider of other medical problems because perphenazine can aggravate many medical conditions.
• Before you have medical tests, tell your health care provider that you're taking perphenazine because it may affect the test results.
• Because perphenazine may make you dizzy, know how you react to it before you drive or perform other activities that require alertness.

✔ Keep in mind
• If you're pregnant or breast-feeding, check with your primary health care provider before taking perphenazine.
• Children and older adults are especially prone to perphenazine's side effects.
• If you're an athlete, be aware that perphenazine is banned and sometimes tested for in shooting events by the U.S. Olympic Committee and the National Collegiate Athletic Association.

Additional instructions
_____
_____
_____

Taking phenazopyridine

Dear Patient,

This medication will help to ease the pain of your infected or irritated urinary tract. Brand names include AZO-Standard, Baridium, or Pyridium.

How to take phenazopyridine
Phenazopyridine comes in tablets. Follow your primary health care provider's directions exactly about how and when to take this medication. If you bought it without a prescription, carefully read the package instructions first.

To prevent stomach upset, take the tablets with meals or a snack.

You may stop using this medication after 3 days if your pain is relieved unless your primary health care provider gives you other instructions.

What to do if you miss a dose
Take the dose as soon as possible. However, if it's almost time for your next dose, skip the missed dose and take your next dose on schedule. Don't double dose.

What to do about side effects
Check with your primary health care provider *right away* if you have bluish skin, shortness of breath or difficulty breathing, a rash, unusual tiredness or weakness, or yellow eyes or skin.

Also let your primary health care provider know if this medication makes you dizzy or nauseated or gives you a headache.

Don't be surprised if phenazopyridine turns your urine reddish orange. This is to be expected and won't harm you. However, it may stain fabrics.

Special directions
• If you have kidney or liver disease, tell your primary health care provider because these medical problems may affect the use of phenazopyridine.

• Before you have medical tests, tell your primary health care provider that you're taking this medication because it may affect the test results.

• Because phenazopyridine may make you dizzy, make sure you know how you react to it before you drive or perform other activities requiring alertness.

• If you have another urinary tract problem in the future, don't use any leftover phenazopyridine without first checking with your primary health care provider.

✔ Keep in mind
Warning: If you have diabetes, this medication may cause false test results with urine glucose or urine ketone tests. Check with your primary health care provider for more information about this, especially if your diabetes isn't well controlled.

Additional instructions
_____
_____
_____
_____
_____
_____
_____
_____
_____
_____
_____

Taking phenobarbital

Dear Patient,

Phenobarbital is used to prevent seizures caused by epilepsy and other disorders. It's also used as a sedative to produce relaxation, such as before surgery. The label may read Barbita, Luminal, or Solfoton.

How to take phenobarbital

Phenobarbital comes in these forms: tablet, capsule, and elixir (oral solution). Follow your primary health care provider's directions exactly. Don't increase your dose because phenobarbital can become habit-forming.

If you're taking the capsule or tablet form, swallow it whole — don't chew or crush it. If you're taking this medication for epilepsy, take it every day in regularly spaced doses, as prescribed.

What to do if you miss a dose

Take the dose as soon as possible. However, if it's almost time for your next dose, skip the missed dose and take your next dose on schedule. Don't double dose.

What to do about side effects

Call for emergency medical help *at once* if you think you may have taken an overdose. Symptoms of overdose include severe drowsiness, weakness, and confusion; slurred speech; and difficulty breathing.

Check with your primary health care provider *right away* if you have any skin problems. Also let him know if this medication makes you feel drowsy, lethargic, or like you're "hung over."

What you must know about alcohol and other drugs

Avoid drinking alcoholic beverages while taking phenobarbital because the combination can lead to excessive drowsiness. For the same reason, don't use other medica-tions that depress the nervous system, including tranquilizers, sleeping pills, and many cold and flu remedies.

To prevent harmful medication interactions, tell your primary health care provider about other medications you're taking. If you take blood thinners, birth control pills, or estrogen, be aware that phenobarbital may decrease the effectiveness of these medications.

Special directions

• Tell your primary health care provider if you have other medical problems, especially asthma, lung disease, or porphyria. Also reveal if you're depressed or in chronic pain.
• Before you have medical tests, tell your primary health care provider that you're taking this medication because it may affect the test results.
• Because phenobarbital may make you drowsy, make sure you know how you react to it before you drive or perform other activities requiring alertness.

☑ Keep in mind

• If you're pregnant or breast-feeding, don't take phenobarbital without specific instructions from your primary health care provider.
• If you're an older adult, you may be especially sensitive to phenobarbital's side effects.
• If you're an athlete, you should know that phenobarbital is banned and sometimes tested for by the U.S. Olympic Committee and the National Collegiate Athletic Association.

Additional instructions

_____

_____

Using nasal phenylephrine

Dear Patient,

This medication will help to relieve your stuffy nose. Phenylephrine is used to relieve nasal congestion caused by hay fever or other allergies, colds, or sinus trouble. The label may read Alconefrin, Neo-Synephrine, or Sinex.

How to use nasal phenylephrine

This medication comes in a nose jelly, nose drops, and a nose spray. Follow your primary health care provider's directions exactly. If you bought your medication without a prescription, carefully read the package directions before using. Also, before you use this medication in any of the following forms, blow your nose gently.

To use the *nose drops,* tilt your head back and squeeze the drops into each nostril. Keep your head tilted back for a few minutes. Rinse the dropper with hot water, dry it with a clean tissue, and recap.

To use the *nose spray,* hold your head upright and spray the medication into each nostril. Sniff briskly while squeezing the bottle. Spray once or twice, then wait a few minutes for the medication to work. Blow your nose and repeat until the complete dose is used.

To use the *nose jelly,* place a pea-size amount of the jelly up each nostril. Sniff it well back into the nose.

Don't use phenylephrine longer than directed because doing so may worsen your runny or stuffy nose.

Don't share the container with anyone else to avoid spreading the infection.

What to do if you miss a dose

Use the medication right away if you remember within 1 hour or so of the missed dose. However, if you don't remember until later, skip the missed dose and take your next dose on schedule. Don't double dose.

What to do about side effects

Check with your primary health care provider if your heart starts to pound irregularly or too rapidly. These symptoms suggest that you've used too much phenylephrine. When you use this medication, your nose may burn, sting, or feel dry. Let your primary health care provider know if these symptoms continue or become bothersome.

Special directions

• Tell your primary health care provider if you have other medical problems, especially heart or blood vessel disease, high blood pressure, glaucoma, diabetes, an overactive thyroid, or diseases of the liver or pancreas.
• Before you have a hearing test, tell your primary health care provider that you're taking phenylephrine because it may affect the test results.

✓ Keep in mind

• If you're giving this medication to a child, check with your primary health care provider first because children are especially prone to side effects from phenylephrine.
• If you're an athlete, you should know that phenylephrine is banned and tested for by the U.S. Olympic Committee. Use of nasal phenylephrine can lead to disqualification in most athletic events.

Additional instructions

_____
_____
_____
_____
_____

Using ophthalmic phenylephrine

Dear Patient,

This medication will relieve the redness of your eyes. Phenylephrine eyedrops also are used to treat some other eye problems and to enlarge the pupils before eye examinations. The label may read AK-Dilate, Neo-Synephrine, and Prefrin Liquifilm.

How to use phenylephrine eyedrops

Follow your primary health care provider's directions exactly. If you bought this medication without a prescription, carefully read the package directions before using. Don't use more of the eyedrops or use them more often than your primary health care provider ordered. To instill the eyedrops, follow these steps.
• First, wash your hands.
• Tilt your head back and pull the lower eyelid away from the eye to form a pouch.
• Squeeze the drops into the pouch and gently close your eye.
• Wash your hands again.

What to do if you miss a dose

Instill the eyedrops as soon as possible. However, if it's almost time for your next dose, skip the missed dose and instill your next dose on schedule. Don't double dose.

What to do about side effects

Check with your primary health care provider if you're told your blood pressure is elevated. When you instill the eyedrops, your eyes may burn, sting, water, or become more sensitive to light. Check with your primary health care provider if these symptoms continue or become bothersome.

What you must know about other drugs

Tell your primary health care provider about other medications you're taking. He may want you to avoid certain medications to prevent harmful interactions. In particular, medications to avoid or use only with your primary health care provider's supervision are those for high blood pressure, Parkinson's disease, and depression or other psychiatric problems. Also, talk to your primary health care provider before taking the herbal product Ma-huang (Ephedra). It may raise your high blood pressure.

Special directions

• Tell your primary health care provider if you have other medical problems, especially heart or blood vessel disease, high blood pressure, glaucoma, diabetes, an overactive thyroid, or diseases of the liver or pancreas.
• Before you have a hearing test, tell your primary health care provider that you're taking phenylephrine because it may affect the test results.
• Because your eyes may be more sensitive to light while you use this medication, wear sunglasses that block ultraviolet light when you're in a bright room or outside on sunny days.

✓ Keep in mind

• If you're giving this medication to a child, check with your primary health care provider first because children are especially prone to side effects from phenylephrine.
• Older adults are also especially prone to its side effects.
• If you're an athlete, you should know that phenylephrine eyedrops are banned by the U.S. Olympic Committee.

Additional instructions

_____
_____
_____
_____

Taking phenytoin

Dear Patient,

This medication is used to control seizures and treat several other medical problems. The label may read Dilantin or Diphenylan.

How to take phenytoin

Phenytoin comes in capsules, chewable tablets, and an oral liquid. Don't take more or less than your primary health care provider orders. Take phenytoin with meals to reduce stomach upset. If you're taking the *liquid* form, use a specially marked measuring spoon (not a household teaspoon) to measure your dose. If you're taking the *capsules,* be sure to swallow them whole.

What to do if you miss a dose

Adjust your dosing schedule as follows.

If you take one dose a day, take the missed dose as soon as possible. But if you don't remember until the next day, skip it and take your next dose on schedule.

If you take more than one dose a day, take the missed dose as soon as possible. However, if it's within 4 hours of your next dose, skip the missed dose and take your next dose on schedule. Don't double dose.

What to do about side effects

Call your primary health care provider *right away* if you have skin problems, heart palpitations, or difficulty breathing. Also call if you have a fever, become extremely weak or tired, or feel very unwell.

Check with your primary health care provider if you experience confusion, dizziness, vision changes, sleeplessness, or slurred speech. Also report uncontrolled movements, nausea, vomiting, and bleeding gums.

What you must know about alcohol and other drugs

Check with your primary health care provider before drinking alcoholic beverages because alcohol may prevent phenytoin from working well.

Tell your health care provider about other medications you're taking. Some medications you may need to avoid or use only with your health care provider's approval are blood thinners, antihistamines (found in cold and allergy medications), the ulcer medication cimetidine (Tagamet), and aspirin.

Special directions

● Tell your primary health care provider if you have other medical problems, especially a heart condition, porphyria, diabetes, and liver, kidney or thyroid disease.
● Make sure you know how you react to phenytoin before you drive or perform other activities requiring alertness. Follow your primary health care provider's orders about driving if you're taking phenytoin for seizures.
● See your dentist regularly, and tell him you're taking phenytoin.

✔ Keep in mind

● If you're pregnant or breast-feeding, check with your primary health care provider before taking this medication.
● If you have diabetes, be aware that phenytoin may affect the results of blood and urine glucose tests.
● If you're an athlete, you should know that phenytoin is banned and sometimes tested for in biathlon and modern pentathlon events by the U.S. Olympic Committee.

Additional instructions

_____

_____

Using pilocarpine

Dear Patient,

Your primary health care provider has ordered pilocarpine to treat your glaucoma or another eye condition. This medication comes in the form of eyedrops, eye gel, and an eye system. Brand names include Adsorbocarpine, Isopto Carpine, Ocu-Carpine, Pilocar, and Pilopine HS.

How to use pilocarpine

Follow your primary health care provider's instructions exactly. Don't use more pilocarpine or use it more often than your primary health care provider orders. Also, before you use pilocarpine, wash your hands. Then follow these steps.

If you're using *eyedrops,* first tilt your head back. Use your index finger to pull the lower eyelid away from the eye, forming a pouch. Squeeze the drops into the pouch and apply pressure to the inner corner of the eye for 1 to 2 minutes. Don't blink.

If you're using *eye gel,* first pull the lower eyelid away to form a pouch. Squeeze a thin strip of gel into the pouch. Gently close your eyes for 1 to 2 minutes.

Right after using the eyedrops or eye gel, wash your hands to remove any pilocarpine that might be on them. Also, take care to keep your medication bottle germfree. Don't let the applicator tip touch any surface, including your eye.

Before you use the *eye system,* read the patient instructions that come with this medication. If you have any questions, check with your primary health care provider.

What to do if you miss a dose

If you forget to use the eyedrops or eye gel, do so as soon as possible. But if it's almost time for your next dose, skip the missed dose and take your next dose on schedule. Don't double dose.

What to do about side effects

This medication may cause brow, head, or eye pain. For a short time after you use pilocarpine, your vision may be blurred or you may notice a change in your near or distant vision, especially at night.

If these symptoms persist or become bothersome, check with your primary health care provider.

What you must know about other drugs

Tell your primary health care provider about other medications you're taking. To prevent harmful interactions, avoid certain other medications, especially some eye medications, such as phenylephrine (for eye redness) and carbachol (Miostat), another glaucoma medication.

Special directions

• Tell your primary health care provider if you have other medical problems, especially asthma, other eye problems, heart disease, urinary difficulty, stomach ulcers, an overactive thyroid, or Parkinson's disease.
• If you're using the eyedrops or eye gel, don't drive or perform other activities that require good vision until your vision clears.

Additional instructions

_____
_____
_____
_____
_____
_____
_____
_____
_____
_____
_____

Taking pirbuterol

Dear Patient,

Your primary health care provider has prescribed pirbuterol to open the air passages in your lungs and help you breathe easier. This medication is used to treat the symptoms of asthma, chronic bronchitis, emphysema, and other lung diseases. The label may read Maxair.

How to take pirbuterol
Pirbuterol comes in an aerosol inhaler. Follow your primary health care provider's instructions for taking pirbuterol. Don't use more of it or take it more often than your primary health care provider directs.

Shake the aerosol canister well before each use. Keep the spray away from the eyes because it may cause irritation. Also, don't take more than two inhalations at any one time unless your primary health care provider gives you other instructions. Hold your breath up to 10 seconds if you can, to give the medication time to settle into your lungs. Wait 1 to 2 minutes after the first inhalation to be sure that a second inhalation is necessary.

What to do if you miss a dose
If you're using the inhaler on a regular schedule, take a missed dose as soon as possible. Then take any remaining doses for that day at regularly spaced times. Don't double dose.

What to do about side effects
Let your primary health care provider know if pirbuterol makes you feel nervous or dizzy or if you have headaches or trouble sleeping. Also tell him if you develop palpitations or a fast heartbeat and if your throat feels dry or sore.

Occasionally, pirbuterol causes changes in smell or taste. Don't worry. These effects are temporary and will go away when you stop using this medication.

What you must know about other drugs
Tell your primary health care provider if you're taking beta blockers, such as propranolol (Inderal), to treat high blood pressure or a heart condition. Taking these medications with pirbuterol may reduce its helpful effects on your lungs.

Before you begin taking any new medication, check first with your primary health care provider.

Special directions
• Tell your primary health care provider if you have other medical problems, especially heart disease, high blood pressure, or a seizure disorder. Other medical problems may affect the use of this medication.
• If pirbuterol makes your throat and mouth feel dry, rinsing your mouth with water after each dose may help.
• If the dosage of pirbuterol you've been using no longer seems to work, check with your primary health care provider. This may mean your condition is getting worse.

✔ Keep in mind
• If you're pregnant, check with your primary health care provider before using this medication.

Additional instructions
_____
_____
_____
_____
_____
_____

Taking piroxicam

Dear Patient,

Your primary health care provider has prescribed piroxicam to treat your arthritis. This medication is used to relieve joint swelling, pain, and stiffness. The label may read Feldene.

How to take piroxicam

Piroxicam comes in capsules. Follow your primary health care provider's instructions for taking this medication. To lessen stomach upset, take your dose with food or an antacid. Also, avoid lying down for 15 to 30 minutes after taking your dose to prevent irritation of your esophagus (food tube).

Take your medication faithfully every day, as directed. Realize that it may take several weeks before you start to feel better.

What to do if you miss a dose

If you remember the missed dose within 1 to 2 hours, take it as soon as possible. Otherwise, skip the missed dose and take your next dose on schedule. Don't double dose.

What to do about side effects

Occasionally, piroxicam can cause serious bleeding from the digestive tract. Call your primary health care provider *at once* if you have warning signs of internal bleeding, such as black, tarry stools; severe abdominal or stomach pain; severe, continuing nausea or heartburn; or vomiting of blood or material that looks like coffee grounds.

Piroxicam also can cause nausea, heartburn, drowsiness, dizziness, and increased light sensitivity. Let your primary health care provider know if these symptoms continue or become bothersome.

What you must know about other drugs

Tell your primary health care provider if you're taking other medications. Don't use aspirin or blood thinners without your primary health care provider's okay because the chance of serious side effects may be increased when used with piroxicam. If you take lithium (Lithane), a medication for manic-depressive disorder, your primary health care provider may need to adjust your lithium dosage.

Special directions

● Tell your primary health care provider if you have other medical problems, especially stomach ulcers or other digestive disorders, diabetes, and heart, kidney, or liver disease. Also reveal if you've ever had an unusual or allergic reaction to aspirin or another medication.
● Because piroxicam may make you more sensitive to sunlight, limit your exposure to bright sun.
● If this medication makes you drowsy or dizzy, don't drive or perform other activities that require alertness.

✔ Keep in mind

● If you're pregnant or breast-feeding, check with your primary health care provider before using this medication.
● If you're an older adult, you may be especially prone to side effects from piroxicam.
● If you have diabetes, check carefully for infection because piroxicam may mask signs.

Additional instructions

_____
_____
_____
_____
_____
_____

Taking potassium chloride

Dear Patient,

Because your body needs additional potassium for good health, your primary health care provider has prescribed potassium chloride supplements. These will help to restore potassium that your body may have lost after illness or treatment with certain medications. Brand names include K+10, Kaochlor 10%, Kaon-Cl, K-Dur, and Micro-K.

How to take potassium chloride

Potassium chloride comes in tablets, extended-release tablets and capsules, an oral liquid, and a soluble powder. If you're taking the *liquid* or *soluble powder,* dilute your dose in at least 4 ounces of cold water or juice. With the soluble powder, wait for any fizzing to stop before you drink the dissolved medication.

If you're taking the *extended-release capsules or tablets,* swallow them whole — don't chew, crush, or break them. Take them with 8 ounces of water. If you have trouble swallowing, check with your primary health care provider or pharmacist.

Take your medication with food or right after meals to prevent stomach upset.

What to do if you miss a dose

If you remember the missed dose within 2 hours, take it with food or liquids as soon as possible. Then go back to your regular dosing schedule. But if you don't remember until later, skip the missed dose and take your next dose on schedule. Don't double dose.

What to do about side effects

Stop taking this medication and call your primary health care provider *right away* if you have:
- confusion
- irregular or slow heartbeat
- "pins and needles" feeling in your hands, feet, or lips
- shortness of breath or difficulty breathing
- unusual tiredness or weakness
- unexplained anxiety
- weakness or heaviness of your legs.

This medication may also cause nausea, vomiting, abdominal pain, or diarrhea. Call your primary health care provider if these effects persist or become bothersome.

What you must know about other drugs

Tell your primary health care provider if you're taking other medications. He may want you to avoid certain medications that slow intestinal movements (including anticholinergic medications, such as atropine) because their use with potassium chloride may increase the risk of side effects.

Make sure your primary health care provider knows if you're taking angiotensin-converting enzyme inhibitors (Vasotec) or potassium-sparing diuretics (Dyrenium) because their combined use may cause potassium levels to rise dangerously high.

Special directions

- Tell your primary health care provider if you have other medical problems, especially Addison's disease, stomach ulcers, severe diarrhea, and kidney or heart disease. Other medical problems may affect the use of this medication.

Warning: Don't use salt substitutes or drink low-salt milk unless your primary health care provider tells you to do so. These products may contain potassium and might cause you to have too much potassium. Also, check for added potassium in the ingredient lists of processed foods.

Additional instructions

_____

_____

_____

Taking pravastatin

Dear Patient,

Your primary health care provider has prescribed pravastatin to lower your cholesterol levels. This medication decreases the level of low-density lipoproteins (LDL) because high LDL levels increase the risk of heart attacks from blocked arteries. The brand name of this medication is Pravachol.

How to take pravastatin

This medication works best if taken at bedtime, since the production of cholesterol is higher at night. Take it with food or on an empty stomach.

What to do if you miss a dose

Take the dose as soon as you remember it. However, if it's close to the time for your next dose, skip the missed dose and take the next scheduled dose. Don't take double doses.

What to do about side effects

Notify your primary health care provider *immediately* if you have a fever, muscle aches or cramps, or unusual tiredness or weakness.

When starting this medication, some patients notice constipation, diarrhea, gas, heartburn, stomach pain, dizziness, blurred vision, headaches, nausea, or rash. Notify your primary health care provider if these continue for longer than a few days or become bothersome.

This medication may also cause liver problems in a small number of patients. Your primary health care provider may order blood tests to check your liver during the first year you take pravastatin.

What you must know about alcohol and other drugs

Ask your health care provider about drinking alcohol when taking this medication.

Tell your health care provider if you're taking other medications, especially immunosuppressive medications, gemfibrozil (Lopid), nicotinic acid (Niacin), or erythromycin. These drugs may cause muscle problems.

Special directions

• Before starting this medication, tell your health care provider if you have a history of alcoholism; of heart, kidney, or liver disease; or of recent major surgery or trauma.
• For this medication to work well, follow the lifestyle changes recommended by your primary health care provider, including regular exercise and a low fat and/or weight loss diet. Visiting a registered dietitian may help you change your diet.
• Your primary health care provider will probably check your blood cholesterol level periodically while you're on this medication. Based on these results, he'll decide whether or not to change your medication dosage. Don't stop the medication or change the dose without talking to him first.
• Don't drive or perform any activities that require alertness until you know how this medication affects you.

✔ Keep in mind

Warning: This medication isn't recommended for use during pregnancy. Notify your primary health care provider immediately if you're pregnant or think you might be.
• Notify your primary health care provider immediately if you wish to breast-feed while on this medication.

Additional instructions

_____

_____

_____

_____

Taking prazosin

Dear Patient,

Your primary health care provider has prescribed prazosin to treat your high blood pressure. This medication works by relaxing blood vessels, allowing blood to pass through them more easily. This helps to lower blood pressure. The label may read Minipress.

How to take prazosin

Prazosin comes in capsules. Your primary health care provider may direct you to take your first dose at bedtime because the first dose of prazosin sometimes causes dizziness and irregular heartbeat. If so, be careful if you need to get up during the night.

Take your doses at the same times every day to help you remember to take your medication.

What to do if you miss a dose

Take the dose as soon as possible. However, if it's almost time for your next dose, skip the missed dose and take your next dose on schedule. Don't double dose.

What to do about side effects

Prazosin may make you feel dizzy, faint, or light-headed, especially when you get up suddenly from a lying or sitting position. Getting up slowly may help.

If this medication makes you feel drowsy, nauseated, or tired or gives you a headache, tell your primary health care provider.

What you must know about alcohol and other drugs

Be careful how much alcohol you drink because it could increase the amount of dizziness or drowsiness you experience.

Tell your primary health care provider if you're taking other medications. If you're taking beta blockers (for high blood pres-

sure or a heart condition), combining them with prazosin may lower your blood pressure too much.

Special directions

• Tell your primary health care provider if you have other medical problems, especially chest pain, kidney disease, or a heart condition. Other medical problems may affect the use of this medication.
• Remember, prazosin won't cure your high blood pressure, but it will help to control it. Therefore, you may have to take high blood pressure medication for the rest of your life.
• Avoid driving or performing other activities requiring alertness until you know how prazosin affects you.
• Keep all appointments for follow-up visits, even if you feel well. This way, your primary health care provider can check your progress and adjust your medication, if necessary.

✓ Keep in mind

• If you're an older adult, you may be especially prone to side effects from prazosin, especially dizziness and light-headedness. Therefore, take care to prevent falls.

Additional instructions

_____
_____
_____
_____
_____
_____
_____
_____
_____

Taking prednisone

Dear Patient,

Prednisone is used to relieve severe inflammation and to treat a number of diseases. Brand names include Deltasone, Orasone, and Sterapred.

How to take prednisone
Prednisone comes in tablet, oral solution, and syrup forms. Take the medication exactly as prescribed. To prevent stomach upset, take your dose with food.

What to do if you miss a dose
Adjust your dosing schedule as follows.

If you take one dose every other day, take the missed dose as soon as possible if you remember it the same morning. If not, wait and take it the next morning. Then skip a day and start your regular dosing schedule again.

If you take one dose daily, take the missed dose as soon as possible. If you don't remember until the next day, skip the missed dose and take your next scheduled dose. Don't double dose.

If you take several doses a day, take the missed dose as soon as possible, then go back to your regular dosing schedule. If you don't remember until your next dose is due, double the next dose.

What to do about side effects
Prednisone can make your potassium level too low or your blood glucose level too high. Call your primary health care provider *at once* if you have symptoms of low potassium: dizziness, tiredness, weakness, leg cramps, nausea, or digestive upset. Also call if you have frequent urination and thirst — symptoms of high blood glucose — or if you have bloody or black, tarry stools or difficulty sleeping.

Prednisone may also affect your mood and cause euphoria.

What you must know about other drugs
Tell your primary health care provider if you're taking other medications. Check with him before you take aspirin or indomethacin (Indocin) because they may cause stomach distress. Also check with your health care provider before you have vaccinations.

If you take barbiturates (sedatives) or medications for seizures or tuberculosis, your primary health care provider may need to adjust your prednisone dosage.

Special directions
Warning: Never stop taking prednisone suddenly without first checking with your primary health care provider. Stopping the drug suddenly could be fatal.
- Tell your health care provider if you have an ulcer, high blood pressure, diabetes, and kidney, liver, or bone disease. Wear a medical identification tag at all times.
- Before you have medical tests, tell your health care provider you're taking prednisone because it may affect the test results.
- Because prednisone may lower your ability to fight infections, call your health care provider if you have a sore throat, fever, sneezing, or coughing.

Keep in mind
- If you're pregnant or breast-feeding, check with your primary health care provider before taking prednisone.
- If you're diabetic, be aware that prednisone may affect your blood sugar level.
- If you're an athlete, be aware that the U.S. Olympic Committee and the National Collegiate Athletic Association have restrictions on prednisone use.

Additional instructions

_____

_____

Taking primidone

Dear Patient,

Your primary health care provider has prescribed primidone to treat your seizure disorder. Brand names include Myidone and Mysoline.

How to take primidone

Primidone comes in tablet and oral suspension forms. Take this medication exactly as your primary health care provider directs. For best results, take it in regularly spaced doses, as ordered.

Don't stop taking primidone suddenly without first checking with your primary health care provider. He may want you to reduce your dosage gradually.

What to do if you miss a dose

Take the dose as soon as possible. But if it's within 1 hour of your next dose, skip the missed dose and take your next dose on schedule. Don't double dose.

What to do about side effects

Occasionally, primidone can make you feel drowsy or cause nausea, vomiting, double vision, or loss of coordination. Check with your primary health care provider if you have any of these side effects, especially if they continue or become bothersome.

What you must know about alcohol and other drugs

Check with your primary health care provider about drinking alcoholic beverages. Alcohol combined with primidone may make you overly drowsy. For the same reason, check with your primary health care provider before you take other medications that slow down your nervous system, such as muscle relaxants, anesthetics, sleeping pills, cold and flu remedies, and Kava Kava, an herbal product.

Tell your primary health care provider if you're taking other medications. In particular, he may need to watch your progress closely if you're taking phenytoin (Dilantin) or carbamazepine (Tegretol), two other medications used to prevent seizures.

Also, tell your health care provider if you're taking birth control pills because the effectiveness may be decreased. You may need to use another form of birth control.

Special directions

• Tell your primary health care provider if you have other medical problems, especially asthma or other lung diseases, porphyria, and liver disease. Other medical problems may affect the use of this medication.
• Before you have diagnostic liver tests, tell your health care provider you're taking primidone because it may affect the test results.
• Primidone can make you drowsy. So know how it affects you before you drive or perform other activities that might be dangerous if you're not fully alert.
• Keep all appointments for follow-up visits, so your primary health care provider can check your progress.

✔ Keep in mind

• If you're pregnant or breast-feeding, don't use primidone unless instructed by your primary health care provider.
• If you're an older adult, you may be especially prone to primidone's side effects.
• If you're an athlete, you should know that primidone is banned and sometimes tested for by the U.S. Olympic Committee and the National Collegiate Athletic Association.

Additional instructions

_____

_____

Taking procarbazine

Dear Patient,

Procarbazine is prescribed to treat cancer. This medication stops the growth of cancer cells by destroying them. The label may read Matulane.

How to take procarbazine

Procarbazine comes in capsules. Follow your primary health care provider's directions exactly. Don't stop taking this medication, even if it makes you feel ill, without first checking with your health care provider.

If you vomit soon after taking a dose, check with your health care provider to find out when you should take another dose.

What to do if you miss a dose

If you remember the missed dose in a few hours, take it as soon as you remember. But if several hours have passed or if it's almost time for your next dose, skip the missed dose and take your next dose on schedule. Don't double dose.

What to do about side effects

Stop taking procarbazine and call your primary health care provider *at once* if you have chest pain, rapid or irregular heartbeat, severe headache, or a stiff neck. Also call *right away* if you become extremely tired or weak or if you start to bruise or bleed easily.

This medication may cause nausea, vomiting, or loss of appetite. Ask your health care provider how to lessen these side effects. Watch for signs of infection, such as fever and sore throat, and report them. Also report hallucinations.

What you must know about alcohol and other drugs

Avoid alcoholic beverages while taking procarbazine because the combination can cause harmful side effects.

Also, tell your health care provider about other medications you're taking. Avoid medications that slow the nervous system, such as tranquilizers, sleeping pills, anesthetics, and cold remedies.

❗ *Warning:* Don't use the pain reliever meperidine (Demerol) with procarbazine because this combination can cause life-threatening low blood pressure.

Also check with your health care provider before you have vaccinations or take new medications — even aspirin.

Taking antidepressants such as amitriptyline (Elavil) or fluoxetine (Prozac) within 2 weeks of procarbazine can cause severe high blood pressure.

Special directions

• Because procarbazine may make you drowsy, know how you react to it before you drive or perform other hazardous activities.

❗ *Warning:* Don't eat foods that have a high tyramine content, such as cheeses and Chianti wine. Ask your primary health care provider for a complete list of foods to avoid.

✓ Keep in mind

• Tell your health care provider if you're pregnant or intend to have children in the future.
• If you're breast-feeding or plan to do so during treatment, check with your health care provider.
• Older adults may be especially sensitive to side effects from procarbazine.
• If you're diabetic, be aware that procarbazine may affect your blood sugar levels.

Additional instructions

_____

_____

Taking prochlorperazine

Dear Patient,

Prochlorperazine is used to relieve or prevent nausea and vomiting. It's also used to manage some psychiatric problems. The label may read Compazine.

How to take prochlorperazine

This medication comes in several forms. Follow your primary health care provider's directions exactly. If you're taking prochlorperazine by mouth, take it with food, water, or milk. If you're taking the *extended-release* capsules, swallow them whole—don't crush, break, or chew them. If you're using the rectal suppository, remove the foil wrapper and moisten with cold water.

What to do if you miss a dose

If you take one dose a day, take the missed dose as soon as possible. But if you don't remember the missed dose until the next day, skip it and go back to your regular dosing schedule.

If you take more than one dose a day, take the missed dose right away if you remember within 1 hour or so. But if you don't remember until later, skip it and take your next dose on schedule. Don't double dose.

What to do about side effects

Call your primary health care provider *right away* if you have a fever, chills, headache, extreme tiredness, or skin problems.

Check with your health care provider if you feel dizzy or have blurred vision, a fast heartbeat, dry mouth, constipation, or difficulty urinating. This medication also can cause a movement disorder called tardive dyskinesia, so be sure to report any uncontrolled movements of your mouth, tongue, or other body parts.

What you must know about alcohol and other drugs

Avoid alcohol or medications that slow down the nervous system, including tranquilizers, sleeping pills, and cold and flu remedies, while taking prochlorperazine because the combination can make you overly drowsy.

Tell your primary health care provider about other medications you're taking. In particular, he may want to watch your progress closely if you're taking medications for Parkinson's disease or depression.

Take antacids at least 2 hours before or after you take prochlorperazine.

Special directions

• Tell your primary health care provider of other medical conditions, especially heart or blood disease, glaucoma, seizure disorder, Parkinson's disease, or kidney or liver problems. Other medical problems may affect the use of this medication.
• Because prochlorperazine may make you dizzy, make sure you know how you react to it before you drive or perform other activities requiring alertness.
• You maybe more sensitive to light, so cover up outdoors and limit your sun exposure.

✓ Keep in mind

• If you're pregnant or breast-feeding, check with your primary health care provider before taking this medication.
• Children and older adults are especially prone to prochlorperazine's side effects.
• Know that this medication is banned and may be tested for by the U.S. Olympic Committee and the National Collegiate Athletic Association.

Additional instructions

Taking propafenone

Dear Patient,

Your primary health care provider has prescribed propafenone to correct your irregular heartbeat to a normal rhythm. The label may read Rythmol.

How to take propafenone

Propafenone comes in tablets. Take this medication exactly as your primary health care provider directs even if you feel well. Don't take more or less of it than prescribed.

For best results, take propafenone at evenly spaced times day and night. To prevent stomach upset, take your medication with food.

What to do if you miss a dose

If you remember the missed dose within 4 hours, take it as soon as possible. But if you don't remember until later, skip it and take your next dose on schedule. Don't double dose.

What to do about side effects

Call your primary health care provider *right away* if you have chest pain, palpitations, a fast or irregular heartbeat, difficulty breathing, or unusual weakness and fatigue.

This medication also may make you dizzy or cause taste changes; let your primary health care provider know if these side effects continue or become bothersome.

What you must know about other drugs

Tell your primary health care provider if you're taking other medications, some of which can interact with propafenone and possibly cause problems. In particular, report if you're taking blood thinners, other heart medications (such as digoxin or quinidine), the ulcer medication cimetidine (Tagamet), high blood pressure medications, or cyclosporine.

Special directions

● Tell your primary health care provider if you have other medical conditions, especially asthma, bronchitis, emphysema, and kidney or liver disease. Also reveal if you've had other heart problems, such as a recent heart attack, or if you have a pacemaker. Other medical problems may affect the use of this medication.
● Because propafenone may make you dizzy, make sure you know how you react to it before you drive or perform other activities that might be dangerous if you're not fully alert.
● This medication may make you more sensitive to light, so cover up outdoors and limit your sun exposure.
● Before you have surgery (including dental surgery) or emergency treatment, tell your primary health care provider or dentist that you're taking propafenone.
● Your primary health care provider may want you to carry a medical identification card or wear a medical identification bracelet stating that you're taking propafenone.

✔ Keep in mind

● If you're pregnant, check with your primary health care provider before taking this medication.

Additional instructions

_____

_____

_____

_____

_____

Taking propantheline

Dear Patient,

Your primary health care provider has prescribed propantheline to help relieve stomach cramps, spasms, and acid stomach. Brand names include Pro-Banthine and Propanthel.

How to take propantheline
Take this medication exactly as the label directs. Take it 30 to 60 minutes before meals. And take your bedtime dose at least 2 hours after your last meal of the day. Swallow the tablets whole; don't chew or crush them.

What to do if you miss a dose
If you forget to take a dose, don't make it up. Just start your schedule all over again with the next dose. Never take a double dose.

What to do about side effects
Call your primary health care provider *right away* if you develop difficulty with urinating or swallowing, dizziness, drowsiness, eye pain, headaches, nervousness, rapid heartbeat or palpitations, or a rash.

Also call him if you have constipation, decreased sweating, heartburn, nausea, or vomiting or if your eyes are unusually sensitive to bright light.

What you must know about alcohol and other drugs
Avoid alcoholic beverages because they may worsen your condition.

Make sure your primary health care provider knows all the medications you're taking including antacids or diarrhea medications. Before you take other medications, consult your primary health care provider. Other medications can interact with propantheline and possibly cause problems.

Special directions
• Tell your primary health care provider if you have other medical problems, especially glaucoma, difficult urination, myasthenia gravis, or diseases of the digestive tract, heart, liver, or kidneys. Other medical problems may affect the use of this medication.
• Propantheline may make you drowsy. So know how you react to it before you drive or perform other activities that might be dangerous if you're not fully alert.

! *Warning:* Your body sweats less while you're taking this medication. To avoid heatstroke, don't exercise too strenuously or stay outside too long in hot weather.
• If your eyes seem unusually sensitive to sunlight, protect them by wearing sunglasses or a wide-brimmed hat.
• While you're taking this medication, avoid eating spicy or acidic foods because they can upset your stomach.
• To prevent constipation, drink lots of extra water or other fluids.

✔ Keep in mind
• If you're pregnant or breast-feeding, check with your primary health care provider before taking this medication.
• Older adults may be especially prone to side effects from propantheline.

Additional instructions
_____
_____
_____
_____
_____
_____
_____
_____

Taking propoxyphene

Dear Patient,

Your primary health care provider has prescribed propoxyphene to help relieve your pain. The label may read Darvocet-N, Darvon, or Dolene.

How to take propoxyphene

A narcotic analgesic, propoxyphene comes in three forms: tablets, capsules, and an oral suspension. Take propoxyphene exactly as the label directs. If you feel your medication isn't working well, don't take more than the prescribed dose. Check with your primary health care provider instead. If you take too much of this medication or take it for too long, it could become habit-forming.

What to do if you miss a dose

Take the dose as soon as you remember. However, if it's almost time for your next dose, skip the missed dose and go back to your regular dosing schedule. Don't double the dose.

What to do about side effects

The most common side effect from propoxyphene is dizziness. This medication may also make you feel drowsy or cause nausea or vomiting. Let your primary health care provider know if these symptoms continue or become bothersome.

What you must know about alcohol and other drugs

Avoid drinking alcoholic beverages while taking propoxyphene because the combination can make you overly drowsy. For the same reason, check with your primary health care provider before using medications that slow down the central nervous system, such as sleeping pills, tranquilizers, sedatives, and many cold, flu, and allergy remedies.

Special directions

! *Warning:* Don't stop taking propoxyphene suddenly. Your primary health care provider may want to reduce your dosage gradually to lessen the chance of withdrawal side effects.

- Tell your primary health care provider if you have other medical problems, especially heart, liver, lung, or kidney disease. Also tell him if you have asthma, a seizure disorder, or a history of medication or alcohol abuse. Other medical problems may affect the use of this medication.
- Propoxyphene may make you dizzy. So know how you react to it before you drive or perform other activities that might be dangerous if you're not fully alert.
- If this medication makes your mouth feel dry, you may use sugarless hard candy or gum, ice chips, or a saliva substitute. If your dry mouth continues for more than 2 weeks, see your dentist.

✓ Keep in mind

- If you're pregnant or breast-feeding, check with your primary health care provider before taking this medication.
- If you're an older adult, you may be especially prone to propoxyphene's side effects.
- If you're an athlete, you should know that propoxyphene is banned and tested for by the U.S. Olympic Committee.

Additional instructions

_____
_____
_____
_____
_____
_____
_____

Taking propranolol

Dear Patient,

Propranolol is prescribed to relieve angina (chest pain) and to treat certain heart conditions and high blood pressure. It may also be used to prevent some kinds of severe headaches. The label may read Betachron E-R, Inderal, or Inderal LA.

How to take propranolol
Propranolol comes in these forms: tablets, extended-release capsules, and an oral solution. Take propranolol exactly as your primary health care provider orders. Take it at the same time each day, with meals, so you're less likely to forget.

Once a day, preferably before the first dose, take your pulse (if instructed by your primary health care provider). If your pulse rate is less than 50 beats a minute, don't take the next dose. Instead, call your primary health care provider as soon as possible.

What to do if you miss a dose
Take the missed dose right away if you remember within 1 hour or so. However, if it's within 4 hours of your next regular dose (or 8 hours of the long-acting form), skip the missed dose and resume your regular dosage schedule. Don't double dose.

What to do about side effects
Call your primary health care provider *right away* if you have a persistent cough, shortness of breath, difficulty breathing, unusual tiredness, lethargy, restlessness, or anxiety.

Check with your health care provider if you're depressed, dizzy, or sleepless, or if you develop a wheeze, a rash, or very slow heart rate.

What you must know about other drugs
To avoid harmful interactions, tell your primary health care provider if you're taking other medications. Also, check with him before you take new medications.

In particular, he needs to know if you're taking insulin or other medications for diabetes; the ulcer medication cimetidine (Tagamet); asthma medications; and medications for heart conditions.

Special directions
Warning: Don't stop taking propranolol suddenly — doing so may increase your angina.
- Tell your health care provider of other medical problems, especially other heart problems, asthma, lung disease, diabetes, low blood glucose, an overactive thyroid, and liver disease. Other medical problems may affect the use of this medication.
- Propranolol may make you dizzy, so know how you react to it before you drive or perform other activities requiring alertness.
- To minimize dizziness, rise slowly from a sitting or lying position and avoid sudden position changes.
- To avoid insomnia, take your last dose no later than 2 hours before bedtime.
- Before you have surgery, tell your health care provider that you're taking propranolol.

✔ Keep in mind
- If you're pregnant or breast-feeding, check with your primary health care provider before taking this medication.
- If you're an athlete, you should know that propranolol is banned and tested for by the U.S. Olympic Committee and the National Collegiate Athletic Association.

Additional instructions
_____
_____
_____

Taking propylthiouracil

Dear Patient,

Because your thyroid gland makes too much thyroid hormone, your primary health care provider has prescribed propylthiouracil. This medication works by making it harder for the body to use iodine to make thyroid hormone. The label may read Propyl-Thyracil.

How to take propylthiouracil

Propylthiouracil comes in tablets. Take your medication exactly as the label directs. Don't take more or less or use it longer or more often than your primary health care provider prescribed.

Take your tablets with meals to prevent stomach upset unless directed otherwise. Also, if you're taking more than one dose a day, try to take your medication at evenly spaced times day and night.

What to do if you miss a dose

Take the dose as soon as you remember. However, if it's almost time for your next dose, take both doses together. Then go back to your regular dosing schedule. If you miss more than one dose, check with your primary health care provider.

What to do about side effects

Call your primary health care provider *right away* if your skin starts to turn yellow, you gain weight unexpectedly, your feet and ankles start to swell, and if you have a fever, chills, a sore throat, or mouth sores.

You may also experience nausea, vomiting, or easy bruising or bleeding. Check with your health care provider, who may adjust the dosage.

What you must know about other drugs

Check with your primary health care provider before you use other prescription or nonprescription medications. He may want you to avoid iodine-containing medications, such as some cough medicines and potassium iodide (Pima). Using these medications with propylthiouracil may lead to a goiter or decrease thyroid activity too much. Tell your primary health care provider if you take blood thinners or digoxin because propylthiouracil may affect the way these medicines work in your body.

Special directions

! *Warning:* Don't stop taking propylthiouracil without first checking with your primary health care provider.

• Call your primary health care provider *right away* if you're injured or get an infection or illness of any kind. He may tell you to stop taking propylthiouracil or change your dosage.

• Tell your primary health care provider if you have other medical problems, especially an infection or liver disease. Other medical problems may affect the use of this medication.

• Before you have medical tests, tell your primary health care provider that you're taking propylthiouracil because it may affect the test results. Also check with him before you have a vaccination.

• Ask your health care provider if you can eat iodine-containing foods, such as iodized salt and shellfish.

✓ Keep in mind

• If you're pregnant or breast-feeding, check with your primary health care provider before using this medication.

Additional instructions

_____

_____

_____

Taking pseudoephedrine

Dear Patient,

Pseudoephedrine is used to relieve stuffiness of your nose or sinuses. It's also used to relieve ear congestion caused by ear infection or inflammation. Brand names include Cenafed, Sudafed, and Sufedrin.

How to take pseudoephedrine

This medication comes in tablets, extended-release tablets and capsules, syrup, and an oral solution. If your primary health care provider prescribed this medication, follow his directions exactly. If you bought the medication without a prescription, carefully read the package instructions before using.

If you're taking the extended-release tablets or capsules, swallow them whole; don't chew, crush, or break them.

To prevent sleeplessness, take your last dose for the day a few hours before bedtime.

What to do if you miss a dose

If you remember the missed dose within 1 hour or so, take it right away. If you don't remember until later, skip the missed dose and take your next dose on schedule. Don't take a double dose.

What to do about side effects

Check with your primary health care provider if this medication makes you feel anxious, nervous, or restless or causes palpitations or trouble sleeping.

What you must know about other drugs

Check with your primary health care provider before you use new prescription or nonprescription medications. Also, tell your primary health care provider about other medications you're taking, especially those for high blood pressure.

Warning: If you're taking a monoamine oxidase (MAO) inhibitor (a medication used to treat depression and other emotional problems), don't use pseudoephedrine because the combination can cause a life-threatening rise in blood pressure.

Special directions

• Tell your primary health care provider if you have other medical problems, especially high blood pressure, heart disease, an overactive thyroid, diabetes, or difficult urination. Other medical problems may affect the use of this medication.
• If pseudoephedrine makes your mouth feel dry, use sugarless gum or hard candy, melt bits of ice in your mouth, or use a saliva substitute.
• If you don't feel better within 5 days or if you also have a high fever, check with your primary health care provider. These signs may mean you have some other medical problem.

✔ Keep in mind

• If you're pregnant or breast-feeding, check with your primary health care provider before using pseudoephedrine.
• If you're an athlete, you should know that pseudoephedrine is banned and tested for by the U.S. Olympic Committee.

Additional instructions

_____
_____
_____
_____
_____
_____
_____
_____

Taking pseudoephedrine with triprolidine

Dear Patient,

This medication contains a decongestant (pseudoephedrine) and an antihistamine (triprolidine) and is used to relieve a stuffy nose caused by colds or hay fever. Brand names include Actifed, Allercon, and Aller-phed.

How to take this medication

This medication comes in tablets, capsules, extended-release capsules, and syrup forms. Follow your primary health care provider's directions exactly. If you bought the medication without a prescription, carefully read the package instructions before using it. If this medication irritates your stomach, take it with food or a full glass (8 ounces) of milk or water.

If you're taking the *extended-release* capsules, swallow them whole. If the capsule is too big to swallow easily, mix its contents with applesauce and swallow without chewing.

If this medication causes trouble with sleeping, take your last dose a few hours before bedtime.

What to do if you miss a dose

Take the dose as soon as possible. But if it's almost time for your next dose, skip the missed dose and take your next dose on schedule. Don't take double doses.

What to do about side effects

Check with your primary health care provider if this medication makes you feel anxious, nervous, or restless or causes palpitations or trouble sleeping.

The antihistamine in this medication may make you feel drowsy, dizzy, or less alert. Tell your health care provider if these symptoms continue or become bothersome.

What you must know about alcohol and other drugs

Avoid alcoholic beverages or medications that slow down the central nervous system, such as sleeping pills, tranquilizers, and medications for colds, flu, and allergies, while taking this medication because the combination may make you overly drowsy.

Check with your health care provider or pharmacist before you take medications for appetite control, high blood pressure, stomach cramps, and depression.

Warning: If you're taking a monoamine oxidase (MAO) inhibitor (a medication used to treat depression, don't use it with pseudoephedrine because a life-threatening rise in blood pressure can occur.

Special directions

• Tell your health care provider if you have other medical problems, especially asthma, diabetes, an enlarged prostate, glaucoma, high blood pressure, an overactive thyroid, or heart or blood vessel disease.
• Make sure you know how you react to this medication before you drive or perform other activities that require alertness.

✔ Keep in mind

• If you're pregnant, check with your primary health care provider before using this medication. Don't use it if you're breast-feeding.
• Children and older adults may be especially sensitive to side effects.
• If you're an athlete, you should know that the U.S. Olympic Committee tests for pseudoephedrine. Athletes may be disqualified if amounts in the urine exceed certain limits.

Additional instructions

_____

_____

Taking psyllium

Dear Patient,

This medication is used to encourage bowel movements to relieve constipation. Brand names include Cillium, Fiberall, Konsyl, Metamucil, Naturacil, Perdiem Fiber, and Prodiem Plain.

How to take psyllium

Psyllium comes in the form of chewable pieces, wafers, and mixable granules and powders. If your primary health care provider prescribed this medication, follow his directions exactly. If you bought psyllium without a prescription, carefully read the package instructions before using it.

If you're using the dry powder or granule forms, always mix your dose with liquid first. Never swallow the dry powder or granules. After mixing, drink your medication immediately or it may congeal.

Drink lots of fluids while taking psyllium. Drink a full glass (8 ounces) of cold water or fruit juice with each dose. Then drink a second glass of water or juice. Throughout the day, try to drink at least 6 to 8 full glasses of liquid. Don't take this medication before meals because you may no longer be hungry.

What to do about side effects

If you take too much psyllium or swallow the dry powder or granules without adequate liquid, this medication may cause choking. Call your primary health care provider *right away* if you experience chest pain, vomiting, or difficulty in swallowing or breathing after taking this product.

Psyllium also may cause some digestive distress, such as nausea, vomiting, abdominal cramps, or diarrhea. Check with your primary health care provider if these symptoms continue or become bothersome. Also tell him if you develop a rash while taking psyllium.

What you must know about other drugs

Psyllium may decrease the effects of blood thinners, digoxin, or antibiotics, such as ciprofloxacin or tetracycline.

Special directions

• Tell your primary health care provider if you have other medical problems, especially ulcers or other digestive disease. Also mention if you're on a low-sodium diet, because this medication is high in sodium, or if you have diabetes, because some products may have a high sugar content. And tell your primary health care provider if you must limit foods that contain phenylalanine.

⚠️ *Warning:* Don't get into the "laxative habit." If you overuse laxatives, you may become dependent on these medications to have a bowel movement. In severe cases, laxative overuse may damage the nerves, muscles, and lining of the digestive tract.

• You may have to wait 2 to 3 days for this medication to work. However, many people have bowel movements within 12 hours after taking psyllium.

• To prevent constipation, eat plenty of whole-grain foods, such as bran and other cereals, as well as vegetables and fresh fruits. Getting regular exercise and drinking lots of fluids also will help to keep you regular.

✔️ Keep in mind

• If you have diabetes, choose a sugar-free brand of psyllium.

Additional instructions

_____
_____
_____
_____

Applying pyrethrins with piperonyl butoxide

Dear Patient,

This medication is used to treat head, body, and pubic lice infections. The lice absorb this medication, which kills them.

If you're using the *shampoo,* the label may read Tisit Shampoo, RID, R & C, or A-200 Shampoo Concentrate. If you're using the *topical gel or solution,* the label may read Tisit or A-200 Pyrinate.

How to apply this medication

If your primary health care provider prescribed this medication, follow his directions exactly. If you bought it without a prescription, carefully read the package instructions before using it.

If you're using the *gel* or *solution,* follow these steps: Apply enough medication to thoroughly wet the skin or dry hair and scalp. Let the medication remain on the treated area for exactly 10 minutes. Wash the treated area with warm water and soap or regular shampoo. Rinse thoroughly and dry with a clean towel.

If you're using the *shampoo,* follow these steps: Apply enough medication to thoroughly wet the dry hair and scalp. Let the medication remain on the treated scalp for exactly 10 minutes. Work the shampoo into a lather, using a small amount of water. Rinse well and dry with a clean towel. After rinsing and drying, use a nit-removal comb to remove dead lice and eggs (nits) from your hair.

Wash your hands right after using this medication. Repeat the treatment 7 to 10 days after the first treatment, as directed.

What to do about side effects

With repeated use, this medication may irritate your skin. Call your primary health care provider if you develop a rash or an infection.

Special directions

Warning: Keep this medication away from your eyes, mouth, and nose. Also, apply it in a well-ventilated room, so you don't inhale the vapors.

• If you have hay fever or are allergic to ragweed, check with your primary health care provider before you use this medication. Also, if you have a skin problem, such as severe inflammation or rawness, see your primary health care provider before applying the medication.

• To prevent the spread of lice, machine wash all clothing, bedding, towels, and washcloths in very hot water. Then dry them using the hot cycle of a dryer for at least 20 minutes. Clothing or bedding that can't be washed should be dry-cleaned and sealed in a plastic bag for 2 weeks.

• Wash all hairbrushes and combs in very hot soapy water for 5 to 10 minutes.

• Clean the house or room by thoroughly vacuuming upholstered furniture, rugs, and floors.

• If more than one person lives in your household, all members should be checked for lice and, if they're infected, treated.

✔ Keep in mind

• If you're pregnant or breast-feeding, check with your primary health care provider before using this medication.

Additional instructions

_____
_____
_____
_____
_____
_____

Taking quinapril

Dear Patient,

Quinapril is used to treat high blood pressure and heart disease and to prevent kidney damage caused by high blood pressure or diabetes. The brand name is Accupril.

How to take quinapril
Quinapril comes in tablet form. Take this medication once or twice a day, as your primary health care provider orders. Take it at the same time every day.

What to do if you miss a dose
Take the dose as soon as possible. However, if it's almost time for the next dose, skip the missed dose and return to your regular schedule. Don't take double doses.

What to do about side effects
Notify your primary health care provider *immediately* if you have these side effects: swelling of your face, lips, throat, or tongue; difficulty swallowing; a fever; or a rash.

Some patients may have dizziness at first and a dry, persistent cough several days to weeks after starting this medication. Diarrhea, headache, and changes in taste are less common. Notify your primary health care provider if any of these continue or are troublesome.

What you must know about other drugs
This medication may decrease the effectiveness of tetracycline antibiotics. Don't take these antibiotics within 2 hours of taking quinapril. Also don't take extra potassium supplements or salt substitutes, unless your primary health care provider prescribes it.

If you're taking this medication for high blood pressure, ask your primary health care provider or pharmacist before taking any nonprescription cough, cold, or allergy medications. Some of these medications may raise your blood pressure.

Special directions
• For this medication to work well, follow the lifestyle changes (such as regular exercise, weight loss, or a low-salt diet) prescribed by your primary health care provider or registered dietitian.
• This medication is used to treat and prevent serious conditions. Don't discontinue it without notifying your primary health care provider.
• Because this medication can cause dizziness at first, use caution when driving, operating heavy machinery, or performing other tasks that require good balance.

✔ Keep in mind
• Notify your primary health care provider if you're pregnant, suspect you're pregnant, or wish to breast-feed.

Additional instructions
_____
_____
_____
_____
_____
_____
_____
_____
_____
_____
_____

Taking quinidine

Dear Patient,

This medication is used to correct an irregular heartbeat to a normal rhythm or to slow an overactive heart. Brand names include Cardioquin, Duraquin, Quinaglute, Quinidex, and Quinora.

How to take quinidine

Quinidine comes in the form of capsules, tablets, and extended-release tablets. Follow your primary health care provider's directions for taking this medication exactly, even if you feel well.

To make sure your medication is well absorbed, take your dose with a full glass (8 ounces) of water on an empty stomach 1 hour before or 2 hours after meals. However, if you have an upset stomach, your primary health care provider may want you to take your dose with food and milk.

If you're taking the extended-release tablets, swallow them whole. Don't chew, crush, or break them.

Don't stop taking quinidine without first checking with your primary health care provider.

What to do if you miss a dose

If you remember the missed dose within 2 hours, take it as soon as possible. However, if you don't remember until later, skip the missed dose and take your next dose on schedule. Don't take a double dose.

What to do about side effects

Call your primary health care provider *at once* if you have blurred vision or other vision changes; dizziness, light-headedness or fainting; fever; severe headache; hearing changes such as buzzing in the ears; or wheezing, shortness of breath, or trouble breathing.

Also report nausea, vomiting, or diarrhea. You may develop a bitter taste in your mouth, but this should go away with continued use.

What you must know about other drugs

Tell your primary health care provider if you're taking other medications. Also check with him before you take new medications. In particular, he needs to know if you use blood thinners, other heart medications, sedatives, seizure medications (such as barbiturates), antacids, the ulcer drug cimetidine (Tagamet), and medications that make the urine less acidic such as acetazolamide (Diamox).

Special directions

• Tell your primary health care provider if you have other medical problems, especially asthma, emphysema, blood diseases, myasthenia gravis, an overactive thyroid, psoriasis, and kidney or liver disease. Other medical problems may affect the use of this medication.
• Keep all appointments for follow-up visits so your primary health care provider can check your progress.
• Before having surgery (including dental surgery), tell your health care provider or dentist that you're on this medication.
• Don't confuse this medication with quinine. Although related to quinidine, it has different medical uses.

✔ Keep in mind

• If you're pregnant, check with your primary health care provider before using quinidine.

Additional instructions

_____

_____

Taking ramipril

Dear Patient,

Ramipril is prescribed to treat high blood pressure and heart disease and to prevent kidney damage caused by high blood pressure or diabetes. Ask your primary health care provider if you're not sure why this medication has been prescribed for you. The brand name is Altace.

How to take ramipril
This medication comes in capsule form. It may be given once or twice a day with or without food. Swallow the capsule whole or sprinkle the contents in about 4 ounces of applesauce, water, or apple juice.

What to do if you miss a dose
Take the dose as soon as possible. However, if it's almost time for the next dose, skip the missed dose and take the next scheduled dose. Don't double dose.

What to do about side effects
Notify your primary health care provider *immediately* and get emergency help if you have swelling of your face, lips, throat or tongue or difficulty swallowing. This is a very rare but potentially serious side effect. Also call *right away* if you have a fever, yellow skin or eyes, and a rash.

Dizziness or light-headedness may also occur when you arise from a sitting or lying position. You may also have a dry, persistent cough; diarrhea; headache; and changes in taste several days to weeks after starting this medication. Call your health care provider if any of these continue or bother you.

What you must know about other drugs
Tell your primary health care provider about other medications you're taking, especially diuretics or lithium. Because this medication may decrease the effectiveness of tetracycline antibiotics, don't take antibiotics within 2 hours of taking ramipril. Also, don't take extra potassium supplements, eat potassium-rich foods, or use salt substitutes without first checking with your health care provider.

If you're taking this medication for high blood pressure, ask your health care provider or pharmacist before taking any nonprescription cough, cold, or allergy medications because some of these may raise your blood pressure. Avoid drinking coffee, tea, colas, and other caffeine-containing foods and beverages.

Special directions
• Tell your primary health care provider if you have other medical problems, such as heart, kidney, or liver disease.
• This medication can cause dizziness. So be cautious when driving or performing other activities that require good balance. Get up slowly from a sitting or lying position. If the dizziness continues, report this to your primary health care provider.
• For best results, follow lifestyle changes (such as regular exercise, weight loss, or a low-salt diet) prescribed by your primary health care provider or registered dietitian. Monitor your blood pressure regularly.
• This medication is used to treat and prevent serious conditions. Don't stop taking it or change the dose without calling your primary health care provider.

✔ Keep in mind
• Don't take ramipril if you're pregnant or breast-feeding. Tell your health care provider right away if you suspect pregnancy.

Additional instructions

_____

_____

Taking ranitidine

Dear Patient,

Ranitidine is prescribed to treat duodenal and gastric ulcers and to prevent their return. It's also used to treat some conditions in which the stomach makes too much acid. The label may read Zantac.

How to take ranitidine

Ranitidine comes in syrup and tablet forms, as well as effervescent granules and tablets. If you're taking one dose a day, take it at bedtime, unless otherwise directed. If you're taking two doses a day, take one in the morning and one at bedtime. If you're taking several doses a day, take them with meals and at bedtime for best results.

If you're using the effervescent granules or tablets, remove the foil wrapping and dissolve the dose in 6 to 8 ounces of water.

If this medication is prescribed by your primary health care provider, take it for the full time of treatment, even after you start to feel better. If you bought ranitidine without a prescription, don't take it for more than 2 weeks unless directed by your primary health care provider.

What to do if you miss a dose

Take the dose as soon as possible. However, if it's almost time for your next dose, skip the missed dose and take your next dose on schedule. Don't double dose.

What to do about side effects

Check with your primary health care provider if you feel dizzy, confused, nauseated, or constipated. Also let your health care provider know if you get a rash or headache or if your heart starts to beat very slowly.

What you must know about other drugs

Tell your primary health care provider if you're taking other medications. Also check with him before you take new medications. If you're using antacids to relieve stomach pain, wait 30 minutes to 1 hour between taking the antacid and ranitidine.

To prevent harmful medication interactions, tell your health care provider if you use blood thinners, muscle relaxants, or medications for diabetes or an irregular heartbeat.

Special directions

- Tell your primary health care provider if you have other medical problems, especially kidney or liver disease.
- Before you have skin tests or tests to determine your stomach acid production, tell your health care provider you're on ranitidine. This medication may affect the test results.
- Because ranitidine may make you drowsy or dizzy, know how you react to it before you drive or perform other activities that might be dangerous if you're not fully alert.
- *Warning:* Don't smoke while taking ranitidine because cigarette smoking reduces its effectiveness.
- Avoid foods and other substances that can irritate your stomach, such as alcohol, aspirin, citrus products, and carbonated drinks.

✓ Keep in mind

- If you're pregnant, check with your primary health care provider before using ranitidine. If you're breast-feeding, don't use this medication unless instructed to do so by your primary health care provider.
- If you're an older adult, you may be especially prone to ranitidine's side effects, particularly confusion and dizziness.

Additional instructions

_____

_____

_____

Taking rifampin

Dear Patient,

Your primary health care provider has prescribed rifampin to treat your tuberculosis. Brand names include Rifadin and Rimactane.

How to take rifampin
Take this medication exactly as directed for as long as your primary health care provider prescribes. Take it 1 hour before or 2 hours after meals. However, if rifampin upsets your stomach, your primary health care provider may tell you to take it with food.

What to do if you miss a dose
Take the dose as soon as possible. But if it's almost time for your next dose, skip the missed dose and take your next dose on schedule. Don't double dose.

What to do about side effects
Call your primary health care provider *immediately* if you have any of the following: appetite loss, bloody or cloudy urine, bone and muscle pain, breathing problems, chills, dizziness, headache, nausea, or vomiting.

Also call him promptly if you experience shivering, sore throat, unusual bleeding or bruising, fever, joint pain and inflammation (especially in the feet), abdominal pain, yellowish skin or eyes (jaundice), dark urine, or light-colored stools.

Some side effects may subside as your body adjusts to the medication. These include diarrhea, itching, reddened skin or a rash, sore mouth or tongue, and stomach cramps.

What you must know about alcohol and other drugs
Avoid drinking alcoholic beverages while taking rifampin because the combination may damage your liver.

Tell your primary health care provider if you're taking other prescription or nonprescription medications because rifampin decreases the effectiveness of many other medications. For instance, if you're taking birth control pills, you may need to use an additional method of birth control. If you're taking a heart or diabetes medication or a blood thinner, your primary health care provider may need to change the dosage.

Special directions
• Tell your primary health care provider if you have other medical problems, especially liver disease or alcoholism, because they may affect the use of this medication.
• Rifampin turns your body fluids and secretions reddish orange or reddish brown. It can permanently discolor soft contact lenses, but it doesn't affect hard lenses.
• Call your primary health care provider if your symptoms seem worse or don't subside after 2 to 3 weeks of therapy.
• Because rifampin may make you drowsy, make sure you know how you react to it before you drive or perform other activities that might be dangerous if you're not fully alert.
• Take precautions to avoid injuries or accidental bleeding because rifampin affects the blood's clotting ability. Be careful when using a regular toothbrush or dental floss.

Warning: Use a reliable form of birth control while taking rifampin.

✔ Keep in mind
• If you're pregnant or breast-feeding, don't use this medication without careful discussion with your primary health care provider.

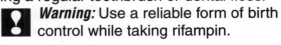

Additional instructions

_____

_____

Taking ritonavir

Dear Patient,

Your primary health care provider has prescribed ritonavir to inhibit the human immunodeficiency virus (HIV). This medication interferes with the virus's ability to multiply itself, helping to slow the progression of the infection. The brand name is Norvir.

How to take ritonavir

Ritonavir is usually given twice a day with food. You can improve the taste of the oral solution by mixing it with chocolate milk within 1 hour of dosing.

What to do about side effects

Notify your primary health care provider *immediately* if you develop a rash; hives; wheezing; swelling of your face, lips, throat or tongue; or difficulty swallowing.

During the first few weeks of treatment, you may experience nausea, diarrhea, vomiting, loss of appetite, changes in taste, muscle weakness, or tingling in your hands or feet. Notify your primary health care provider if these side effects continue or become bothersome.

What you must know about other drugs

Ritonavir may interact with many medications. So tell your primary health care provider about all the prescription and nonprescription medications you're taking, and don't start any new medications without notifying him. For example, talk to him before taking sedatives or sleeping pills (such as alprazolam, diazepam, or flurazepam) and pain medications (such as ibuprofen and naproxen).

Special directions

• Tell your primary health care provider if you have other medical problems, especially liver disease.

• Keep ritonavir in its original bottle to protect it from light. Although you may keep it at room temperature for up to 30 days, refrigerating it as much as possible is recommended.

• Ritonavir is commonly used in combination with other medications for the treatment of HIV infection. To get the full benefit from this medication, follow your primary health care provider's instructions carefully. Ask questions if you're unsure about something, and don't stop the medication or change the dosage without first discussing it with your primary health care provider.

• Your primary health care provider may request blood samples periodically to monitor the effect of this medication on your blood cells, liver function, and the course of the HIV infection.

✓ Keep in mind

• Before starting ritonavir, notify your primary health care provider if you're pregnant or suspect you're pregnant. Women with HIV infection shouldn't breast-feed.

• If you also have diabetes, ritonavir may increase your blood sugar level. Ask your health care provider how frequently you should check and record your blood sugar at home. Report any symptoms of high blood sugar, such as weight loss, fatigue, or increased thirst, hunger, or urination.

Additional instructions

_____

_____

_____

_____

_____

_____

_____

Taking salmeterol

Dear Patient,

Salmeterol is a medication that relaxes smooth muscles in the lungs and improves your breathing. It's used to prevent asthma attacks, not to treat an acute episode that's already started. The brand name is Serevent.

How to take salmeterol

This medication is available as an inhaler. Take it at 12-hour intervals to increase its effectiveness and decrease side effects. Rinse your mouth after each use.

Ask your primary health care provider or pharmacist to teach you the correct technique for delivering medication through this inhaler. Shake the inhaler well before using. Rinse the plastic case and cap under warm water daily and air dry. Store the canister at room temperature with the nozzle end down.

What to do if you miss a dose

If you miss a dose, take it as soon as possible. If it's almost time for your next dose, skip the missed dose and go back to your regular schedule. Don't take double doses.

What to do about side effects

Call your primary health care provider *at once* if still have trouble breathing or if your breathing gets worse after using salmeterol. You may experience increased heart rate, increased or decreased blood pressure, headache, abnormal heart rhythm, nervousness, insomnia, dizziness, pharyngitis, and cough. If these side effects continue or worsen, call your primary health care provider.

What you must know about other drugs

Tell your primary health care provider if you're taking beta blockers (such as atenolol, timolol, labetalol, propranolol, or metoprolol), monoamine oxidase (MAO) inhibitors (such as phenelzine, selegiline, or tranylcypromine), antidepressants, weight reduction medications, or other asthma medications.

Special directions

Warning: Don't stop this medication or change the dose without first consulting your primary health care provider.
- Tell your primary health care provider if you have thyroid disease, heart disease, high blood pressure, epilepsy, diabetes, or any medication allergies.
- If you begin wheezing after using the inhaler, notify your primary health care provider.
- You may take salmeterol 30 to 60 minutes before exercising to prevent exercise-induced bronchospasm. But don't space the doses less than 12 hours apart.

✔ Keep in mind

- Consult your primary health care provider about using salmeterol during pregnancy. Its use should be restricted to patients for whom benefit outweighs risk. It's not known whether salmeterol occurs in breast milk.

Additional instructions

_____
_____
_____
_____
_____
_____
_____
_____
_____
_____

Taking saquinavir

Dear Patient,

Saquinavir is used alone or in combination with other medications to treat human immunodeficiency virus (HIV) infection. This medication won't cure or prevent HIV infection. The brand name is Invirase.

How to take saquinavir

This medication is available as a capsule. Take it by mouth exactly as prescribed, usually three times a day. It's best to take it with food or within 2 hours after a full meal.

What to do if you miss a dose

If you miss a dose, take it as soon a possible. If it's almost time for your next dose, skip the missed dose and go back to your regular schedule. Don't double dose.

What to do about side effects

You may experience nausea, abdominal pain, yellow skin or eyes, muscle or joint pain, cough, diarrhea, rash, weakness, tingling or loss of feeling in your fingers and toes, headache, bleeding, or easy bruising. Tell your primary health care provider if any of these side effects continue or become intolerable.

What you must know about alcohol and other drugs

Tell your primary health care provider about all the over-the-counter and prescription medications you're taking, particularly rifampin (Rifadin), phenytoin (Dilantin), carbamazepine (Tegretol), dexamethasone (Decadron), ketoconazole (Nizoral), astemizole (Hismanal), ritonavir (Norvir), calcium channel blockers (such as Verapamil or Procardia), clindamycin (Cleocin), quinidine, (Quinaglute) and triazolam (Halcion).

Special directions

• Drink grapefruit juice — it may increase the benefits of saquinavir.
• Keep all appointments with your primary health care provider and appointments for laboratory tests. This is how your condition will be monitored.
• Avoid direct sunlight and use a sunscreen when outdoors.

Warning: Don't increase, decrease, or stop taking this medication without first consulting your primary health care provider.

Keep in mind

• This medication may not be safe during pregnancy. Also, don't breast-feed while taking it — HIV can be transmitted to the infant through breast milk. Discuss these issues with your primary health care provider.

Additional instructions

_____
_____
_____
_____
_____
_____
_____
_____
_____
_____

Using ophthalmic scopolamine

Dear Patient,

Your primary health care provider has prescribed scopolamine eyedrops to dilate your pupils. This medication is used before eye examinations, before and after eye surgery, and to treat certain eye conditions. The label on your eyedrop container may read Isopto Hyoscine.

How to use scopolamine eyedrops

First, wash your hands. Then follow these steps: Tilt your head back. With your middle finger, apply pressure to the inside corner of the eye. (And continue to apply pressure for 2 to 3 minutes after you've instilled the drops.) Using your index finger, pull the lower eyelid away from the eye to form a pouch. Squeeze the drops into the pouch. Gently close your eyes. Don't blink. To help the eyedrops become absorbed, keep your eyes closed for 1 to 2 minutes. Wash your hands again.

To keep your eyedrop bottle as germfree as possible, take care not to touch the applicator tip to any surface, including your eye. Close the bottle tightly between uses.

What to do if you miss a dose

Instill the drops as soon as possible. However, if it's almost time for your next dose, adjust your dosing schedule as follows.

If you instill one dose daily, skip the missed dose. Instill the next day's dose on schedule.

If you instill more than one dose daily, skip the missed dose and instill the next dose on schedule. Don't double dose.

What to do about side effects

If you begin to have blurred vision or irritated eyes, check with your primary health care provider, especially if these symptoms continue or become bothersome. You may also notice that your eyes are unusually sensitive to bright lights.

Special directions

• Tell your primary health care provider if you have other medical problems, especially glaucoma and other eye problems, Down syndrome, or spastic paralysis because they may affect the use of this medication.
• Because scopolamine eyedrops may blur your vision, make sure you can see clearly before you drive or perform other activities that might be dangerous if you can't see well.
• Expect your eyes to be more sensitive than usual to light while using this medication. Wear sunglasses to protect your eyes when you're outdoors or in a brightly lighted room.

✓ Keep in mind

• If you're an older adult, you may be especially prone to side effects from scopolamine eyedrops. If your vision becomes blurred, take extra care to prevent slips and falls.

Additional instructions

_____
_____
_____
_____
_____
_____
_____
_____
_____
_____
_____

Applying the scopolamine patch

Dear Patient,

Your primary health care provider has prescribed scopolamine to prevent nausea and vomiting caused by your motion sickness. The label may read Transderm-Scōp.

How to apply the scopolamine patch

This medication comes in the form of a small patch, called a transdermal disk, that you wear behind your ear. First, carefully read the directions that come with the transdermal disk. Wash and dry your hands well before and after handling the disk to avoid accidental contact with your eyes. Apply the disk to a hairless skin area behind the ear.

Apply the disk the night before or at least 4 hours before your trip. Don't place it over any cuts or irritations on your skin. Wear only one disk at a time. If the disk loosens, remove it and replace it with a new disk on another area behind the ear.

When you no longer need the medication, remove and discard it. Wash your hands and the skin that was beneath the disk. The disks are designed to deliver medication for up to 3 days.

What to do about side effects

Check with your primary health care provider if this medication makes you drowsy or dries your mouth, especially if these symptoms continue or bother you.

Also, while using the disk or even after removing it, your eyes may be more sensitive than usual to light. You may also notice the pupil in one eye is larger than the pupil in the other eye. Call your primary health care provider if this side effect persists or troubles you.

Special directions

- Tell your primary health care provider if you have other medical problems, especially glaucoma, asthma, lung disease, myasthenia gravis, or intestinal disease because they may affect the use of this medication.
- Because scopolamine may make you drowsy, know how you react to it before you drive or perform other activities that might be dangerous if you're not fully alert.
- This product comes with a brochure containing helpful information. Request this brochure from your pharmacist.
- If scopolamine makes your mouth feel dry, use sugarless gum or hard candy, ice chips, or a saliva substitute. If your mouth still feels dry after 2 weeks, see your dentist.

✔ Keep in mind

- If you're breast-feeding, check with your primary health care provider before using scopolamine.
- If you're an athlete, you should know that scopolamine is banned and sometimes tested for in biathlon and modern pentathlon events by the U.S. Olympic Committee.

Warning: Don't use the transdermal disk on children.

Additional instructions

_____
_____
_____
_____
_____
_____
_____
_____
_____
_____
_____

Taking a seizure medication

Dear Patient,

Your primary health care provider has prescribed medication to treat your seizures. This medication is called an anticonvulsant.

This information sheet contains general information about seizure medications. It's not meant to replace the sheet describing the particular medication you're taking.

How to take a seizure medication
This medication is available as a tablet, capsule, or solution. Take it exactly as directed by your primary health care provider. If this medication upsets your stomach, take it with food or milk unless otherwise directed by your primary health care provider.

What to do if you miss a dose
If you miss a dose, adjust your schedule as follows:

If you take one dose a day, take the missed dose as soon as possible. However, if you don't remember until the next day, skip the missed dose and take your next dose on schedule. Don't double dose.

If you take more than one dose a day, take the missed dose as soon as possible. However, if it's within 4 hours of your next dose, skip the missed dose and take your next dose on schedule. Don't double dose.

What to do about side effects
Call your primary health care provider *immediately* if you have seizures, skin problems, bleeding problems, dark urine, abdominal pain, sore throat, heart palpitations, or difficulty breathing.

Check with your primary health care provider as soon as possible if you experience confusion, dizziness, eye problems, uncontrolled movements, nausea and vomiting, fever, or an unwell feeling.

What you must know about alcohol and other drugs
Check with your primary health care provider before drinking alcoholic beverages because alcohol may prevent this medication from working.

Tell your primary health care provider about other medications you're taking because many of them may interact with the anticonvulsant. Also check with him before taking any nonprescription medications.

Special directions
• Tell your primary health care provider if you have other medical problems, especially heart, liver, and kidney disease; porphyria; or asthma.
• Know how you react to this medication before you drive or perform other activities requiring alertness.
• *Warning:* Don't stop taking this medication unless your primary health care provider says to — you may have seizures.
• When you refill a prescription of this medication, check the bottle carefully to make sure it's the correct medication.

✔ Keep in mind
• If you're pregnant or breast-feeding, check with your primary health care provider before taking this medication.
• Older adults and children are usually more sensitive to the effects of this medication.

Additional instructions
_____
_____
_____
_____
_____

Taking sertraline

Dear Patient,

Your primary health care provider has prescribed sertraline to treat your depression or obsessive-compulsive disorder. This medication increases the concentration of the chemical serotonin, thought to be deficient in people with those disorders. The brand name is Zoloft.

How to take sertraline
This medication is available as a tablet. The dosage schedule varies from patient to patient, but generally, take the medication with food at the same time every day, to make sure it's absorbed in the same way.

What to do if you miss a dose
Before starting sertraline, talk to your primary health care provider about what to do if you miss a dose. This medication may be given to different patients at different times of the day.

What to do about side effects
Tell your primary health care provider *immediately* if you experience weight loss, anxiety, nervousness, decreased sexual desire or ability, fast or irregular heartbeat, or blurred vision.

You may also experience dizziness, drowsiness, diarrhea, constipation, loss of appetite, nausea, fatigue, headache, dry mouth, sweating, or tremors as you adjust to the medication. Tell your primary health care provider if these problems continue or become bothersome.

What you must know about alcohol and other drugs
Check with your primary health care provider before drinking alcoholic beverages because the combined effects of alcohol and sertraline may increase drowsiness.

Tell your primary health care provider about any over-the-counter or prescription medications you're taking, including other medications for depression, monoamine oxidase (MAO) inhibitors (such as Parnate and Nardil), diazepam (Valium), warfarin (Coumadin), cough medications containing dextromethorphan, and any medication that causes drowsiness.

Special directions
• You may not see any improvement in your condition for 4 weeks.

Warning: Don't stop taking this medication or change your dosage without first consulting your primary health care provider.

• Tell your primary health care provider if you have any other medical problems, such as kidney disease, liver disease, or a history of seizures.

• Avoid driving and other activities requiring alertness until you know how you react to this medication.

✔ Keep in mind
• This medication shouldn't be used during pregnancy unless absolutely necessary. Discuss the risks and benefits with your primary health care provider. It isn't known if this medication occurs in breast milk.

Additional instructions

_____

_____

_____

_____

_____

_____

Taking simvastatin

Dear Patient,

Your primary health care provider has prescribed simvastatin for your high cholesterol. This medication blocks the production of cholesterol and reduces the level in the blood. The brand name is Zocor.

How to take simvastatin

This medication is available as a tablet. It works better if taken with your evening meal.

What to do if you miss a dose

Take the dose as soon as you remember. If it's almost time for the next dose, skip the missed dose and go back to your regular dosing schedule. Don't take double doses.

What to do about side effects

Tell your primary health care provider *right away* if you have unexplained muscle pain, tenderness, or weakness; an unwell feeling; a fever; vision changes; or yellowing of the eyes or skin.

During the first few days of treatment, you may experience an upset stomach, heartburn, diarrhea, constipation, a rash, dizziness, or blurred vision. These problems should subside once your body adjusts to the medication. Call your primary health care provider if they don't go away or if they get worse.

What you must know about other drugs

Tell your primary health care provider about any prescription or over-the-counter medications you're taking, including warfarin (Coumadin), cyclosporine (Neoral), digoxin (Lanoxin), erythromycin (E-Mycin), gemfibrozil (Lopid), cholestyramine (Questran), niacin (Niac), and azole antifungal medications (such as Sporanox or Nizoral).

Special directions

• Tell your primary health care provider if you have other medical problems, such as liver disease, seizures, or kidney failure, or if you've had an organ transplant.
• Carefully follow the diet your primary health care provider gives you.
• You may notice the full effect of this medication for weeks or even months. Check your progress by making regular visits to your primary health care provider.
• Tell your primary health care provider or dentist that you're taking this medication before having emergency treatment, surgery, or dental surgery.

✔ Keep in mind

Warning: Don't take this drug if you're pregnant or if you plan to become pregnant in the near future. Breast-feeding is also not recommended because of the possible side effects to the infant.

Additional instructions

_____
_____
_____
_____
_____
_____
_____
_____
_____
_____

Applying a skin disorder medication

Dear Patient,

Your primary health care provider has prescribed a medication for your skin condition. In general, these medications are applied topically (to the skin); they're not taken internally. They usually work by being absorbed through the skin to treat a specific condition, such as acne or rash.

This information sheet contains general information about skin disorder medications. It's not meant to replace the sheet describing the particular medication you're taking.

How to apply skin disorder medication

This medication is available as a cream, lotion, or ointment. Carefully follow the directions on the label as well as those of your primary health care provider. Apply the medication on a regular basis, but don't use more than prescribed because this may cause skin irritation. Generally speaking, keep these medications away from your mouth, nose, and eyes. Before applying the medication, wash and dry the area to be treated. Don't cover the area with a dressing unless instructed to do so.

What to do if you miss a dose

Try not to miss any doses. But if you do, skip the missed dose and apply the next one at the scheduled time.

What to do about side effects

Topical medication can cause burning, blistering, peeling, and redness of the skin. If these problems become severe or your condition seems to be worsening, call your primary health care provider.

What you must know about other drugs

Most topical medications can be used along with other types of medications. However, if you're applying two or more topical medica-tions to the same area, talk to your primary health care provider to make sure that the medications won't interfere with each other.

Special directions

• If your condition doesn't improve after 1 week, call your primary health care provider. Some topical medications, such as tretinoin for acne, take 2 to 3 weeks to take effect and may even seem to worsen your condition at first.
• If you apply too much of some topical medications, they can cause effects throughout your body. For example, diphenhydramine (Benadryl) cream can cause some drowsiness. So use these medications only as directed.

✔ Keep in mind

• If you're pregnant or breast-feeding, check with your primary health care provider before using topical medications.

Additional instructions

_____

_____

_____

_____

_____

_____

_____

_____

_____

_____

Taking spironolactone

Dear Patient,

Spironolactone is used to treat high blood pressure and a condition called hyperaldosteronism. This diuretic (water pill) makes you urinate more, while also increasing the amount of potassium in your body. The label may read Aldactone.

How to take spironolactone

Spironolactone comes in tablets. Take this medication exactly as directed. For better absorption, take the tablets with meals.

What to do if you miss a dose

Take the dose as soon as possible. However, if it's almost time for your next dose, skip the missed dose and take your next dose on schedule. Don't double dose.

What to do about side effects

Call your primary health care provider if you experience abdominal cramps, diarrhea, loss of appetite, or nausea; confusion, drowsiness, fatigue, headache, loss of coordination, or weakness; a rash; or excessive thirst. Also call if you have breast enlargement (in men) or, in women, breast soreness, deepening voice, increased facial hair, or menstrual irregularities.

What you must know about other drugs

Tell your primary health care provider about other medications you're taking. Also, check with him before you take new medications.

Don't take aspirin or aspirin-containing medications (except if specifically prescribed by your primary health care provider) because spironolactone may not work well. Your primary health care provider also needs to know if you take the heart medication digoxin (Lanoxin), potassium pills, high blood pressure pills, or other water pills.

Special directions

• Tell your primary health care provider if you have other medical problems, especially diabetes, urinary problems, and kidney or liver disease because they may affect the use of this medication.

Warning: Don't use salt substitutes (which contain a lot of potassium) or eat potassium-rich foods (for example, bananas, carrots, and nonfat dry milk) without first checking with your primary health care provider. Spironolactone can cause you to retain too much potassium.

• Spironolactone may make you drowsy. So know how it affects you before you drive or perform other activities that might be dangerous if you're not fully alert.

• Keep all appointments for follow-up examinations so your primary health care provider can check your progress. He may order a higher dose of spironolactone at first and then reduce the amount as your body adjusts.

✔ Keep in mind

• If you're pregnant, don't use spironolactone unless your primary health care provider instructs you to do so.

• If you're an athlete, you should know that diuretics are banned and tested for by the U.S. Olympic Committee and the National Collegiate Athletic Association.

Additional instructions

_____
_____
_____
_____
_____
_____
_____

Taking stavudine

Dear Patient,

Your primary health care provider has prescribed stavudine for the treatment of acquired immunodeficiency syndrome (AIDS). This medication inhibits the replication of the human immunodeficiency virus (HIV), but it won't cure or prevent HIV infections or AIDS. The brand name is Zerit.

How to take stavudine
This medication is available as a capsule. Take it exactly as prescribed, usually twice daily with or without food.

What to do if you miss a dose
If you miss a dose, take it as soon as possible. If it's almost time for your next dose, skip the missed dose and return to your regular dosing schedule. Don't take double doses.

What to do about side effects
Tell your primary health care provider *right away* if you experience abdominal pain, nausea, vomiting, or yellowing of your eyes. Also report numbness, tingling, burning or pain of the hands or feet, chills, fever, sore throat, or rash.

What you must know about other drugs
Tell your primary health care provider if you're taking any of the following medications: chloramphenicol (Chloromycetin), cisplatin (Platinol), didanosine (Videx), ethambutol (Myambutol), ethionamide (Trecator-SC), hydralazine (Apresoline), isoniazid (Laniazid), lithium (Lithobid), metronidazole (Flagyl), nitrofurantoin (Macrodantin), phenytoin (Dilantin), vincristine (Navelbine) or zalcitabine (Hivid).

Special directions
• Keep taking stavudine for the full course of treatment even if you begin to feel better.
• Don't take any other medications without first checking with your primary health care provider.
• Inform your primary health care provider if you have liver disease, kidney disease, or peripheral neuropathy.

✓ Keep in mind
• If you're pregnant, don't use this medication unless it's absolutely necessary. Discuss the risks and benefits with your primary health care provider. It's not known if this medication occurs in breast milk.

Additional instructions

Taking a steroid

Dear Patient,

Your primary health care provider has prescribed a steroid medication for you. Steroids are used to treat inflammation, itching, swelling, redness, and allergic reactions. They're also used to treat or prevent symptoms caused by diseases such as asthma and arthritis.

This information sheet contains general information about steroids. It's not meant to replace a sheet describing the particular medication you're taking.

How to take steroids

Steroids come in the form of tablets and solutions to be taken by mouth, and inhalants to be inhaled into the lungs or nose. Follow your primary health care provider's orders or the directions on the label exactly. Never take more or less than what is prescribed for you.

If you're taking steroids *by mouth,* take them with food or milk.

If you're taking steroids by *lung inhalation,* follow these steps. Shake the inhaler. Place the mouthpiece in your mouth and close lips around it. Press the metal canister down with a finger, while you inhale slowly and deeply. Hold your breath as long as possible, and then exhale slowly. Wait 1 minute before repeating. Gargle and rinse your mouth with water after each dose.

Using a special device called a spacer may help the medication get into your lungs. To prevent asthma attacks, use this medication every day in regularly spaced doses. You may not notice an improvement in your condition for 4 weeks.

If you're taking steroids by *nasal inhalation*, blow your nose to clear your nasal passages. Then insert the nosepiece into your nostril, aiming the spray toward the inner

corner of your eye. After 1 to 3 weeks of regular usage, you'll feel the effects.

What to do if you miss a dose

By mouth: If you take one dose every other day, take the missed dose as soon as possible if you remember it the same morning. If not, take it the next morning. Then skip a day and resume your regular schedule.

If you take one dose daily, take the missed dose as soon as possible. If you don't remember until the next day, skip the missed dose and take your next dose on schedule. Don't double dose.

If you take several doses a day, take the missed dose as soon as possible, then go back to your regular schedule. If you don't remember until your next dose is due, double the next dose.

By lung inhalation: If you miss a dose, use it as soon as possible. Then take the remaining doses for that day at regularly spaced times.

By nasal inhalation: If you miss a dose and remember it within an hour, take it right away. If you don't remember until later, skip the missed dose and go back to your regular schedule.

What to do about side effects

By mouth: Call your primary health care provider *right away* if you have a sore throat, fever, or coughing (signs of infection). Also call if you have blurred vision, any type of bleeding, increased thirst or urination, or confusion. Steroids may also cause increased appetite, nervousness, or restlessness, but these problems usually go away once your body adjusts to the medication.

By lung inhalation: Call your primary health care provider *immediately* if you have trouble breathing or tightness in the chest.

(continued)

Taking a steroid *(continued)*

Also report if you develop white, curd-like patches in your mouth or throat (signs of a fungal infection). Other side effects that go away after your body adjusts to the medication are coughing, dry mouth, and hoarseness.

By nasal inhalation: Call your primary health care provider *as soon as possible* if you have nosebleeds, crusty white patches or sores in your nose, eye pain, headache, and loss of smell, or if you smell something bad. Burning, dryness, and irritation of the nose usually go away with time.

What you must know about alcohol and other drugs

Avoid alcohol while taking steroids because the combination can cause increased stomach irritation. Also avoid aspirin, nonsteroidal anti-inflammatory medication (such as ibuprofen), and cigarette smoking because they can increase your risk of stomach problems.

Special directions

Warning: If you're taking steroids by mouth for more than 1 week, don't stop taking them abruptly. Your primary health care provider will decrease the dosage gradually.

● Keep active to prevent osteoporosis (bone loss). Your primary health care provider should periodically monitor your bone status with X-rays.

● Avoid contact with anyone who has an infection, especially chickenpox, measles, or a respiratory infection.

● Long-term therapy can cause changes in your physical appearance, such as acne, fat deposits in the face, hirsutism (abnormal hairiness), or a change in your body shape.

● Tell your primary health care provider if you're having skin tests or surgery (including dental surgery), or if you get a serious infection or injury.

● Wear medical identification at all times.

● Practice good oral hygiene with inhalation therapy to prevent fungal infections in the mouth.

✔ Keep in mind

● Tell your primary health care provider if you're pregnant or planning to becoming pregnant.

● If you're breast-feeding, you may have to stop or take another medication.

● If you are diabetic, you may need to take more insulin to keep your blood sugar under control.

Additional instructions

_____
_____
_____
_____
_____
_____
_____
_____
_____
_____

Taking sucralfate

Dear Patient,

Your primary health care provider has prescribed sucralfate to treat your stomach ulcer. This medication works by forming a barrier over you ulcer. This protects the ulcer from stomach acid and allows it to heal. Another name for this medication is Carafate.

How to take sucralfate

Sucralfate is available in tablet and liquid form. Take the medication 1 hour before meals and at bedtime because it works best on an empty stomach. For this reason, take the medication only with water. Shake the liquid well before use.

Continue taking the medication for as long as your primary health care provider has prescribed, even after you've begun to feel better.

What to do if you miss a dose

Take the dose as soon as possible. But if it's almost time for your next dose, skip the missed dose and take the next one at the regular time. Don't take two doses at once.

What to do about side effects

You may become constipated while you're taking this medication. If you do, call your primary health care provider. He may prescribe a laxative to relieve the problem.

What you must know about alcohol and other drugs

Don't drink alcoholic beverages or take aspirin while taking sucralfate because these substances can increase stomach irritation. Also, don't smoke because it increases acid production in your stomach and could worsen your ulcer.

Antacids can keep sucralfate from working properly. So don't take them for 30 minutes before or after a scheduled dose of sucralfate.

Check with your primary health care provider or pharmacist before taking any other medications because sucralfate can interfere with the way they work. In particular, be sure to report if you're taking an antibiotic.

Special directions

• If you have a history of kidney failure or an intestinal obstruction, let your primary health care provider know. He may want to change your medication.
• While you're taking sucralfate, don't eat foods that irritate your stomach.
• Store the medication in a cool, dry place—not in your bathroom medicine cabinet or near the kitchen sink. Protect the medication from direct light, and don't put it in the refrigerator.
• Don't take this medication for more than 8 weeks.

✓ Keep in mind

• If you're pregnant or breast-feeding, check with your primary health care provider before taking this medication.

Additional instructions

_____
_____
_____
_____
_____
_____
_____
_____
_____
_____

Using sulfacetamide

Dear Patient,

Your primary health care provider has prescribed sulfacetamide to treat your eye infection. This medication has several brand names, including Bleph-10, Cetamide, and Sodium Sulamyd.

How to use sulfacetamide

If you're using sulfacetamide *eyedrops,* follow these steps. First wash your hands. Then tilt your head back and pull your lower eyelid away from your eye to form a pouch. Without touching your eye with the applicator, instill the prescribed amount of drops into the pouch. Then gently close your eye and don't blink. Keep your eye closed for 1 to 2 minutes to give the medication time to saturate the area. If you think you didn't get the drop of medication into your eye properly, use another drop.

If you're using sulfacetamide *eye ointment,* follow these steps. Wash your hands. Pull your lower eyelid away from your eye to form a pouch. Without touching your eye with the applicator tip, squeeze a thin strip of ointment, about ½ inch to 1 inch long, into the pouch. Gently close your eye. Keep your eye closed for 1 to 2 minutes to give the medication time to saturate the area.

After you finish using the medication, wash your hands again.

Use all of the medication as prescribed by your primary health care provider, even if your symptoms subside after a few days.

What to do if you miss a dose

Take the medication as soon as possible. However, if it's almost time for your next dose, skip the missed dose and take the next dose on schedule.

What to do about side effects

Call your primary health care provider *right away* if you develop a rash, if blisters form in your mouth or on your eyelids, or if your skin turns red and starts to peel. Also call if your eyelids swell, itch, and burn constantly.

You may notice that your eyes sting or burn for a few minutes after you use the drops or ointment. This is to be expected. Also expect your vision to blur briefly after applying eye ointment.

What you must know about other drugs

Sulfacetamide isn't compatible with any type of silver eye preparation. If you're using silver nitrate or a mild silver protein for the eye, tell your primary health care provider or pharmacist.

Special directions

• Tell your primary health care provider if you've ever had an allergic reaction to any type of sulfa medication.
• Don't share your medication with anyone. If someone in your family develops the same symptoms that you have, call your primary health care provider.

☑ Keep in mind

• Check with your primary health care provider before using this medication if you are pregnant or breast-feeding.

Additional instructions

_____
_____
_____
_____
_____
_____

Taking sulfamethoxazole

Dear Patient,

Your primary health care provider has prescribed sulfamethoxazole to treat your infection. The label on your medication bottle may read Bactrim or Gantanol.

How to take sulfamethoxazole
This medication is available in tablet and oral suspension form. Take it just as prescribed by your primary health care provider. Take it at the same times every day so that the amount of medication in your bloodstream remains constant. Keep taking your medication even if you feel better after a few days.

With each dose, drink a full glass (8 ounces) of water. Also drink several more glasses of water throughout the day to help prevent unwanted side effects.

What to do if you miss a dose
Take the dose as soon as you can. But if it's almost time for your next dose, you'll need to adjust your schedule. If your primary health care provider has prescribed two doses a day, wait 5 to 6 hours after taking the missed dose and then take your next dose. After that, resume your regular dosing schedule.

If your primary health care provider has prescribed three or more doses a day, wait 2 to 4 hours after taking the missed dose and then take the next dose. After that, resume your regular dosing schedule.

What to do about side effects
Call your primary health care provider *right away* if your skin itches, develops a rash, blisters, turns red, or starts to peel. Also report if you have increased sensitivity to the sun, a sore throat, a fever, or pallor while taking this medication.

Right after you start taking the medication, you may experience diarrhea, headaches, dizziness, loss of appetite, nausea or vomiting, and fatigue. If these symptoms continue for more than a day or so, tell your primary health care provider.

What you must know about other drugs
Before you take any other medication, check with your health care provider because sulfamethoxazole can interfere with the way some other medications work.

Tell your health care provider if you're taking blood thinners or any oral medication to control diabetes. Sulfamethoxazole may increase the effects of these medications, making it necessary to adjust your dose.

Special directions
● Tell your primary health care provider if you've ever had a reaction to any type of sulfa medication or any medication containing sulfur, such as the water pill furosemide (Lasix) or oral diabetes medication.
● Tell your health care provider if you have a history of anemia, glucose-6-phosphate dehydrogenase deficiency, urinary obstruction, kidney or liver disease, severe allergies, asthma, blood disorders, or porphyria.
● Because sulfamethoxazole may make your skin more sensitive to the sun, limit your exposure while you're taking the medication and use sunscreen if exposed.
● Because this medication makes some people dizzy, don't drive or operate any machinery until you know how you respond to it.

✔ Keep in mind
● If you're pregnant or breast-feeding, tell your health care provider. He can determine if it's safe for you to take this medication.

Additional instructions

_____

_____

Taking sulfasalazine

Dear Patient,

Your primary health care provider has prescribed sulfasalazine to help treat rheumatoid arthritis or ulcerative colitis (a bowel condition). This medication works by helping to reduce inflammation inside the bowel and other symptoms. Other names for this medication are Azulfidine and Azulfidine EN-Tabs.

How to take sulfasalazine

This medication comes in tablets, enteric-coated tablets, or an oral suspension. Take each dose with a full glass (8 ounces) of water. Also drink several more glasses of water during the day. This will help prevent certain side effects.

Because sulfasalazine may upset an empty stomach, take the medication after meals or with food. Take the enteric-coated tablets whole — don't crush or break them.

Follow your primary health care provider's directions exactly. Take the entire prescription even if you feel better after a few days.

What to do if you miss a dose

Take the dose as soon as possible. But if it's almost time for your next dose, skip the missed dose and take your next dose as scheduled.

What to do about side effects

Call your primary health care provider *right away* if you develop aching joints and muscles; a continuous headache; a rash or blisters; red, peeling skin; itching; or difficulty breathing.

Also tell your health care provider if you develop nausea, vomiting, diarrhea, dizziness, or increased sensitivity to sunlight.

Don't worry if you notice that the medication turns your urine or skin an orange-yellow color. This symptom will disappear after you've finished your medication.

What you must know about other drugs

Sulfasalazine may affect your response to other medications. For example, it may change the effects of oral medications for diabetes, birth control pills, blood thinners (Coumadin and aspirin), and folic acid. Tell your health care provider or pharmacist if you're taking these medications.

Special directions

• Tell your primary health care provider if you've ever had an allergic reaction to a sulfa medication, a diuretic (a water pill, such as Lasix), or an oral medication for diabetes. Also mention if you've ever had an allergic reaction to aspirin or an oral medication for glaucoma.
• Also tell your primary health care provider if you have a history of anemia, glucose-6-phosphate dehydrogenase deficiency, urinary or intestinal tract obstruction, kidney or liver disease, severe allergies, asthma, blood disorders, or porphyria.
• Because sulfasalazine may make your skin more sensitive to sunlight, limit your sun exposure while you're taking the medication and use sunscreen.
• This medication makes some people dizzy, so don't drive or perform activities that require alertness until you know how you respond to it.

✔ Keep in mind

• Tell your primary health care provider if you're pregnant or breast-feeding.

Additional instructions

_____

_____

Using ophthalmic sulfisoxazole

Dear Patient,

Your primary health care provider has prescribed sulfisoxazole to treat your eye infection. The label may read Gantrisin.

How to use ophthalmic sulfisoxazole

This medication comes as an eyedrop and an eye ointment.

If you're using the *eyedrop* form of the medication, follow these steps. First wash your hands. Then tilt your head back and pull your lower eyelid away from your eye to form a pouch. Without touching your eye with the applicator, instill the prescribed amount of drops into the pouch. Then gently close your eye and don't blink. Keep your eye closed for 1 to 2 minutes to give the medication time to saturate the area.

If you're using the *eye ointment* form of the medication, follow these steps. Wash your hands. Pull your lower eyelid away from your eye to form a pouch. Without touching your eye with the applicator tip, squeeze a thin strip of ointment, about ½ inch to 1 inch long, into the pouch. Gently close your eye. Keep your eye closed for 1 to 2 minutes to give the medication time to saturate the area. After applying the medication, wash your hands again.

Use all of the medication as prescribed by your primary health care provider even if your symptoms subside after a few days.

What to do if you miss a dose

Take the medication as soon as possible. However, if it's almost time for your next dose, skip the missed dose and take the next dose on schedule.

What to do about side effects

Call your primary health care provider *right away* if you develop a rash, if blisters form on your mouth or on your eyelids, or if your skin turns red and starts to peel. Also call if your eyelids swell, itch, and burn constantly.

You may notice that your eyes sting or burn for a few minutes after you use the drops or ointment. This is to be expected. Also expect your vision to blur briefly after applying eye ointment.

What you must know about other drugs

Sulfisoxasole isn't compatible with any type of silver eye preparation. If you're using silver nitrate or a mild silver protein for the eye, tell your primary health care provider or pharmacist.

Special directions

● Tell your primary health care provider if you've ever had an allergic reaction to any type of sulfa medication.
● Don't share your medication with anyone. If someone in your family develops the same symptoms that you have, call your primary health care provider.

✔ Keep in mind

● If you're pregnant or breast-feeding, check with your primary health care provider before using this product.

Additional instructions

_____
_____
_____
_____
_____
_____
_____
_____
_____
_____

Taking oral sulfisoxazole

Dear Patient,

Your primary health care provider has prescribed sulfisoxazole to help treat your infection. Another name for this medication is Gantrisin or Pediazole.

How to take oral sulfisoxazole

This medication comes in tablet or liquid form. Take it exactly as prescribed, at the same times every day. Continue to take the medication even after you start to feel better.

Drink a full glass of water with each dose. Also drink several more glasses of water throughout the day to help prevent unwanted side effects.

What to do if you miss a dose

Take the dose as soon as you can. But if it's almost time for your next dose, you need to adjust your dosing schedule. For example, if your primary health care provider has prescribed two doses a day, wait 5 to 6 hours after taking the missed dose before taking the next dose. Then resume your regular dosing schedule.

If your primary health care provider has prescribed three or more doses a day, wait 2 to 4 hours after taking the missed dose before taking the next dose. After that, resume your regular dosing schedule.

What to do about side effects

Call your primary health care provider *right away* if you notice itching or a rash; red, blistering, or peeling skin; decreased urine output; or difficulty swallowing.

Right after you start taking the medication, you may experience diarrhea, headaches, dizziness, loss of appetite, nausea or vomiting, and fatigue. If these symptoms continue for more than a day or so, tell your primary health care provider.

What you must know about other drugs

Sulfisoxazole may change how your body responds to certain medications. Don't take it with medications containing ammonium chloride (such as some cough medications); para-aminobenzoic acid (PABA), which is found in some multivitamins; or vitamin C.

Sulfisoxazole may also change the effects of birth control pills, oral medications for diabetes (such as Glucotrol), blood thinners (such as Coumadin or aspirin), the heart medication digoxin (Lanoxin), and folic acid. If you're taking any of these medications, let your primary health care provider know.

Special directions

• Tell your primary health care provider if you've ever had a reaction to a sulfa medication or any medication containing sulfur, a diuretic (a water pill such as Lasix), or an oral medication for diabetes.
• Because sulfisoxazole may make your skin more sensitive to sunlight, limit your exposure to the sun and use sunscreen if exposed.

✓ Keep in mind

• Don't give sulfisoxazole to children under 2 months. Pregnant women at term and nursing mothers of infants under 2 months also shouldn't take this medication.

Additional instructions

_____
_____
_____
_____
_____
_____
_____

Taking sulindac

Dear Patient,

Your primary health care provider has prescribed sulindac to help treat your condition. Sulindac helps control inflammation and relieve pain. It's often called a *nonsteroidal anti-inflammatory medication.* The label on your medication bottle may read Clinoril.

How to take sulindac
This medication is available as tablets. Follow your primary health care provider's instructions exactly. Take sulindac with milk, meals, or an antacid. This will help prevent stomach upset, which could occur if you take the medication on an empty stomach.

Also drink a full glass (8 ounces) of water with each dose. Don't lie down for 15 to 30 minutes after taking the medication. This will help prevent irritation that could cause you to have difficulty swallowing.

What to do if you miss a dose
If your primary health care provider has prescribed this medication on a regular schedule and you miss a dose, take it as soon as you remember. But if it's almost time for your next dose, skip the missed dose and take your next dose as scheduled.

What to do about side effects
Tell your primary health care provider *immediately* if you notice any of these side effects:
• stomach pain or burning
• bloody or black, tarry stools
• easy bruising and bleeding
• changes in vision
• swelling in your face, feet, or lower legs
• persistent nausea.

Mild stomach upset may be treated with antacids.

What you must know about alcohol and other drugs
Avoid alcohol while taking this medication because alcohol may increase stomach irritation.

Because sulindac may affect the action of other medications, tell your primary health care provider or pharmacist about any medications you're taking at the same time. In particular, mention if you're taking aspirin, a blood thinner (such as Coumadin), or medications for seizures (such as Dilantin or Tegretol), for thyroid problems, or for inflammation.

Special directions
• Tell your primary health care provider if aspirin or another anti-inflammatory medication has ever caused you to have difficulty breathing, a tight sensation in your chest, a runny nose, or itching.
• Also tell your primary health care provider if you have a history of stomach or intestinal bleeding, liver or kidney disease, asthma, heart disease, or high blood pressure.
• This medication makes some people drowsy or dizzy, so don't drive or perform any activities that require alertness until you know how you react to it.

✔ Keep in mind
• This medication can hide the symptoms of an infection. If you have diabetes, be especially careful about your feet and watch for problems, such as redness or sores.
• Because sulindac can cause you to retain fluid, have your blood pressure checked when your health care provider recommends.

Additional instructions

Taking sumatriptan

Dear Patient,

Sumatriptan is used to treat migraine headaches. It's not effective in preventing migraines or in treating other types of headaches. Sumatriptan affects chemicals in the brain associated with migraine headaches. The brand name is Imitrex.

How to take sumatriptan

Sumatriptan is available as a tablet, nasal spray, and subcutaneous (just under the skin) injection.

If you're taking the *tablets,* take one by mouth at the first sign of a migraine. Don't take another tablet for the same migraine without first talking to your primary health care provider. He'll probably tell you to wait at least 2 hours after the first dose before taking the second dose. Don't take more than 300 mg of this medication in a 24-hour period. Also, don't crush or chew the tablets — swallow them whole with a full glass (8 ounces) of water.

If you're taking the *nasal spray,* spray once into one nostril when the headache occurs. If the headache returns, you can use a second spray at least 2 hours after the first dose. But don't use more than 40 mg in 1 day.

If you're giving yourself a *subcutaneous injection,* do so as soon as migraine symptoms appear. Don't give yourself more than two injections daily, with at least 1 hour between injections.

What to do if you miss a dose

This medication is used to treat migraines, not to prevent or reduce their occurrence. It's not for routine use.

What to do about side effects

Tell your primary health care provider *at once* if you develop chest pain, tightness in your chest or throat, an irregular or fast heart rate, a rash, or swelling of the face or lips.

At first, this medication may cause flushing, dizziness, weakness, nausea, drowsiness, and a feeling of warmth. Tell your primary health care provider if these side effects continue or become bothersome.

What you must know about alcohol and other drugs

Don't drink alcohol while on this drug; the combination may make you overly drowsy.

Tell your health care provider of nonprescription or prescription medications that you start or stop while being treated with sumatriptan.

⚠ *Warning:* Stop taking monoamine oxidase inhibitors (such as Nardil or Parnate) at least 2 weeks before starting sumatriptan. Don't take ergotamine and sumatriptan within 24 hours of each other.

Special directions

- You can buy an auto-injector for giving subcutaneous sumatriptan. Ask your primary health care provider or pharmacist for instructions on how to use it.
- Tell your health care provider if you have heart disease, high blood pressure, an abnormal heart rhythm, kidney disease, liver disease, or allergies to medications.
- Don't drive or perform any activities that require alertness while taking sumatriptan.

✔ Keep in mind

- Tell your primary health care provider if you're pregnant or breast-feeding before taking this medication.

Additional instructions

_____

_____

Taking tamoxifen

Dear Patient,

Your primary health care provider has prescribed tamoxifen to help treat your breast cancer. Tamoxifen blocks the effects of the hormone estrogen which, in turn, may improve your condition. Another name for this medication is Nolvadex.

How to take tamoxifen

Follow your primary health care provider's instructions exactly. Don't take more of the medication than has been prescribed, and be careful not to miss a dose. Take the medication even if it makes you feel nauseated.

If you're taking enteric-coated tablets, swallow the tablet whole. Don't crush or break up the tablet before taking.

What to do if you miss a dose

Skip the missed dose entirely, and take your next regular dose as scheduled. Call your primary health care provider to let him know you missed a dose.

If you vomit shortly after taking a dose of tamoxifen, call your primary health care provider. Depending on the circumstances, he may tell you to take the dose again or to wait until the next scheduled dose.

What to do about side effects

Tamoxifen may cause easy bruising or bleeding. If these symptoms develop, call your primary health care provider. The medication may also cause nausea, vomiting, hot flashes, weight gain, bone pain, and changes in your menstrual cycle. Let your primary health care provider know if these symptoms become a problem.

Tamoxifen causes women to become more fertile. But, because you shouldn't become pregnant while taking the medication, use a barrier contraceptive (condom or diaphragm).

What you must know about other drugs

Birth control pills may change the effects of tamoxifen. So while you're taking this medication, use a barrier method of birth control.

Special directions

- Before taking tamoxifen, tell your primary health care provider if you've ever had cataracts or another eye problem.
- To help control hot flashes, don't drink alcoholic beverages or smoke while you're taking the medication. Also, drink lots of fluids, wear layers of clothing that you can easily remove if you get too warm, and use fans or an air conditioner to control indoor temperature.
- Try to eat a high-calorie diet. If you become nauseated, sip fluids throughout the day.

✔ Keep in mind

❗ *Warning:* Tell your primary health care provider *immediately* if you think you've become pregnant while taking tamoxifen.

Additional instructions

_____
_____
_____
_____
_____
_____
_____
_____
_____
_____
_____

Taking temazepam

Dear Patient,

Your primary health care provider has prescribed this sedative to help treat your condition. Temazepam helps relieve nervousness and tension to help you sleep. The name on the label may read Restoril.

How to take temazepam

This drug comes in capsule form. Follow your primary health care provider's instructions exactly. Don't increase your dose even if you think your current one isn't effective. Instead, call your primary health care provider. Because temazepam can be habit-forming, don't take it for a longer time than prescribed.

What to do about side effects

Temazepam may make you feel tired, drowsy, or dizzy. If the symptoms are severe, or if you feel very tired or "hung over" the day after you've taken the medication, your dose may be too high. Call your primary health care provider so he can adjust your dosage.

What you must know about alcohol and other drugs

Don't drink any alcoholic beverages — beer, wine, or liquor — while you're taking temazepam because the combination can cause extreme drowsiness and an overdose.

For the same reason, avoid taking other medications that can slow down your nervous system unless your primary health care provider says otherwise. Examples include many allergy or cold medications, narcotics, muscle relaxants (such as Flexaril or Soma), sleeping pills (such as Halcion or Restoril), and medications for seizures (such as Dilantin or Tegretol).

Tell your primary health care provider if you're taking the medication zidovudine (also called AZT). Temazepam could cause your body to absorb more zidovudine, so your primary health care provider may need to lower your zidovudine dosage.

Special directions

• Temazepam can make some medical problems worse. For this reason, tell your primary health care provider if you have glaucoma, a history of alcohol or drug abuse, mental depression, myasthenia gravis, Parkinson's disease, chronic obstructive pulmonary disease, kidney or liver disease, or porphyria.
• Check with your primary health care provider every month to make sure you still need to be taking this medication.
• Temazepam may make you drowsy or light-headed. So don't drive or perform other activities that require alertness until you know how you respond to it.

✔ Keep in mind

• Don't take temazepam if you think you might be pregnant or if you're breast-feeding.
• If you're an older adult, this medication could make you feel drowsy during the day, which could lead to falls.
• If you're an athlete, you should know that temazepam is banned and in some cases tested for by the U.S. Olympic Committee and the National Collegiate Athletic Association.

Additional instructions

_____
_____
_____
_____
_____

Taking terazosin

Dear Patient,

Your primary health care provider has prescribed terazosin to help treat your high blood pressure. This medication works by relaxing your blood vessels so that blood passes through them more easily. This helps to lower your blood pressure.

Terazosin is also used for a condition called benign prostatic hyperplasia. The label on your medication bottle may read Hytrin.

How to take terazosin
Follow your primary health care provider's instructions exactly. This medication won't cure your high blood pressure; it will only help control it. That's why you need to continue to take it even if you feel well. You may even need to take it for the rest of your life.

What to do if you miss a dose
Take the dose as soon as you remember, as long as it's the same day as the missed dose. But, if you don't remember until the next day, skip the missed dose and take the next dose as scheduled. If you miss several doses, call your primary health care provider before resuming your medication.

What to do about side effects
Terazosin causes some people to feel dizzy or light-headed, especially when getting up after sitting or lying down. Other possible side effects include an irregular heartbeat, swelling in the feet and lower legs, stuffy nose, and nausea. Call your primary health care provider if any of these symptoms become bothersome.

What you must know about other drugs
Avoid alcoholic beverages because they increase dizziness.

Don't take any medications — even non-prescription ones — without first talking with your primary health care provider. This is especially true for diet, asthma, cold, cough, hay fever, and sinus medications because these medications may increase your blood pressure.

Special directions
• Because your first dose of terazosin will most likely make you drowsy or dizzy, take it at bedtime. For this same reason, be careful if you get up during the night. Don't drive or operate any machinery until you know how you're going to respond to the medication.
• To lessen dizziness, get up slowly. If you begin to feel light-headed once you're standing, lie down so you don't faint. Then sit up for a few moments before standing.
• You're more likely to feel dizzy if you drink alcoholic beverages, stand for a long period of time, or exercise or when the weather is hot.
• Keep all your appointments with your primary health care provider, even if you feel well. Check your blood pressure frequently.

✔ Keep in mind
• Tell your primary health care provider if you think you're pregnant or if you're breast-feeding.

Additional instructions
_____
_____
_____
_____
_____
_____
_____

Taking terbutaline

Dear Patient,

Your primary health care provider has prescribed terbutaline to help treat your breathing problem. Terbutaline opens the air passages in your lungs, which will help you to breathe easier. The label on your medication may read Brethaire, Brethine, or Bricanyl.

How to take terbutaline

If your primary health care provider has prescribed the *oral* form of this medication, follow his instructions exactly.

If your primary health care provider has prescribed the *aerosol* form of this medication, follow these steps. Blow your nose and clear your throat. Breathe out, emptying your lungs as much as possible. Hold the medication canister in an upright position. Place the mouthpiece well inside your mouth and close your lips around it. Press down on the top of the medication canister. At the same time, breathe in deeply. Hold your breath for several seconds. Remove the mouthpiece from your mouth and breathe out slowly. If your primary health care provider has ordered more than one inhalation, wait at least 2 minutes before you use the inhaler the second time. Never use the inhaler more than twice in a row.

What to do if you miss a dose

If you're using terbutaline regularly, take your missed dose as soon as you remember. Then take any remaining doses that day at regularly spaced intervals. Don't take two doses at the same time.

What to do about side effects

If your wheezing gets worse or your breathing becomes more difficult after taking terbutaline, stop the medication and call your primary health care provider *immediately.*

You may feel nervous, develop a tremor, or get a headache while taking terbutaline. These symptoms are common, but if they become bothersome, call your primary health care provider.

What you must know about other drugs

Don't take terbutaline if you're taking a type of antidepressant called a monoamine oxidase (MAO) inhibitor. Taking them together could cause severe high blood pressure.

If you're taking a beta blocker (such as Tenormin or Lopressor), tell your primary health care provider or pharmacist. These medications could keep terbutaline from working properly.

Also tell your primary health care provider if you're taking the heart medication digitalis (Lanoxin).

Special directions

● Because terbutaline can make certain medical problems worse, tell your primary health care provider if you have a history of seizures, brain damage, diabetes, mental illness, heart disease, high blood pressure, an overactive thyroid, or Parkinson's disease.

✔ Keep in mind

● If you're an athlete, you should know that oral forms of terbutaline are banned and tested for by the U.S. Olympic Committee. However, the committee permits the use of terbutaline in aerosol or inhalation form.

Additional instructions

_____
_____
_____
_____
_____

Using terconazole

Dear Patient,

Your primary health care provider has ordered terconazole to treat your vaginal fungal infection. It works by killing fungus or preventing its growth. The medication is also called Terazol.

How to use terconazole

This medication comes as a cream or vaginal suppository. With either form of medication, you should find an applicator in the carton. Use the applicator to insert the medication into your vagina at bedtime. If you're inserting a suppository, remain lying down for at least 30 minutes after each dose to allow your vagina time to absorb the terconazole.

Use the medication for the number of nights prescribed by your primary health care provider. Don't stop before then, even if your symptoms subside. If you stop using the medication too soon, your symptoms may return.

What to do if you miss a dose

Take the dose as soon as possible. But if it's almost time for your next dose, skip the missed dose and take your next dose as scheduled.

What to do about side effects

If your vagina becomes irritated or burns after using this medication, and you didn't have these problems before, call your primary health care provider as soon as possible.

Some women develop a headache after using terconazole. If this occurs, take acetaminophen (Tylenol) or another mild pain reliever.

Special directions

• Tell your primary health care provider if you've ever had an allergic reaction to terconazole or another antifungal medication. Also tell him if you're using a douche or another type of vaginal medication.

• Keep using the medication, even if your period starts. But don't use tampons because they'll absorb some of the medication in your vagina.

• To keep the medication from soiling your clothes, wear a minipad or sanitary napkin.

• If your symptoms don't subside or if they worsen after using the medication for several days, call your primary health care provider.

• To keep your infection from returning, wear all-cotton panties or panties with a cotton crotch and pantyhose with a cotton crotch.

! *Warning:* You can spread your infection to your sexual partner during intercourse. Or, he could be carrying the fungus in his genital tract. To prevent spreading the infection or becoming reinfected, have your partner wear a condom during intercourse. However, if you're using a suppository, it's best to avoid intercourse because the medication may weaken the latex in condoms.

✓ Keep in mind

• If you're pregnant or breast-feeding, check with your primary health care provider before using terconazole.

Additional instructions

_____
_____
_____
_____
_____
_____
_____
_____

Taking oral and topical tetracycline

Dear Patient,

Your primary health care provider has prescribed tetracycline to help treat your infection. If you're taking the *oral* form of this medication, such as a tablet or capsule, the label may read Achromycin, Panmycin, or Tetracyn. If you're applying *topical* tetracycline, the label may read Topicycline.

How to take tetracycline

If you're taking *oral* tetracycline, take the medication 1 hour before or 2 hours after meals because foods can decrease your body's ability to absorb the medication. For the same reason, don't take the medication with milk or other dairy products. To help prevent stomach irritation, drink a full glass of water with each dose.

If you're using *topical* tetracycline, control the rate of application by adjusting the pressure of the applicator against your skin. Avoid contact with your eyes, nose, and mouth.

What to do if you miss a dose

Take the dose as soon as possible. But if it's almost time for your next dose, adjust your dosing schedule as follows.

If you're taking *one dose a day,* space the missed dose and your next dose 12 hours apart.

If you're taking *two doses a day,* space the missed dose and the next dose 5 to 6 hours apart.

If you're taking *three or more doses a day,* space the missed dose and the next dose 2 to 4 hours apart.

Then resume your regular dosing schedule.

What to do about side effects

Call your primary health care provider if you develop a sore throat, diarrhea, reddened skin, rash, or hives, or skin changes after being in the sun.

Also tell your health care provider if you have difficulty swallowing, indigestion, loss of appetite, or nausea and, if you're female, if you have a vaginal infection.

What you must know about other drugs

Don't take tetracycline with antacids, iron preparations, or sodium bicarbonate. Tell your primary health care provider if you're taking anticoagulant medication because your dosage may need to be changed.

Warning: Because tetracycline may keep birth control pills from working properly, use a second form of birth control.

Special directions

• Before taking tetracycline, tell your primary health care provider if you have diabetes insipidus. Tetracycline could make this condition worse. Also tell him if you have kidney or liver disease because you may have a greater risk of developing side effects.
• If you're using topical tetracycline, use up the solution within 2 months and be careful when applying it because it may stain your clothing.
• Because tetracycline may make your skin more sensitive to sunlight, limit your exposure to the sun and use sunscreen.

✔ Keep in mind

Warning: Avoid tetracycline if you're pregnant. It could stain your baby's teeth or cause other problems.
• Don't give tetracycline to children under age 8.

Additional instructions

_____

_____

Taking theophylline

Dear Patient,

Your primary health care provider has prescribed theophylline to help treat and prevent the symptoms of your asthma. This medication works by opening up the bronchial tubes and increasing the flow of air through them. If you're taking the *liquid* form of the medication, the label may read Aquaphyllin, Elixicon, or Slo-Phyllin. If you're taking a *tablet* or *capsule,* the label may read Constant-T, Theo-Dur, or Slo-bid.

How to take theophylline
Follow your primary health care provider's instructions exactly. Don't take more or less of the medication than prescribed, and don't take it more often or for a longer time. Take it at the same time every day.

In general, take theophylline 30 minutes to 1 hour before meals or 2 hours after meals, unless your primary health care provider directs you otherwise. Theophylline works best on an empty stomach.

If you're taking the *extended-release* form of the medication, don't crush or break the capsules or tablets. If it's difficult to swallow, talk to your primary health care provider.

What to do if you miss a dose
For the medication to work properly, you need to take every dose on time. If you do miss a dose, though, take it as soon as possible. If it's almost time for your next dose, skip the missed dose and take your next dose on schedule.

What to do about side effects
Call your primary health care provider *immediately* if you develop diarrhea or have a seizure. Also let him know if you feel nervous or dizzy, have difficulty sleeping, have a rapid heartbeat, become nauseated or vomit, or lose your appetite.

What you must know about other drugs
Theophylline can interfere with the way some other drugs work, and vice versa. So tell your primary health care provider if you're taking birth control pills; medications for seizures, heart problems, tuberculosis, or a stomach ulcer; or nonprescription medications.

Also tell him if you've smoked tobacco or marijuana within the last 2 years. Smoking may affect the theophylline dose.

Special directions
• Tell the primary health care provider if you've ever had an allergic reaction to theophylline or any medication for asthma.
• Because theophylline can make some medical problems worse, tell your primary health care provider if you have heart or circulatory problems, diabetes, glaucoma, high blood pressure, an overactive thyroid, stomach ulcers, or indigestion.
• *Warning:* Don't consume large amounts of foods or liquids containing caffeine, such as chocolate, tea, coffee, and colas. The extra caffeine may increase the stimulant effects of theophylline.
• Call your health care provider right away if you develop a fever or think you have the flu.
• A blood test may be used to determine if you're taking the correct dose.

Keep in mind
• If you're pregnant or breast-feeding, check with your primary health care provider before taking theophylline.
• If you're an older adult, you may be especially prone to side effects.

Additional instructions
_____
_____
_____

Taking thioridazine

Dear Patient,

Your primary health care provider has prescribed thioridazine to treat your condition. The label may read Mellaril.

How to take thioridazine

Thioridazine comes in tablet and liquid form.

If it comes in a bottle with a dropper, use the dropper to measure each dose. Dilute the dose in half a glass (4 ounces) of fruit juice, soda, milk, water, or semisolid food.

If the medication is in *liquid* form, shake the bottle well before use. Avoid touching your skin with thioridazine because rash may occur.

To prevent stomach irritation, take your medication with food or a glass of water. Also, don't stop taking your medication unless your primary health care provider tells you to or you develop a severe reaction.

What to do if you miss a dose

If you take one dose a day and you remember the missed dose the same day, take it as soon as possible. Otherwise, skip the missed dose and resume your regular dosing schedule.

If you take more than one dose a day and you remember the missed dose within an hour, take it right away. Otherwise, skip the missed dose and take your next dose as scheduled.

What to do about side effects

Call your primary health care provider *right away* if you have uncontrolled movements of your mouth, tongue, cheeks, jaw, or arms and legs. Also report if fever, sore throat, fast heartbeat, rapid breathing, profuse sweating, fainting or dizziness, difficult urination, or blurred vision occurs.

Check with your health care provider if you become constipated or unusually tired; also report if you have dry mouth or changes in skin color after being in the sun.

What you must know about alcohol and other drugs

Don't drink alcohol because you could become overly drowsy.

Tell your health care provider if you're taking barbiturates, lithium (Lithane), or high blood pressure medication. For your body to fully absorb thioridazine, don't take an antacid 2 hours before or after your dose.

Special directions

• Tell your health care provider if you've had an allergic reaction to a phenothiazine, such as Thorazine. Also report if you have a history of a blood or bone marrow disorder, heart disease, encephalitis, respiratory disease, seizures, glaucoma, an enlarged prostate, urine retention, Parkinson's disease, a low calcium level, or stomach ulcers.
• Avoid direct exposure to the sun and use sunscreen. Thioridazine reduces sweating, so be careful not to become overheated.
• Because the medication may make you drowsy, don't drive or perform any activities that require alertness. The drowsiness should become less noticeable after several weeks.

✔ Keep in mind

• If you're breast-feeding or pregnant, talk with your primary health care provider before taking this medication.
• If you're an athlete, you should know that thioridazine is banned and sometimes tested for by the U.S. Olympic Committee and the National Collegiate Athletic Association.

Additional instructions

_____

_____

Taking thiothixene

Dear Patient,

Your primary health care provider has prescribed thiothixene to treat your condition. The label may read Navane.

How to take thiothixene
Take only the amount ordered by your primary health care provider. You may need to take the medication for several weeks before you notice its full effect.

If you're taking the *liquid concentrate,* use the bottle dropper to measure the exact dose. Then dilute the dose in half a glass (4 ounces) of water, milk, soda, or tomato or fruit juice. Don't let thiothixene touch your skin; it could cause a rash.

Don't suddenly stop taking thiothixene unless told by your primary health care provider or you have a severe reaction.

What to do if you miss a dose
Take the dose as soon as possible. But if it's within 2 hours of your next dose, skip the missed dose and take your next dose as scheduled.

What to do about side effects
Call your primary health care provider *right away* if you have uncontrolled movements of your mouth, tongue, cheeks, jaw, or arms and legs. Also call if you have a fever, a sore throat, a fast heartbeat, rapid breathing, profuse sweating, fainting or dizziness, difficult urination, or blurred vision.

Tell your health care provider if you become constipated, have a dry mouth, or have changes in skin color after being in the sun.

What you must know about alcohol and other drugs
Warning: Don't drink alcoholic beverages while taking this medication because you could become dangerously drowsy. For the same reason, avoid allergy medications, pain relievers, and muscle relaxants. Call your primary health care provider before taking any other medications.

So that your body can absorb thiothixene completely, don't take an antacid 2 hours before or 2 hours after your dose.

Special directions
● Tell your primary health care provider if you're allergic to any medications. Because thiothixene may make some medical problems worse, tell him if you have a history of a blood or bone marrow disorder. Also tell him if you've ever been in a coma, had a head injury, or had a circulation problem.
● Tell your primary health care provider if you have heart or lung problems, seizures, glaucoma, an enlarged prostate, Parkinson's disease, urine retention, tumors, a low calcium level, or kidney or liver disease.
● Because this medication makes your skin more sensitive to sunlight, avoid direct exposure to the sun and use sunscreen. Thiothixene also reduces sweating, so try not to become overheated.
● This medication may make you drowsy, so don't drive or perform any activities that require alertness. The drowsiness should become less noticeable after several weeks.

✔ Keep in mind
● If you're breast-feeding or think you're pregnant, talk with your primary health care provider before taking this medication.
● Thiothixene is banned by the U.S. Olympic Committee and the National Collegiate Athletic Association.

Additional instructions
_____
_____

Taking a thyroid supplement

Dear Patient,

Your primary health care provider has prescribed thyroid hormone to supplement the amount of hormone produced by your thyroid gland. The label may read Levothyroxine, Liothyronine, or Liotrix.

How to take thyroid supplements

Take this medication exactly as your primary health care provider has prescribed. Don't take more or less of it, and don't take it more or less often than prescribed. Also, don't stop taking this medication without first talking with your primary health care provider.

If you're taking this medication for an underactive thyroid gland, it may take several weeks before you notice any change in your condition.

What to do if you miss a dose

Take the dose as soon as possible. But if it's almost time for your next dose, skip the missed dose and take your next dose as scheduled. Don't take two doses at the same time.

If you miss two or more doses in a row, call your primary health care provider.

What to do about side effects

Call your primary health care provider *right away* if you develop any of these symptoms:
- nervousness
- inability to sleep
- hand tremor
- rapid heartbeat or palpitations
- nausea
- headache
- fever
- sweating.

Also let your primary health care provider know if you experience a change in your appetite, changes in your menstrual period, diarrhea, increased sensitivity to heat, leg cramps, irritability, or weight loss.

What you must know about other drugs

Some medications, when taken with thyroid supplements, can cause undesirable effects. Let your primary health care provider know if you're taking amphetamines, blood thinners, diet pills, medication for a high cholesterol level, medication for asthma or other breathing problems, or allergy or cold medication.

Before you take any other medications, check with your primary health care provider or pharmacist.

Special directions

- Because other medical problems may affect how much thyroid hormone your primary health care provider prescribes, let him know if you have diabetes, hardening of the arteries, heart disease, high blood pressure, an underactive adrenal or pituitary gland, or a history of an overactive thyroid.
- If you have heart disease, this medication may cause you to develop chest pain or shortness of breath when you exert yourself. If this occurs, don't overdo physical exercise.

✓ Keep in mind

- Tell your primary health care provider right away if you become pregnant or if you're breast-feeding.

Additional instructions

_____
_____
_____
_____
_____

Using timolol

Dear Patient,

Your primary health care provider has prescribed timolol eyedrops to treat your glaucoma. Timolol helps lower eye pressure by reducing the amount of fluid produced by the eye. The label on your medication may read Timoptic.

How to use timolol

To instill your eyedrops, follow these steps. First wash your hands. Then tilt your head back. Using your middle finger, apply pressure to the inside corner of your eye. Then, with the index finger of your same hand, pull the lower eyelid away from your eye to form a pouch. Instill the prescribed number of drops into the pouch. Don't touch the applicator to your eye or surrounding tissue. Gently close your eyes, but don't blink. With your eyes closed, keep your middle finger pressed against the inside corner for 1 minute. This will help the medication stay in your eye and keep your body from absorbing it. Wash your hands again.

If your primary health care provider has ordered another eyedrop to be used with this one, wait at least 5 minutes before using the second medication. This will help keep the second medication from washing away the first.

What to do if you miss a dose

If you take one dose a day, take the missed dose as soon as possible. But if you don't remember until the next day, skip the missed dose and take your next dose as scheduled.

If you take more than one dose a day, take the missed dose as soon as possible. But if it's almost time for your next dose, skip the missed dose and take your next dose as scheduled.

What to do about side effects

Call your health care provider *right away* if you develop any of these side effects:
- dizziness or feeling faint
- irregular, slow, or pounding heartbeat
- wheezing or trouble breathing
- swelling of feet or lower legs
- unusual tiredness or weakness
- rash or itching
- severe eye irritation, vision disturbances.

What you must know about other drugs

Because timolol may affect how some other medications work, tell your primary health care provider if you're taking a beta blocker, such as Inderal. Because timolol may interact with some anesthetics, tell him you're taking timolol before you undergo any kind of surgery or emergency treatment.

Special directions

● Because timolol may make some medical problems worse, tell your primary health care provider if you have a history of asthma, diabetes, heart or blood vessel disease, myasthenia gravis, kidney or liver disease, or an overactive thyroid.

✔ Keep in mind

Warning: If you have diabetes, timolol may affect your blood glucose (sugar) levels. It may also cover up some signs of low blood glucose, such as trembling and increased heart rate and blood pressure. If you notice a change in your blood or urine glucose tests, call your health care provider.
● Timolol eyedrops are banned by the National Collegiate Athletic Association.

Additional instructions

_____

_____

Using tobramycin

Dear Patient,

Your primary health care provider has prescribed tobramycin to treat your eye infection. The medication works by killing bacteria. The label on your medication may read Tobrex.

How to use tobramycin

If you're using the *eyedrop* form of the medication, follow these steps. First, wash your hands. Tilt your head back. With your middle finger, press on the inside corner of your eye. At the same time, use your index finger to pull your lower eyelid away from your eye, forming a pouch. Without touching your eye with the applicator, instill the prescribed amount of drops into the pouch. Gently close your eye and don't blink. Keep your eye closed and your finger pressed against the inside corner for 1 minute to give the medication time to saturate the area.

If your primary health care provider has ordered another solution to be used with this one, wait at least 5 minutes before using the second medication. This will help keep the second medication from washing away the first.

If you're using the *eye ointment* form of the medication, follow these steps. Wash your hands. Pull your lower eyelid away from your eye to form a pouch. Without touching your eye with the applicator tip, squeeze a thin strip of ointment, about ½ inch long, into the pouch. Gently close your eye. Keep your eye closed for 1 to 2 minutes. After you finish applying the medication, wash your hands again.

Use all of the medication as prescribed by your primary health care provider, even if your symptoms improve after a few days.

What to do if you miss a dose

Take the medication as soon as possible. However, if it's almost time for your next dose, skip the missed dose and take the next dose on schedule.

What to do about side effects

Call your primary health care provider *immediately* if your eyelids swell, itch, or burn constantly. This may signal that you're allergic to the medication.

Your eyes may sting or burn for a few minutes after you apply the drops or ointment. This is to be expected. Also expect your vision to blur briefly after applying eye ointment.

What you must know about other drugs

Don't use this medication if you're using an eye medication containing tetracycline. The two medications don't work well together.

Special directions

• Tell your primary health care provider if you've ever had an allergic reaction to tobramycin. Also tell him if you have a history of kidney disease; ear problems, such as ringing or hearing loss; myasthenia gravis; Parkinson's disease; or low calcium levels.

Additional instructions

_____

_____

_____

_____

_____

_____

_____

_____

_____

_____

Taking tocainide

Dear Patient,

Your primary health care provider has prescribed tocainide to correct your irregular heartbeat. This medication works by slowing nerve impulses in the heart and making the heart tissue less sensitive. The label on your medication may read Tonocard.

How to take tocainide
This medication comes in tablet form. Take the exact amount prescribed by your primary health care provider. The medication works best when you have a constant amount in your bloodstream. So try to take it at the same time every day, and space your doses evenly throughout the day and night. If the medication upsets your stomach, take it with food or milk.

Continue to take the medication as directed, even if you feel well.

What to do if you miss a dose
If you remember your missed dose within 4 hours, take it as soon as possible. But if you don't remember it until later, skip the missed dose and take your next dose as scheduled. Don't take two doses at the same time.

What to do about side effects
Call your primary health care provider *right away* if you develop any of the following side effects:
- trembling or shaking
- coughing or shortness of breath
- fever or chills
- unusual bleeding or bruising
- unusual tiredness.

Also let your primary health care provider know if you experience nausea, vomiting, stomach pain, dizziness, or light-headedness.

What you must know about other drugs
Tocainide may interfere with how some other medications work. For this reason, tell your primary health care provider if you're taking a beta blocker, such as Inderal or Lopressor. Also talk with your primary health care provider or pharmacist before beginning any new medications.

Tell your primary health care provider or dentist you're taking tocainide before having any kind of surgery (including dental surgery) or emergency treatment.

Special directions
- Tocainide may make some medical conditions worse. Tell your primary health care provider if you have a history of kidney or liver disease, a bone marrow disorder, heart failure, or some other heart problem.
- Also tell your primary health care provider if you've ever had an allergic reaction to an anesthetic.
- Because this medication may make you dizzy, don't drive or do anything else that requires you to be alert until you know how you react to this medication.

✔ Keep in mind
- If you're pregnant or breast-feeding, talk with your primary health care provider before taking this medication.
- If you're an older adult, be careful when walking or first getting up out of a chair. You may be especially prone to dizziness, and you could fall.

Additional instructions
_____
_____
_____
_____
_____

Taking tolazamide

Dear Patient,

Your primary health care provider has prescribed tolazamide tablets to help control your diabetes. Taken by mouth, tolazamide works by stimulating the pancreas to produce more insulin. The label on your medication may read Tolamide or Tolinase.

How to take tolazamide
Take each dose with food. If your primary health care provider has prescribed one dose a day, take it with breakfast. If he's prescribed two doses a day, take one dose with breakfast and the second dose with your evening meal.

Keep taking the medication, even if you feel well. Tolazamide doesn't cure diabetes; it only relieves the symptoms.

What to do if you miss a dose
Take it as soon as you remember. But if it's almost time for your next dose, skip the missed dose and take your next dose as scheduled. Don't take two doses at once.

What to do about side effects
Taking too much tolazamide may cause a condition called hypoglycemia, which can produce symptoms such as drowsiness, headache, nervousness, cold sweats, and confusion. If these symptoms occur, eat or drink something sweet, such as orange juice, and call your primary health care provider.

What you must know about alcohol and other drugs
Avoid drinking alcoholic beverages while you're taking tolazamide because this can cause unpleasant side effects. Keep in mind that many foods and medications contain alcohol.

Tell your primary health care provider if you're taking other medications. Tolazamide may interfere with the way some medications work, and vice versa. Especially report if you're taking a blood thinner; diet pills; medication for asthma, colds, allergies, high blood pressure, or tuberculosis; sulfa medication; aspirin; steroids; or a thiazide diuretic (a type of water pill).

Special directions
• Tell your primary health care provider if you've ever had an allergic reaction to an oral medication used for treating diabetes or to a diuretic.
• Because some medical conditions may prevent you from taking tolazamide, tell your primary health care provider if you have a disorder that affects your liver, kidneys, adrenal glands, pituitary gland, or thyroid gland.
• Follow your primary health care provider's instructions for testing your blood or urine for glucose. Also closely follow your instructions for diet and exercise.
• This medication may increase your sensitivity to sunlight. Take precautions to protect your skin when outdoors.
• At all times, wear a medical identification bracelet stating you have diabetes and listing your medication.

✔ Keep in mind
• Tell your primary health care provider if you're breast-feeding or pregnant. He may need to prescribe a different medication.

Additional instructions
_____
_____
_____
_____

Taking tolbutamide

Dear Patient,

Your primary health care provider has prescribed tolbutamide to help control your diabetes. Taken by mouth, tolbutamide works by stimulating the pancreas to produce more insulin. The label on your medication may read Oramide or Orinase.

How to take tolbutamide
Take each dose with food. If your primary health care provider has prescribed one dose a day, take it with breakfast. If he's prescribed two doses a day, take one dose with breakfast and the second dose with your evening meal.

Keep taking the medication, even if you feel well. Tolbutamide relieves the symptoms of diabetes; it doesn't cure it.

What to do if you miss a dose
Take the dose as soon as you remember. But if it's almost time for your next dose, skip the missed dose and take your next dose as scheduled. Don't take two doses at once.

What to do about side effects
Taking too much tolbutamide may cause hypoglycemia, which can produce symptoms such as drowsiness, headache, nervousness, cold sweats, and confusion. If these symptoms occur, eat or drink something sweet, such as orange juice, and call your primary health care provider.

What you must know about alcohol and other drugs
Avoid drinking alcoholic beverages while you're taking tolbutamide. If you do, you could have unpleasant side effects. Remember that many foods and medications contain alcohol.

Tell your primary health care provider if you're taking any other medication. Tolbutamide may interfere with the way some medications work, and vice versa. Especially report if you're taking a blood thinner; diet pills; medication for asthma, colds, allergies, high blood pressure, or tuberculosis; sulfa medication; aspirin; steroids; or a thiazide diuretic (a type of water pill).

Special directions
• Tell your primary health care provider if you've ever had an allergic reaction to an oral medication used for treating diabetes or to a diuretic.
• Because some medical conditions may prevent you from taking tolbutamide, tell your primary health care provider if you have a disorder that affects your liver, kidneys, adrenal glands, pituitary gland, or thyroid gland.
• Follow your primary health care provider's instructions for testing your blood or urine for glucose. Also closely follow his prescribed diet and exercise regimen.
• This medication may increase your sensitivity to sunlight. Take precautions to protect your skin when outdoors.
• Always wear a medical identification bracelet stating that you have diabetes and listing your medication.

✔ Keep in mind
• Tell your primary health care provider if you're breast-feeding or pregnant. He may need to prescribe a different medication.

Additional instructions
_____
_____
_____
_____

Taking tolmetin

Dear Patient,

Your primary health care provider has prescribed tolmetin to treat your condition. Tolmetin helps control both inflammation and pain. The label on your medication may read Tolectin or Tolectin DS.

How to take tolmetin

Tolmetin comes in tablet and capsule forms. Take it with milk, meals, or an antacid. This will help prevent stomach upset, which could occur if you take the medication on an empty stomach. If you use an antacid, choose one containing magnesium and aluminum hydroxides, such as Maalox.

Also drink a full glass (8 ounces) of water with each dose. Don't lie down for 15 to 30 minutes after taking the medication. This will help prevent irritation that could cause you to have difficulty swallowing.

What to do if you miss a dose

If your primary health care provider has prescribed this medication on a regular schedule and you miss a dose, take it as soon as you remember. But if it's almost time for your next dose, skip the missed dose and take your next dose as scheduled.

What to do about side effects

Notify your primary health care provider *immediately* if you notice any of these side effects:
• stomach pain or burning
• bloody or black, tarry stools
• easy bruising and bleeding
• changes in vision
• swelling in your face, feet, or lower legs
• persistent nausea or vomiting
• loss of appetite or weight loss.

What you must know about alcohol and other drugs

Avoid alcoholic beverages because they can increase stomach irritation.

Because tolmetin may interact with other medications, tell your primary health care provider or pharmacist about other medications you're taking. In particular, mention aspirin, phenytoin (Dilantin), thyroid medication, another anti-inflammatory medication (such as Motrin), or a blood thinner (such as Coumadin).

Special directions

• Tell your primary health care provider if aspirin or another anti-inflammatory medication has ever caused you to experience asthma-like symptoms, a runny nose, or itching.
• Also tell your primary health care provider if you have a history of stomach or intestinal bleeding, liver or kidney disease, asthma, heart disease, or high blood pressure.
• Although the medication should begin working in 1 week, you may not feel its full effects for 2 to 4 weeks. But if your pain persists or worsens, let your primary health care provider know.

✔ Keep in mind

Warning: This medication can hide the symptoms of an infection. Therefore, if you have diabetes, you need to be especially careful about caring for your feet and watching for any problems that might be caused by an infection.

Additional instructions

_____
_____
_____
_____

Using tolnaftate

Dear Patient,

Your primary health care provider has prescribed tolnaftate to treat your fungal skin infection. Available without a prescription, the label may read Aftate, Tinactin, or Genaspor.

How to use tolnaftate

Before using any form of the medication, wash the affected area and dry it thoroughly. Then apply enough medication to cover the area. Usually, a ¼-inch to ½-inch ribbon of *cream* or three drops of *lotion* will cover an area the size of your hand.

If you're using a *powder* on your feet, sprinkle it between your toes, on your feet, and in your socks and shoes.

If you're using an *aerosol powder or solution,* shake the can well. Then, holding the can 6 to 10 inches away, spray the affected area. Don't inhale the vapor or powder from the spray. Also, don't use it near heat, an open flame, or while you're smoking.

If you're using a *pump-spray liquid,* hold the container 4 to 6 inches away from the area and spray.

Keep using the medication for 2 weeks after burning, itching, or other symptoms have disappeared. This will help you clear up the infection completely.

What to do if you miss a dose

Take the dose as soon as possible. Then return to your regular dosing schedule.

What to do about side effects

Check with your primary health care provider or pharmacist if skin irritation occurs that wasn't present before you used this medication. If you're using the spray solution form of tolnaftate, you may experience a mild, temporary stinging sensation.

Special directions

• If you have a fungal infection of your hair or nails, see your primary health care provider. This medication alone won't cure these types of infections.

• If you're treating athlete's foot and your symptoms haven't subsided after using the medication for 10 days, call your primary health care provider. If you're treating another type of fungal infection and you've used the medication for 4 weeks without improvement, or if your symptoms have worsened, call your primary health care provider.

• To help prevent reinfection after you've finished your treatment, use the powder or spray powder each day after bathing. Also sprinkle the powder or spray the aerosol inside your socks and shoes.

✔ Keep in mind

Warning: Don't use tolnaftate on a child under age 2, unless ordered by your primary health care provider.

Additional instructions

_____

_____

_____

_____

_____

_____

_____

_____

_____

_____

Taking trazodone

Dear Patient,

Your primary health care provider has prescribed trazodone tablets to help treat your depression. The label may read Desyrel, Trazon, or Trialodine.

How to take trazodone

Take your medication after a meal or light snack, even if you're taking a dose at bedtime. This will help your body absorb the medication better and will lessen your risk of becoming dizzy or developing an upset stomach.

Continue taking the medication, even if you don't feel any different. You need to take it for 2 weeks before you feel any effect at all, and for 4 weeks before you feel the full effect.

What to do if you miss a dose

Take it as soon as possible. However, if you don't remember until it's less than 4 hours until your next dose, skip the missed dose and take your next dose on schedule. Don't take two doses at once.

What to do about side effects

If you're male, stop taking the medication and call your primary health care provider *at once* if you develop a painful, inappropriate erection. For both sexes, call your primary health care provider if you have confusion, muscle tremor, nausea and vomiting, loss of muscle coordination, or extreme drowsiness.

The most common side effects are drowsiness and dizziness. These should subside after a few weeks.

What you must know about alcohol and other drugs

Avoid drinking alcoholic beverages or taking depressant medications. Trazodone will add to the effects of alcohol and depressants, placing you at risk for oversedation. Examples of depressant medications include cold or allergy medications, sleeping pills, pain medications, muscle relaxants, or anesthetics.

Trazodone may also alter how your body uses other medications. Before taking it, tell your primary health care provider if you're taking high blood pressure medication, heart medication, medication for seizures, or another type of antidepressant called a monoamine oxidase (MAO) inhibitor.

Special directions

• Tell your primary health care provider if you're allergic to trazodone or another medication used to treat depression.
• Because this medication can make certain medical conditions worse, inform your primary health care provider if you have a history of heart, liver, or kidney disease or a problem with ejaculation.
• Don't stop taking this medication without talking with your primary health care provider first. He may want you to reduce your dose gradually.
• This medication may make you drowsy or less alert than normal. So don't drive or perform any activities that require alertness. Also, to prevent dizziness and protect yourself against a fall, get up slowly after you've been lying down.

✔ Keep in mind

• If you're pregnant or breast-feeding, don't take this medication until you talk with your primary health care provider.

Additional instructions

_____

_____

Applying tretinoin

Dear Patient,

Your primary health care provider has prescribed tretinoin for your condition. Primarily used to treat acne, it may also be used to treat fine wrinkles resulting from sun damage. The label may read Retin-A or Renova.

How to apply tretinoin

Before using any form of this medication, wash your skin with a mild, nonallergenic soap and water and gently pat it dry. Then wait 20 to 30 minutes to allow your skin to dry completely.

If you're applying the *cream* or *gel*, apply enough medication to cover the affected areas and rub in gently.

If you're applying the *solution*, use your fingertips, a gauze pad, or a cotton swab to cover the affected areas.

What to do if you miss an application

Skip the missed dose and apply your next dose as scheduled.

What to do about side effects

If you have severe burning or redness, swelling, blisters, or crusting, or if your skin darkens or lightens noticeably, check with your primary health care provider *right away.*

When you first start using tretinoin, your skin may turn red and you may notice a slight stinging or feeling of warmth. After a few days, your skin may scale or peel.

Special directions

● Tell your primary health care provider if you're allergic to vitamin A or retinoic acid. Also mention whether you've had eczema.
● Avoid applying tretinoin close to your eyes or mouth, at the angles of your nose, on your mucous membranes, in an open wound, or to windburned or sunburned skin.

! *Warning:* While you're using tretinoin, don't use any of the following, unless your primary health care provider tells you otherwise: abrasive or perfumed soaps or cleansers; other topical acne medications, especially those that make the skin peel; cosmetics or soaps that dry the skin; medicated cosmetics; or skin products containing high concentrations of alcohol (such as skin freshener or aftershave lotion), menthol, spices, or lime (in some perfumes). These products can interact with tretinoin and irritate your skin.
● Don't wash your face more than two or three times a day to keep from drying out your skin. You may, however, wear cosmetics.
● Tretinoin increases your skin's sensitivity to sunlight. So wear a sunscreen, a hat, and protective clothing. If your face becomes sunburned, stop using the medication until the burn heals.
● This medication may also increase your sensitivity to wind and cold. Protect yourself by covering all exposed skin when you go out.

✔ Keep in mind
● If you're pregnant or breast-feeding, talk with your primary health care provider before using this medication.

Additional instructions

_____
_____
_____
_____
_____
_____
_____

Taking a triamcinolone inhaler

Dear Patient,

Your primary health care provider has prescribed a triamcinolone inhaler to make your breathing easier. This medication, called a corticosteroid, works in the lungs and nasal passages to reduce inflammation.

The *oral inhaler* is used to prevent wheezing caused by asthma, bronchitis, or emphysema. The *nasal inhaler* is used to relieve symptoms of seasonal or perennial allergic rhinitis. The brand name for the oral inhaler is Azmacort and for the nasal inhaler, Nasacort.

How to take triamcinolone

If you're using the *oral inhaler*, shake the canister and exhale. Place the mouthpiece in your mouth, and depress the canister as you inhale deeply. Hold your breath for a few seconds and exhale. Wait at least 1 minute before the next dose. Gargle and rinse your mouth after each dose to prevent yeast infections.

If you're using the *nasal inhaler,* shake the canister. Then blow your nose to clear it. Tilt your head slightly forward and insert the nozzle into one nostril so it points away from the middle of your nose. Hold your nostril closed, and then gently breathe in and spray. Repeat in the other nostril.

What to do if you miss a dose

If you miss a dose but remember within 1 or 2 hours, take the dose right away. If more than 2 hours has elapsed, skip the missed dose and go back to your regular dosing schedule. Don't double dose.

What to do about side effects

Tell your primary health care provider *immediately* if you have an allergic reaction, such as a rash, swelling of your face and lips, or labored breathing.

You may also have a dry cough, an irritated throat, an unpleasant taste, nasal congestion, a headache, and a nosebleed. If these side effects worsen or become bothersome, call your primary health care provider.

If you're using an oral inhaler, gargle and rinse your mouth after each use to prevent a yeast infection.

What you must know about other drugs

Before using triamcinolone, inform your primary health care provider of any nonprescription or prescription medications that you're taking. Because only small amounts of this medication reach the blood, interactions are unlikely.

Special directions

• Tell your primary health care provider if you've had a recent fungal, bacterial, or viral infection; chickenpox; glaucoma; allergies; tuberculosis; or ocular herpes infections.
• Use this medication cautiously if you've recently had nasal septal ulcers, nasal surgery, or nasal trauma
• Watch for signs of nasal or oral infections.

! *Warning:* This medication is used to prevent an acute asthma attack — it's not used to relieve one.

✔ Keep in mind

• Tell your primary health care provider if you're pregnant or breast-feeding before using this medication.

Additional instructions

_____

_____

_____

_____

Taking triazolam

Dear Patient,

Your primary health care provider has prescribed triazolam tablets to help you sleep. The label may read Halcion.

How to take triazolam
Follow your primary health care provider's instructions exactly. Don't increase your dose, even if you think your current dose isn't effective. Instead, call your primary health care provider.

Also, because triazolam can be habit-forming, don't take the medication for a longer time than your primary health care provider recommends.

What to do about side effects
This medication may make you feel tired, drowsy, or dizzy. If the symptoms are severe, or if you feel very tired or "hung over" the day after you've taken the medication, your dose may be too high. Call your primary health care provider so he can adjust your dosage.

What you must know about alcohol and other drugs
Don't drink alcoholic beverages while you're taking triazolam because you could become dangerously drowsy and overdose. For the same reason, avoid taking narcotic medications unless told otherwise by your primary health care provider.

Inform your primary health care provider if you're taking cimetidine (Tagamet) or erythromycin (E-Mycin). Either of these medications could cause triazolam to stay in your bloodstream for a prolonged period of time.

Also tell your primary health care provider if you're taking zidovudine (also called AZT). Triazolam could cause your body to absorb a greater amount of zidovudine.

Therefore, the dosage may need to be decreased.

Special directions
• Triazolam could aggravate certain medical problems. For this reason, be sure to tell your primary health care provider if you have glaucoma, a history of alcohol or medication abuse, a mental disorder, myasthenia gravis, Parkinson's disease, or kidney or liver disease.
• Because this medication may make you drowsy or light-headed, don't drive or perform any activities that require alertness until you know how you respond.
• After you stop taking triazolam, you may have difficulty sleeping for the next few nights. This is not unusual and should stop on its own.

✔ Keep in mind
• Don't take this medication if you think you might be pregnant or if you're breast-feeding.
• If you're an older adult, this medication could make you drowsy during the day, which could lead to falls.
• If you're an athlete, be aware that triazolam is banned and in some cases tested for by the U.S. Olympic Committee and the National Collegiate Athletic Association.

Additional instructions

_____
_____
_____
_____
_____
_____
_____
_____

Taking trimethobenzamide

Dear Patient,

Your primary health care provider has prescribed trimethobenzamide to help treat your nausea and vomiting. The label may read Tigan or Trimazide.

How to take trimethobenzamide

Follow your primary health care provider's instructions exactly. Don't use more of this medication, or take it more often, than your primary health care provider has ordered.

If you're using a *rectal suppository*, remove the foil wrapper and moisten the suppository with cold water. Lie down on your side and use your finger to push the suppository well up into your rectum. If the suppository is too soft to insert, place it in the refrigerator for 30 minutes, or run cold water over it before removing the wrapper. Wash your hands before and after inserting the suppository.

What to do if you miss a dose

Take the dose as soon as possible. But if it's almost time for your next dose, skip this dose and take your next dose as scheduled. Don't take two doses at once.

What to do about side effects

Call your primary health care provider *immediately* if you develop any of the following uncommon side effects:
- rash
- shakiness or tremor
- unusual tiredness
- severe or continued vomiting
- yellow eyes or skin.

This medication commonly causes drowsiness.

What you must know about alcohol and other drugs

Avoid alcohol while taking this medication because the combination may cause you to be overly drowsy. For the same reason, don't use other medications that slow the nervous system, such as sleeping pills, sedatives, tranquilizers, and cold, flu, and allergy medications.

Special directions

- Tell your primary health care provider if you've ever had an allergic reaction to this medication, to benzocaine, or to a local anesthetic. Also mention whether you have other medical problems, particularly a high fever or an intestinal infection.
- Because this medication may make you dizzy or light-headed, don't drive or perform any activities that could be dangerous if you're dizzy or not alert.

✓ Keep in mind

Warning: Don't give this medication to a child unless you know the cause of vomiting. When given to a child with a viral illness (a common cause of vomiting), this medication may lead to Reye's syndrome, a potentially fatal brain disorder.
- If you're pregnant or breast-feeding, don't take this medication without first talking with your primary health care provider.

Additional instructions

_____
_____
_____
_____
_____
_____

Taking troglitazone

Dear Patient,

Troglitazone is used to treat diabetes (high blood sugar). It helps the body's own insulin to lower blood sugar levels. The brand name for this medication is Rezulin.

How to take troglitazone

This medication is available as a tablet. Take it once a day with a meal or as directed by your primary health care provider.

What to do if you miss a dose

If you miss a dose, take it with the next meal. If it's near the time of the next dose, skip the missed dose and resume your normal dosing schedule. Don't double dose.

What to do about side effects

Tell your primary health care provider *right away* if you have pain, back pain, an infection, increased or painful urination, swelling of your feet or legs, or yellow eyes or skin.

You may also initially experience dizziness, headache, and weakness, but these effects usually go away with continued treatment.

What you must know about alcohol and other drugs

Drink alcoholic beverages in moderation, if at all. Alcohol increases your chance of feeling dizzy or light-headed while taking this medication.

Tell your primary health care provider if you're taking cholestyramine (Questran), oral contraceptives (birth control pills), and other diabetic medications (such as insulin or Glucotrol).

Special directions

● Notify your primary health care provider if you have symptoms of low blood sugar (sweating, shakiness, hunger, or a fast heart rate). Carry glucose tablets to treat symptoms of low blood sugar.
● Know the symptoms of high blood sugar (thirst, increased urination, and hunger).
● Treatment of diabetes involves diet modifications, regular exercise, and close monitoring.
● Before taking this medication, inform your primary health care provider if you have allergies or liver or heart disease.

Warning: Birth control pills may lose their effectiveness when taken along with troglitazone. Use another method of birth control.

✓ Keep in mind

● Tell your primary health care provider if you're breast-feeding or if you're pregnant or plan to become pregnant.

Additional instructions

_____
_____
_____
_____
_____
_____
_____
_____
_____
_____
_____

Taking valacyclovir

Dear Patient,

Valacyclovir is used to treat the symptoms of herpes zoster (shingles) and genital herpes. It inhibits the growth of the herpes virus. The brand name for this medication is Valtrex.

How to take valacyclovir
This medication is available as a tablet and may be taken with meals.

What to do if you miss a dose
If you miss a dose, take it as soon as you remember. If it's almost time for your next dose, skip the missed dose and go back to your regular dosing schedule. Don't double dose.

What to do about side effects
You may experience headaches, nausea, constipation, diarrhea, dizziness, or weakness. Contact your primary health care provider if these symptoms persist or become severe.

What you must know about other drugs
Tell your primary health care provider if you're taking any prescription or nonprescription medications because they might interact with valacyclovir.

Special directions
• Keep taking valacyclovir for the full course of treatment even if your symptoms improve.
• Valacyclovir works best if used within 2 days after the symptoms of shingles or genital herpes appear. Symptoms include pain, blisters, and burning.
• Valacyclovir isn't a cure for genital herpes, so take precautions so you don't transmit the infection to your sexual partner.
• Notify your primary health care provider if

you have kidney disease or have had a kidney transplant.

 Keep in mind
• Tell your primary health care provider if you're breast-feeding or if you become pregnant while taking this medication. It's not known if valacyclovir passes into breast milk.
• If you have an advanced HIV infection or have had a bone marrow or organ transplant, don't take this medication.

Additional instructions

_____
_____
_____
_____
_____
_____
_____
_____
_____
_____

Taking valproic acid

Dear Patient,

Valproic acid is used to treat your seizures. The label may read Depakene, Depakote, or Myproic Acid.

How to take valproic acid

Swallow your medication (whether in tablet or capsule form) whole, without breaking or chewing it. Take it with food or water to keep it from upsetting your stomach. Don't take it with milk.

If you're taking the *syrup* form of the medication, you may mix it with food or a beverage. However, don't mix it with a carbonated beverage, like soda. Doing so may irritate your mouth and throat.

What to do if you miss a dose

If you take one dose a day, take the missed dose as soon as possible. If you don't remember until the next day, take your next dose as scheduled.

If you take two or more doses a day, and you remember the missed dose within 6 hours, take it right away. Then equally space your remaining doses for the day. Never take two doses at once.

What to do about side effects

Call your primary health care provider *immediately* if you develop any of the following side effects:
● unusual bleeding or bruising
● extreme drowsiness, tiredness, or weakness
● loss of appetite
● continued nausea and vomiting
● yellow eyes or skin
● trembling
● fever
● visual problems.

What you must know about alcohol and other drugs

Avoid alcohol while taking this medication. Alcohol may decrease the effectiveness of the medication and cause drowsiness.

Don't take antacids or aspirin without first talking with your health care provider. If taken while you're taking valproic acid, these medications could cause undesirable side effects. Also tell him if you're taking a blood thinner, other medications to control seizures, or other medications or herbs.

Special directions

● Tell your health care provider if you have a history of liver disease; it may affect your body's ability to break down valproic acid.
● Don't drive or perform any activities that require mental alertness until you know how this medication affects you.

Warning: Don't stop taking this medication suddenly — you might have a seizure. Because valproic acid may affect how quickly your blood clots, take precautions to keep from cutting yourself. For example, use an electric razor and a soft toothbrush.

Keep in mind

● If you have diabetes, this medication may make urine tests for ketones unreliable.
● If you're pregnant or breast-feeding, don't take this medication until you talk with your primary health care provider.
● If you're an athlete, you should know that valproic acid is banned and in some cases tested for by the U.S. Olympic Committee and the National Collegiate Athletic Association.

Additional instructions

_____

_____

Taking vancomycin

Dear Patient,

Your primary health care provider has prescribed vancomycin to treat your bacterial infection. The label may read Vancocin.

How to take vancomycin
Vancomycin comes in oral liquid and injection forms. Take it only as your primary health care provider directs.

If you're taking the *oral liquid* form of the medication, use a specially marked measuring spoon to accurately measure each dose. A household teaspoon may not hold the correct amount.

If you're taking the *injection* form by mouth, dissolve the powder in each vial in 1 ounce of water. Then drink the liquid.

Continue to take this medication even after you begin to feel better. Stopping too soon allows your infection to return.

What to do if you miss a dose
Take the dose as soon as possible. However, if it's almost time for your next dose, skip the missed dose and take your next dose as scheduled. Don't double dose.

What to do about side effects
Call your primary health care provider *right away* if you develop any of the following side effects:
- ringing or buzzing in your ears
- a feeling of fullness in your ears
- a rash or itching
- difficulty breathing.

Also check with your primary health care provider if you experience nausea and vomiting after taking the medication.

What you must know about other drugs
Taking certain medications at the same time you're taking vancomycin may increase your risk for side effects. So be sure to tell your primary health care provider if you're taking any of these medications: aminoglycosides (a type of antibiotic), amphotericin B (Fungizone), cisplatin (Platinol), or pentamidine (NebuPent or Pentam 300).

If you're taking *oral* vancomycin, tell your primary health care provider if you're taking cholestyramine (Questran) or colestipol (Colestid). Both of these medications may prevent vancomycin from working properly. He may have you space the medications every 3 to 4 hours.

Special directions
- Tell your primary health care provider if you've ever had an allergic reaction to vancomycin. Also, because certain medical conditions may prevent your using this medication, tell your primary health care provider if you have a history of kidney disease, hearing loss, or an inflammatory bowel disorder.
- Check with your primary health care provider if you don't feel better in a few days or if you get worse.
- Before using new a medication, or if you develop a new medical problem while you're taking vancomycin, check with your primary health care provider.

✓ Keep in mind
- If you're pregnant or breast-feeding, check with your primary health care provider before taking vancomycin.

Additional instructions

_____
_____
_____
_____
_____

Taking venlafaxine

Dear Patient,

Your primary health care provider has prescribed venlafaxine for your depression. This medication increases the chemicals in the brain that are associated with improvement of depression. The brand name is Effexor.

How to take venlafaxine

This medication is available as a tablet. Take it with food to avoid stomach upset.

What to do if you miss a dose

If you miss a dose, take it as soon as your remember. If it's within 2 hours of your next dose, skip the missed dose and resume your regular dosing schedule. Don't double dose.

What to do about side effects

Tell your primary health care provider *right away* if you experience drowsiness, dizziness, nausea, sweating, loss of appetite, dry mouth, anxiety, tremor, blurred vision, high blood pressure, seizures, constipation, or changes in sexual function or desire.

You may become dizzy or light-headed when you get up quickly from a lying or sitting position. Getting up slowly may help.

What you must know about alcohol and other drugs

Avoid drinking alcoholic beverages while taking venlafaxine because the combination may make you overly drowsy. For the same reason, don't use other medications that slow down your nervous system including pain medications, many cough and cold preparations, sleeping medications, muscle relaxants, and seizure medications.

Check with your primary health care provider before taking any nonprescription medications and any of the following pre-scription medications: cimetidine (Tagamet), monoamine oxidase (MAO) inhibitors (such as Parnate and Nardil), other antidepressants, and lithium (Lithobid).

Special directions

• You may have to take venlafaxine for a month or longer to see improvement in symptoms of depression.
• Don't drive or perform any activities that require mental alertness until you know how the medication affects you.
• Tell your primary health care provider if you have high or low blood pressure, kidney or liver disease, or a history of seizures.

✔ Keep in mind

• Tell your primary health care provider if you're pregnant or breast-feeding.
• If you are an older adult, you may be more sensitive to the effects of this medication.

Additional instructions

_____
_____
_____
_____
_____
_____
_____
_____
_____
_____
_____
_____

Taking verapamil

Dear Patient,

Your primary health care provider has prescribed verapamil tablets to treat your condition. Verapamil helps relax blood vessels, which increases the flow of blood to your heart. In turn, this helps relieve chest pain, heart irregularities, and high blood pressure. The brand names are Calan and Isoptin.

How to take verapamil

Take verapamil only as your primary health care provider directs. If you're taking an extended-release tablet, swallow it whole, without crushing or chewing it.

Take verapamil on an empty stomach. Taking extended-release tablets with food may decrease your body's ability to absorb the medication.

Take your medication even if you feel well. Stopping suddenly could cause your condition to worsen.

What to do if you miss a dose

Take the dose as soon as possible. However, if it's almost time for your next dose, skip the missed dose and take your next dose as scheduled.

What to do about side effects

Call your primary health care provider *immediately* if you develop any of the side effects listed here:
• breathing difficulty, coughing, or wheezing
• irregular or fast, pounding heartbeat
• swelling of ankles, feet, or lower legs.

Also notify your primary health care provider if you become constipated or faint, feel unusually tired, or continue to have chest pain.

What you must know about other drugs

Some medications may affect how verapamil works. At the same time, verapamil may interfere with another medication's actions. Therefore, be sure to tell your primary health care provider about any medications you're taking, particularly lithium (Lithobid), heart medications, or medications for high blood pressure, seizures, tuberculosis, or glaucoma.

Special directions

• Because verapamil may cause certain medical conditions to worsen, tell your primary health care provider if you have a history of kidney or liver disease or some other heart or blood vessel disorder.
• Eat foods high in fiber and be sure to drink plenty of fluids (unless your primary health care provider tells you otherwise) to help prevent constipation.
• If fatigue is a problem, remember to allow yourself several rest periods during the day.

✓ Keep in mind

• If you're pregnant or breast-feeding, check with your primary health care provider before taking verapamil.

Additional instructions

_____

Taking zalcitabine (ddC)

Dear Patient,

Your primary health care provider has prescribed zalcitabine (ddC), which is used in the treatment of acquired immunodeficiency syndrome (AIDS). It works by inhibiting the replication of the human immunodeficiency virus (HIV). This medication won't cure or prevent HIV infection or AIDS. The brand name is Hivid.

How to take zalcitabine
This medication is available as a tablet. Take it on an empty stomach because food will decrease its absorption. Take this medication exactly as prescribed by your primary health care provider.

What to do if you miss a dose
If you miss a dose, take it as soon as you remember. If it's nearly time for your next dose, skip the missed dose and resume your regular dosing schedule. Don't double dose.

What to do about side effects
Tell your primary health care provider *immediately* if you experience numbness, tingling, burning, or pain in your hands or feet. Also report if you have abdominal pain, nausea, and vomiting.

During the first week of treatment you may experience headaches, diarrhea, rash, stomach upset, mouth sores, and fever. Tell your primary health care provider if these continue or become more severe.

This medication may also cause anemia and the need for blood transfusions.

What you must know about other drugs
Check with your primary health care provider if you're taking any of the following medications: antacids (such as Mylanta), chloramphenicol (Chloromycetin), didanosine (Videx), cisplatin (Platinol), foscarnet (Foscavir), valproic acid (Depakene), Bactrim, Septra, disulfiram (Antabuse), glutethimide, gold salts (such as Myochrysine), hydralazine (Apresoline), isoniazid (Laniazid), metronidazole (Flagyl), nitrofurantoin (Macrodantin), phenytoin (Dilantin), ribavirin (Virazole), or vincristine (Navelbine). Also check before starting any prescription or nonprescription medications.

Special directions
• Your primary health care provider may order blood tests to monitor you for anemia.
• Keep taking zalcitabine for the full course of treatment, even if you begin to feel better.
• Tell your primary health care provider if you have other medical problems, especially liver disease or alcoholism. Zalcitabine may increase liver damage.

✔ Keep in mind
• Don't breast-feed when taking zalcitabine. Also tell your primary health care provider if you're pregnant or trying to become pregnant before taking this medication.

Additional instructions
_____
_____
_____
_____
_____
_____
_____
_____
_____
_____
_____

Taking zidovudine

Dear Patient,

Your primary health care provider has prescribed zidovudine, also known as AZT or Retrovir. Zidovudine helps slow the progress of the human immunodeficiency virus (HIV). In turn, this helps slow HIV's destruction of the immune system. Zidovudine doesn't cure HIV infection or acquired immunodeficiency syndrome (AIDS). It also won't keep you from spreading HIV to others.

How to take zidovudine

Take zidovudine only as your primary health care provider directs. Don't take more or less of it, and don't take it more often or longer than he directs. Take it for the full length of treatment, even if you begin to feel better. Don't stop taking it without checking with your health care provider first.

You need to take the medication as prescribed, without missing doses, even during the night. Take your medication at the same times every day.

If you're taking the *syrup* form of the medication, measure your dose in a specially marked spoon. A household teaspoon may not hold the correct amount.

What to do if you miss a dose

Take the missed dose as soon as possible. But if it's almost time for your next dose, skip the missed dose and take your next dose as scheduled. Don't double dose.

What to do about side effects

! *Warning:* Zidovudine may cause some serious side effects, including bone marrow problems. Call your primary health care provider *right away* if you develop fever, chills, sore throat, pale skin, unusual tiredness or weakness, or unusual bleeding or bruising.

Also let your health care provider know if you develop a severe headache, muscle soreness, nausea, or trouble sleeping.

What you must know about other drugs

Taking certain medications while you're taking zidovudine may increase your risk for dangerous side effects. That's why you need to tell your primary health care provider of all other medications you're taking — prescription and nonprescription.

Special directions

• Because other medical problems may affect the use of zidovudine, tell your primary health care provider if you have anemia, other blood disorders, or liver disease.
• Remember to keep follow-up appointments with your primary health care provider. You need to have your blood checked frequently — at least every 2 weeks — to make sure that the medication is working properly and that you're not developing any dangerous side effects.
• If the medication makes you dizzy, don't drive or perform any activities that could be dangerous if you're not fully alert.
• Because zidovudine may cause blood problems and slow healing, be careful not to injure yourself. Use a soft toothbrush, and use toothpicks or dental floss cautiously so you don't injure your gums.

✔ Keep in mind

• If you become pregnant, let your primary health care provider know at once. If you're breast-feeding, you should stop while you're taking the medication.

Additional instructions

_____

_____

Taking zolpidem

Dear Patient,

Your primary health care provider has prescribed zolpidem because of insomnia (trouble sleeping). The brand name for this medication is Ambien.

How to take zolpidem
This medication is available as a tablet. Take it just before bedtime when you're ready to sleep. Zolpidem may be taken with or without food, but it works faster on an empty stomach.

What to do if you miss a dose
If you miss a dose, skip the missed dose and go back to your regular schedule. Don't take this medication the next morning or any time other than bedtime, or you'll become drowsy. Don't double dose.

What to do about side effects
Tell your primary health care provider if you experience daytime drowsiness or if you're dizzy, light-headed, or less alert than normal. He may want to change your dosage. Other effects include double vision, memory loss, behavior changes, nausea, vomiting, labored breathing, and a slow heart rate. Call your primary health care provider if these continue or become more severe.

What you must know about alcohol and other drugs
Don't drink alcoholic beverages while taking zolpidem because the combination may make you overly drowsy. For the same reason, don't use other medications that slow down your nervous system, including pain medication, many cough and cold preparations, sleeping medications, muscle relaxants, and seizure medications.

Special directions
- You may have trouble sleeping for a few nights after stopping zolpidem.
- Don't use this medication more often or for a longer time than prescribed by your primary health care provider.
- Note your reaction to zolpidem before driving or performing any activity that requires mental alertness.
- Zolpidem may become habit forming if it's used for a long time.
- Keep this medication out of the reach of children.

! *Warning:* If you're taking this medication for a long time, don't stop taking it abruptly without first checking with your primary health care provider.

✔ Keep in mind
- Tell your primary health care provider if you're breast-feeding or if you become pregnant while taking this medication.
- If you are an older adult, you may be more sensitive to this medication.

Additional instructions

_____
_____
_____
_____
_____
_____
_____
_____
_____
_____
_____
_____
_____

Supportive measures

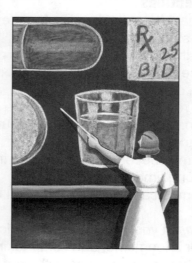

Medication therapy often requires measures to support and enhance a medication's effectiveness. Your patient may have to adjust his diet, learn to take his blood pressure, or remember to take his medication. Changes like these require patient teaching; the aids in this section can help.

Divided into four groups, these supportive teaching aids address comfort and dietary measures, health monitoring, and health promotion. Step-by-step organization, illustrations, large print, and lists make these teaching aids easy to read and understand.

The teaching aids in *Comfort measures* help your patient to learn relaxation techniques to relieve pain and reduce stress. Also included are guidelines on controlling chemotherapy's side effects, selecting cold medications, and using pain relief equipment at home.

Because patients may mistakenly rely on medications alone to resolve their health problems, they may not realize the role of diet in their treatment. Medications may cause vitamin and mineral deficiencies or other side effects, such as constipation, that require changes in the patient's diet. *Dietary measures* includes teaching aids that cover common diet changes, such as reducing salt and cholesterol or adding fiber, calories, or other nutrients.

The tips and memory aids suggested in *Health monitoring* may help the patient who has a hard time remembering to take his medication. His medication regimen may require that he check his temperature, pulse rate, blood pressure, and prothrombin time. These teaching aids spell out the proper procedures for your patient in simple terms.

By making your patient aware of *Health promotion* issues, such as infection control, you can reduce the risk of reinfection or contagion. Included in this section are aids telling your patient about medication-induced photosensitivity and alerting him to avoid allergy triggers.

Performing relaxation breathing

Dear Patient,

Relaxation breathing can help you cope with stress or pain. You can use it anywhere and at any time. You can also combine it with other techniques to help control pain. Try to practice these simple breathing techniques daily. Now, get yourself comfortable and begin.

1 Close your eyes. Inhale slowly and deeply through your nose as you count silently: "In, 2, 3, 4." Notice how your stomach expands first, then your rib cage, and finally your upper chest.

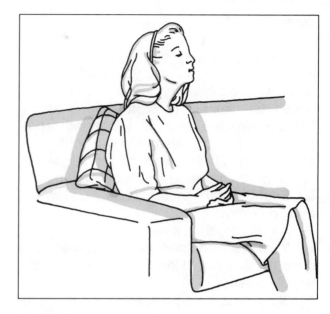

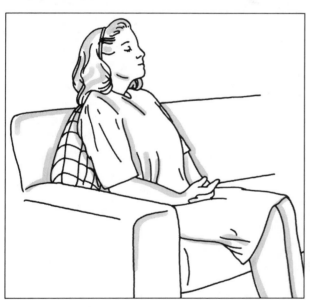

Now exhale slowly through your mouth as you count silently: "Out, 2, 3, 4, 5, 6." Pretend you're breathing out through a straw to lengthen exhalation. Let your shoulders drop slightly as your upper chest, rib cage, and stomach gently deflate. Repeat this exercise four or five times.

2 Inhale for 4 seconds. Hold your breath for the count of 4, but don't strain. Then exhale through your mouth for 6 to 8 seconds. Practice this exercise four or five times.

A few tips

Use these breathing exercises for as long as you need to during painful periods. You may vary the rhythm, but always exhale for 2 to 4 seconds longer than you inhale.

If you feel light-headed or your fingers tingle, you may be breathing too deeply or too fast. Reduce the depth and speed of your breathing, or breathe into a paper bag until the feeling goes away.

Additional instructions

_____
_____
_____
_____
_____
_____
_____
_____
_____
_____
_____

Using imagination to relieve pain

Dear Patient,

With guided imagery, you learn to create mental images that make your pain less intense. Guided imagery affects how your body perceives and responds to pain and helps control the message your mind sends to your body. It can also help you control stress. Here's how to use this technique.

1 Begin by focusing on your breathing. Spend a few minutes breathing slowly and smoothly.

2 As you breathe, slowly count backward from 5, sinking deeper and deeper into a state of relaxation. Repeat to yourself, "I feel deeply relaxed."

3 Next, imagine a pleasant place that you can return to in your mind whenever you need relaxation or pain relief. For example, imagine a warm, quiet beach or a tranquil, fragrant garden. Close your eyes to help you concentrate.

4 Use all your senses — sight, touch, smell, hearing, and taste — to experience the place you've imagined. Remain there for at least 5 minutes, and let your imagination run free. Name the colors you see, trace the shapes of the flowers blooming in the garden, breathe in the sweet fragrance of the blossoms, listen to the birds chirping, and feel the sun warm your skin.

5 When your pain is relieved and you feel relaxed, slowly let the image fade from the center of your attention. Focus again on your breathing. Stay relaxed, and when you're ready, count slowly to 5 and open your eyes.

Additional instructions

_____
_____
_____
_____
_____
_____
_____
_____
_____
_____
_____

Relaxing your muscles

Dear Patient,

No matter where you are, you can relax your muscles with a technique called progressive muscle relaxation. This technique helps to relieve the muscle tension that accompanies pain. By learning to tense and relax your muscles one by one, you'll find you can relax your entire body. Here's how.

1 Get comfortable, and close your eyes. Starting at the top of your body, tense your forehead and face. Do you notice how these muscles feel tight and strained? Hold this tension for 5 to 10 seconds.

2 Next, relax your forehead and face. Do you notice the relief you feel? Hold and enjoy this relaxation for 10 to 15 seconds.

3 Now work down your body toward your feet. First, tense and relax your jaw muscles. Proceed to the muscles in each shoulder, arm, and hand, then to your stomach, buttocks, each thigh, each lower leg, and finally to each ankle and foot.

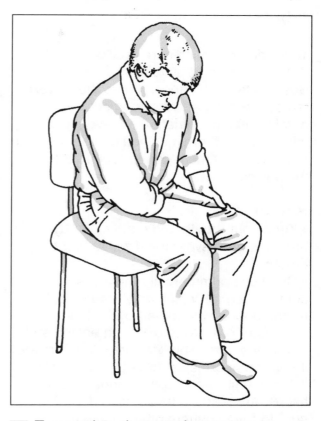

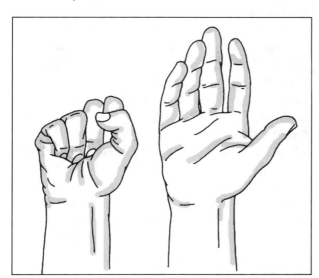

If you have trouble relaxing some muscles, or if the tension brings on pain, try gently massaging that body part until the muscles relax and feel comfortable.

4 To complete the exercise, open your eyes, stretch, and relax your entire body. Take a few deep breaths as if you're waking up from a deep sleep. Don't engage in any activity until you're fully alert.

Additional instructions

_____

_____

_____

_____

_____

_____

_____

_____

_____

Controlling side effects of chemotherapy

Dear Patient,

Your primary health care provider has ordered chemotherapy to treat your cancer. Besides treating cancer, these therapies often cause unpleasant side effects. Fortunately, you can sometimes prevent or minimize them. Other times you can do things to make yourself more comfortable. Just follow the advice below.

Mouth sores
• Keep your mouth and teeth clean by brushing after every meal with a soft toothbrush.
• Don't use commercial mouthwashes that contain alcohol, which may irritate your mouth during chemotherapy. Instead, rinse with water or water mixed with baking soda or use a suspension of sucralfate (Carafate) if your primary health care provider orders it. Floss daily, and apply fluoride if your dentist recommends it. If you have dentures, be sure to remove them often for cleaning.
• Until your mouth sores heal, avoid foods that are difficult to chew (such as apples) or irritating to your mouth (such as acidic citrus juices). Also avoid drinking alcohol, smoking, and eating extremely hot or spicy foods.
• Eat soft, bland foods, such as eggs and oatmeal, and soothing foods, such as popsicles. Your primary health care provider might also prescribe medication for mouth sores.

Dry mouth
• Frequently sip cool liquids and suck on ice chips or sugarless candy.
• Ask your primary health care provider about artificial saliva. Use water, juices, sauces, and dressings to soften your food and make it easier to swallow. Don't smoke or drink alcohol, which can further dry your mouth.

Nausea and vomiting
• Before a chemotherapy treatment, try eating a light, bland snack, such as toast or crackers. Or don't eat anything—some patients find that fasting controls nausea better.
• Keep unpleasant odors out of your dining area. Avoid strong-smelling foods. Also brush your teeth before eating to refresh your mouth.
• Eat small, frequent meals and avoid lying down for 2 hours after you eat. Try small amounts of clear, unsweetened liquids, such as apple juice, and then progress to crackers or dry toast. Stay away from sweets and fried or other high-fat foods. It's best to stay with bland foods.
• Take antiemetic drugs, as your primary health care provider orders. Be sure to notify him if vomiting is severe or lasts longer than 24 hours or if you urinate less, feel weak, or have a dry mouth.

Diarrhea
• Stick with low-fiber foods, such as bananas, rice, applesauce, toast, or mashed potatoes. Stay away from high-fiber foods, such as raw vegetables and fruits and whole-grain breads. Also avoid milk products and fruit juices. Cabbage, coffee, beans, and sweets can increase stomach cramps.
• Because potassium may be lost when you have diarrhea, eat high-potassium foods, such as bananas and potatoes. Check with your primary health care provider to see if you need a potassium supplement.
• After a bowel movement, clean your anal area gently and apply petroleum jelly (Vaseline) to prevent soreness.
• Ask your primary health care provider about antidiarrheal medications. Notify him if your diarrhea doesn't stop or if you urinate less, have a dry mouth, or feel weak.

(continued)

Controlling side effects of chemotherapy *(continued)*

Constipation
• Eat high-fiber foods unless your primary health care provider tells you otherwise. They include raw fruits and vegetables (with skins on, washed well), whole-grain breads and cereals, and beans. If you're not used to eating high-fiber foods, start gradually to let your body get accustomed to the change — or else you could develop diarrhea.
• Drink plenty of liquids — unless your primary health care provider tells you not to.
• If changing your diet doesn't help, ask your primary health care provider about stool softeners or laxatives. Check with your primary health care provider before using enemas.

Heartburn
• Avoid spicy foods, alcohol, and smoking. Eat small, frequent meals.
• After eating, don't lie down right away. Avoid bending or stooping.
• Take oral medications with a glass of milk or a snack.
• Use antacids, as your primary health care provider orders.

Muscle aches or pain, weakness, numbness, or tingling
• Take acetaminophen (Tylenol). Or ask your primary health care provider for acetaminophen with codeine.
• Apply heat where it hurts or feels numb.

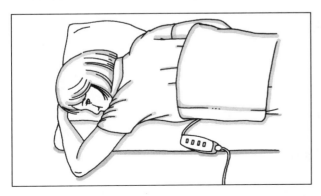

• Be sure to rest. Also, avoid activities that aggravate your symptoms.
• If symptoms don't go away and pain focuses on one area, notify your primary health care provider.

Hair loss
• Wash your hair gently. Use a mild shampoo and avoid frequent brushing or combing.
• Get a short haircut to make thinning hair less noticeable.
• Consider wearing a wig or toupee during therapy. Buy one before chemotherapy begins. Or use a hat, scarf, or turban to cover your head during therapy.

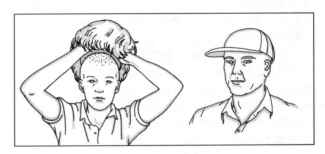

Skin problems
• For sensitive or dry skin, ask your primary health care provider or nurse to recommend a lotion.

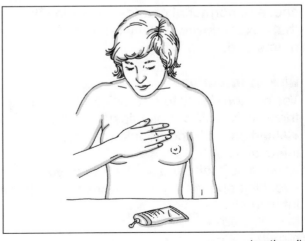

(continued)

Controlling side effects of chemotherapy *(continued)*

• Use cornstarch to absorb moisture, and avoid tight clothing over the treatment area. Be sure to report any blisters or cracked skin to your primary health care provider.
• Stay out of the sun during the course of therapy. You may even have to avoid the sun for several months afterward, so check with your primary health care provider, especially if you're planning a vacation to a sunny area. When you *can* go out in the sun again, wear light clothes over the treated area, and wear a hat, too. Cover all exposed skin with a good sunblock lotion (skin protection factor [SPF] 15 or above).

Tiredness
• Limit activities, especially sports.
• Get more sleep.
• Try to reduce your work hours until the end of treatments. Discuss your therapy schedule with your employer.
• If at all possible, schedule chemotherapy treatments at your convenience.
• Ask for help from family and friends, whether it's pitching in with daily chores or driving you to the hospital. Most people are glad to help out—they just need to be asked.
• If you lose interest in sex during treatments, either because you're too tired or because of hormonal changes, bear in mind that sexual desire usually returns after treatments end.

Risk of infection
You're more likely to get an infection during therapy, so follow these tips:
• Avoid crowds and people with colds and infections.
• Use a soft toothbrush. It will help you avoid injuring your gums—a frequent site of infection.

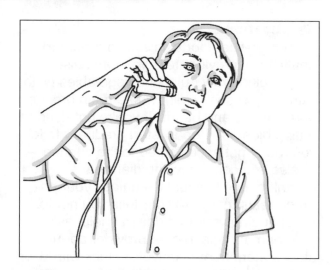

• Use an electric shaver instead of a razor.
• Tell your primary health care provider if you have a fever, chills, a tendency to bruise easily, or any unusual bleeding.

Additional instructions

_____
_____
_____
_____
_____
_____
_____
_____
_____
_____
_____
_____

Learning about TENS

Dear Patient,

Your primary health care provider has ordered transcutaneous electrical nerve stimulation (also called TENS) to help relieve your pain.

How TENS works

A small, battery-operated device sends safe electrical signals through wires and into your body by way of electrodes, which you attach to your skin.

Where to place the electrodes

Your TENS therapist will show you where to attach the electrodes. Ask him to label the sites with a marker. If necessary, use a mirror to help you see them. Ask a friend or a family member to note the sites, too. That way he can give you reassurance if you feel nervous the first few times you use the TENS unit. Or if needed, he can help you place the electrodes another time.

If your electrodes require conductive jelly, spread it in a thin layer across each electrode before applying the electrode.

Placing your electrodes on the wrong sites probably won't harm you, but avoid placing them on your belly if you're pregnant, on the sides of the neck, or on the voice box area.

Using TENS

The knobs on your unit are adjustable:
• Set the AMP/A at _____.
• Set the rate at _____.
• Set the pulse-width at _____.
• Turn your TENS unit *on* for _____ minutes and *off* for _____ minutes throughout the day.

You should feel a pleasant sensation while the machine is working. If you develop muscle spasms, contact the TENS therapist. The AMP may be set too high, or you

may have placed the electrodes in the wrong places.

If your pain is increasing, follow the directions your TENS therapist gave you to change the settings on your TENS unit.

Safety tips

Follow your therapist's instructions carefully for the amount of time you should leave your TENS unit on. Don't get into water with the unit on, and don't sleep with it on.

Skin care

Take good care of your skin. Prevent local skin irritation — redness and rash — by cleaning your skin before attaching the electrodes. Watch for signs of irritation.

If your skin becomes irritated, don't place electrodes on those areas. Keep the skin clean and dry until it heals. If it's still irritated after a week, contact your primary health care provider.

If you repeatedly develop local skin irritation from the electrodes, contact your TENS therapist to discuss an alternative wearing schedule or another type of electrode.

Caring for the TENS unit

Clean your TENS unit weekly by lightly wiping it with rubbing alcohol.

Additional instructions

_____
_____
_____
_____
_____
_____
_____
_____

Selecting cold remedies

Dear Patient,

The only real cure for a cold is time. After 7 to 10 days, a cold and its symptoms have usually run their course. But during this period, a cold can make you feel miserable. Cold remedies offer temporary relief from aches, sniffles, and sneezes. Learn about ingredients. Then pick your product carefully and use it as directed.

Safety first

You want to avoid undesirable side effects from any cold remedy, so take only one cold remedy at a time. Taking more than one could cause an overdose if the products contain the same ingredients. Also, don't take both a cold remedy and a prescription medication without asking your primary health care provider or pharmacist if it's safe to combine them.

Pain relievers

Most cold remedies contain pain relievers, such as aspirin or acetaminophen (Tylenol), to decrease fever, muscle soreness, and headaches. Avoid taking these medications if you're taking painkillers for another condition.

Antihistamines

These medications have a drying effect on your body's tissues. That's why they relieve a runny nose and watery eyes. But most of them also make you sleepy. If you take them, avoid activities that require alertness, such as driving or using power tools. Check the labels of any medications for insomnia or diarrhea. They may contain antihistamines, too. Taking both remedies increases your chances for such side effects as constipation, urine retention, dry mouth, and blurred vision.

Decongestants

By narrowing the blood vessels in your nose, decongestants reduce stuffiness. If you use a decongestant, take only the amount directed because it can raise your blood pressure. Check the label for *phenylpropanolamine,* a stimulant and diet pill ingredient, which can produce unwanted side effects.

Consider using decongestant nasal sprays or drops. They're safer than liquids or tablets because little of the medication enters your bloodstream when applied directly into your nose. Don't overuse the spray, though. If you do, stuffiness may continue after your cold goes away.

Cough medications

These products may contain a cough suppressant, an expectorant, or both. Use suppressants if you have a dry hacking cough. Don't use them if your cough brings up mucus. A "wet" cough helps clear your breathing passages.

Expectorants loosen mucus to produce a wet cough. Drink plenty of fluids to make your mucus easier to expel.

Other ingredients

Many liquid medications contain alcohol to dissolve the other ingredients and caffeine to neutralize the effects of alcohol or antihistamines. Avoid these medications if you can't tolerate them.

Additional instructions

_____
_____
_____
_____
_____

Adding fiber to your diet

Dear Patient,

Here are four easy ways to add fiber to your diet.

Eat whole-grain breads and cereals
For the first few days, eat one serving daily of whole-grain breads (1 slice), cereal (½ cup), pasta (½ cup), or brown rice (⅓ cup). Examples of whole-grain breads are whole wheat and pumpernickel. Examples of high-fiber cereals are bran or oat flakes and shredded wheat. Gradually increase to four or more servings daily.

Eat fresh fruits and vegetables
Begin by eating one serving daily of raw or cooked, unpeeled fruit (one medium-size piece; ½ cup cooked) or unpeeled vegetables (½ cup cooked; 1 cup raw). Gradually increase to four servings daily. Examples of high-fiber fruits include apples, oranges, and peaches. Some high-fiber vegetables are carrots, corn, and peas.

Eat dried peas and beans
Begin by eating one serving (⅓ cup) a week. Increase to at least two to three servings a week.

Eat unprocessed bran
Add bran to your food. Start with 1 teaspoon a day, and over a 3-week period work up to 2 to 3 tablespoons a day. Don't use more than this. Remember to drink at least six 8-ounce (oz) glasses of fluid a day.

A small amount of bran can be beneficial, but too much can irritate your digestive tract, cause gas, interfere with mineral absorption, and even lodge in your intestine.

Note: Crisp fresh fruits and vegetables, cooked foods with husks, and nuts must be chewed thoroughly so that large particles don't pass whole into the intestine and lodge there, causing problems.

A sample menu
Breakfast
½ grapefruit
Oatmeal with milk and raisins (add bran if desired)
Bran muffin
8 oz liquid
Lunch
Cabbage slaw
Tuna salad sandwich on whole-wheat bread
Fresh pear with skin
8 oz liquid
Dinner
Vegetable soup
Broiled fish with almond topping
Baked potato with skin
Carrots and peas
Canned crushed pineapple
8 oz liquid
Snack
Dried fruit and nut mix
8 oz liquid

Additional instructions

_____

Adding calories to your diet

Dear Patient,

Here are some tips to help add calories to your diet.

Eat high-calorie snacks
Good choices include dried fruits, such as raisins and apricots; peanut butter or cheese spread on crackers, bread, fresh fruit, or raw vegetables; milk shakes made with ice cream, cream, powdered milk, or instant breakfast powders; and breakfast bars.

Add fat and sugar to food
• Put margarine or butter on bread, rice, noodles, potatoes, and vegetables. Use mayonnaise or margarine on sandwiches.
• Add sour cream to casseroles, or serve it with potatoes, vegetables, meat, and fruit.
• Serve meat, vegetables, and casseroles with cream sauces or gravy.
• Mix extra amounts of salad dressing in salads.
• Add whipped cream to hot chocolate, fruit, and desserts.
• Top ice cream with syrup or preserves.
• Spread bread, muffins, biscuits, or crackers with jam, jelly, or honey.
• Substitute half-and-half or cream for milk in coffee or tea.
• Add cheese to scrambled eggs, sauces, vegetables, casseroles, and salads.
• Use extra eggs in sauces, casseroles, sandwich spreads, and salads. Add powdered eggs or "Eggbeaters" brand eggs to milk shakes. (Don't use raw eggs — they can cause food poisoning.)
• Sprinkle chopped or ground nuts on ice cream, yogurt, frozen yogurt, pudding, breads, and desserts. (Children under age 4 shouldn't eat whole nuts because they might choke.)

Use high-calorie supplements
If you've experienced lung damage, repeated infections, or weight loss, try adding commercial, high-protein, high-calorie supplements to your daily diet. Typical commercial supplements include Ensure, Ensure Plus, Meritene, Nu Basics, Resource, and Sustacal. Or use instant breakfast powders mixed with whole milk to get about the same number of calories and nutritional value as the supplements at half the cost.

Additional instructions

_____
_____
_____
_____
_____
_____
_____
_____
_____
_____
_____
_____

Cutting down on salt

Dear Patient,

Your primary health care provider may recommend cutting down on salt because too much salt can affect your health. Reducing your salt intake isn't hard to do. The following information and suggestions will help you get started.

Facts about salt
• Table salt is about 40% sodium.
• Americans consume about 20 times more salt than their bodies need.
• About three-fourths of the salt you consume is already in the foods you eat and drink.
• One teaspoon (tsp) of salt contains about 2 grams (2,000 milligrams [mg]) of sodium.
• You can reduce your intake to this level simply by not salting your food during cooking or before eating.

Tips for reducing salt intake
Reducing your salt intake to a teaspoon or less a day is easy if you:
• read labels on medications and foods.
• put away your salt shaker; or, if you must use salt, use "light salt" that contains half the sodium of ordinary table salt.
• buy fresh meats, fruits, and vegetables instead of canned, processed, and convenience foods.
• substitute spices and lemon juice for salt.
• watch out for sources of hidden sodium — for example, carbonated beverages, nondairy creamers, cookies, and cakes.
• avoid salty foods, such as bacon, sausage, pretzels, potato chips, mustard, pickles, and some cheeses.

Know your sodium sources
Canned, prepared, and "fast" foods are loaded with sodium; so are condiments such as ketchup. Some foods that don't taste salty contain high amounts of sodium. Consider the values below:

Food	mg sodium
1 can tomato soup	872
1 cup canned spaghetti	1,236
1 hot dog	639
1 cheeseburger	709
1 slice pepperoni pizza	817
1 tablespoon ketchup	156
1 tsp salt	1,955
1 dill pickle	928
1 cup corn flakes	256
3 ounces lean ham	1,128
2½ oz dried chipped beef	3,052

Other high-sodium sources include baking powder, baking soda, barbecue sauce, bouillon cubes, celery salt, chili sauce, cooking wine, garlic salt, onion salt, softened water, and soy sauce.

Surprisingly, many medications and other nonfood items contain sodium, such as alkalizers for indigestion, laxatives, aspirin, cough medication, mouthwash, and toothpaste.

Additional instructions

_____
_____
_____
_____
_____
_____
_____
_____
_____
_____
_____

Cutting down on cholesterol

Dear Patient,

By changing your diet, you can help lower your cholesterol level and ensure better health. You also need to reduce the amount of saturated fats you eat. This means cutting down drastically on eggs, dairy products, and fatty meats. Rely instead on poultry, fish, fruits, vegetables, and high-fiber breads.

Use this list as a basis for your new diet. If you do a lot of home baking, adapt your recipes by using modest amounts of unsaturated oils. Remember that one whole egg can be replaced with two egg whites.

Additional instructions

_____

_____

FOOD	ELIMINATE	SUBSTITUTE
Bread and cereals	Breads with whole eggs listed as a major ingredient	Oatmeal, multigrain, and brain cereal; whole-grain breads; rye bread
	Egg noodles	Pasta, rice
	Pies, cakes, doughnuts, biscuits, high-fat crackers and cookies	Angel food cake; low-fat cookies; crackers; and home-baked goods
Eggs and dairy products	Whole milk, 2% milk, imitation milk	Skim milk, 1% milk, buttermilk Low-fat/nonfat whipped cream, evaporated skim milk, light cream
	Cream, half-and-half, most nondairy creamers, whipped toppings	None
	Whole milk yogurt and cottage cheese	Nonfat or low-fat yogurt, low-fat (1% or 2%) cottage cheese
	Cheese, cream cheese, sour cream, light cream cheese, light sour cream	Cholesterol-free sour cream alternative, such as King Sour; fat-free cream cheese
	Egg yolks	Egg whites
	Ice cream	Sherbet, frozen tofu, fat-free frozen yogurt, popsicles
Fats and oils	Coconut, palm, and palm kernel oils, and any oils that have been hydrogenated or partially hydrogenated	Unsaturated vegetable oils (corn, olive, canola, safflower, sesame, soybean, and sunflower)
	Butter, lard, bacon fat	Unsaturated margarine and shortening, diet margarine
	Dressings made with egg yolks	Mayonnaise, unsaturated or low-fat salad dressings
	Chocolate	Baking cocoa
Meat, fish, and poultry	Fatty cuts of beef, lamb, or pork	Lean cuts of beef, lamb, or pork
	Organ meats, spare ribs, cold cuts, sausage, hot dogs, bacon	Poultry
	Sardines, roe	Sole, salmon, mackerel

Learning about potassium-rich foods

Dear Patient,

If you're taking medication that decreases the level of potassium in your body, your primary health care provider may recommend adding potassium to your diet.

How much potassium do you need?

Primary health care providers recommend 300 to 400 milligrams (mg) of potassium daily. Not enough potassium can cause leg cramps, weakness, paralysis, and spasms. Too much can cause heart problems and fatigue.

The chart below lists potassium-rich foods along with their potassium content (the number of milligrams in a 3½-ounce serving). Because some of these foods are also high in calories, check with your primary health care provider or dietitian if you're on a weight-reduction diet.

Additional instructions

_____
_____
_____
_____

POTASSIUM CONTENT OF COMMON FOODS

Meats	mg
Beef	370
Chicken	411
Lamb	290
Liver	380
Pork	326
Turkey	411
Veal	50

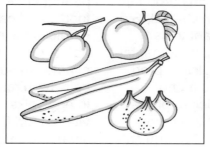

Fish	mg
Bass	256
Flounder	342
Haddock	348
Halibut	525
Oysters	203
Perch	284
Salmon	421
Sardines, canned	590
Scallops	476
Tuna	301

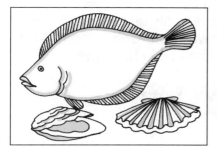

Fruits	mg
Apricots	281
Bananas	370
Dates	648
Figs	152
Nectarines	294
Oranges	200
Peaches	202
Plums	299
Prunes	262
Raisins	355

Vegetables	mg
Asparagus	238
Brussels sprouts	295
Cabbage	233
Carrots	341
Endive	294
Lima beans	394
Peppers	213

	mg
Potatoes	407
Radishes	322
Spinach	324
Sweet potatoes	300

Juices	mg
Orange, fresh	200
reconstituted	186
Tomato	227

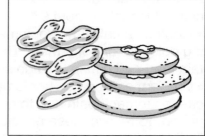

Other foods	mg
Gingersnap cookies	462
Graham crackers	384
Oatmeal cookies with raisins	370
Ice milk	195
Milk, dry (nonfat solids)	1,745
Molasses (light)	917
Peanuts	674
Peanut butter	670

Choosing a calcium supplement

Dear Patient,

Your body needs calcium to keep your bones and teeth strong, to prevent excessive bleeding, and to keep your muscles, brain, and nerves functioning well. If your primary health care provider recommends a nonprescription calcium supplement for you, here are some guidelines you need to know.

Choosing a supplement

• Read the bottle label to learn how much *elemental calcium* the supplement contains. Elemental calcium is the amount that's actually used by your body. Different supplements contain different amounts of elemental calcium. For example, calcium carbonate products, such as Caltrate 600, Os-Cal, Bio-Cal, oyster shell calcium, and antacids (such as Tums), contain the most elemental calcium — about 40%. Other calcium products contain less: dibasic calcium phosphate (about 36%), tribasic calcium phosphate (about 29%), calcium citrate (about 24%), calcium lactate (about 13%), and calcium gluconate (about 9%).

• Don't take calcium supplements containing dolomite or bone meal. They may contain lead and cause lead poisoning.

• Calcium carbonate supplements may cause stomach pain due to gas and constipation. To relieve these effects, drink more liquids, such as juice or water, or eat more foods that are liquids at room temperature, such as ice cream, gelatin, or pudding. Eating more high-fiber foods, such as bran cereal or whole-wheat crackers, may also help. Just be sure to eat them between meals — extra fiber with meals interferes with your body's absorption of calcium.

Other calcium sources

Besides taking a calcium supplement, try to include calcium-rich foods in your daily diet.

Good sources of calcium include collards, turnip greens, broccoli, dried peas and beans, sardines, salmon, tofu, and dairy products (milk, cheese, yogurt, and ice cream).

If you have trouble digesting milk, most large grocery stores carry lactose-reduced milk or acidophilus milk. Or ask your pharmacist about products that can be added to milk to make it easier to digest.

More tips

These additional suggestions will help you get the most from the calcium you eat and take in vitamin form.

• Consume less red meat, chocolate, peanut butter, rhubarb, sweet potatoes, fatty foods, and caffeine-containing drinks.

• Calcium is most effective when your body has enough vitamin D. Spending just 15 minutes in sunshine every day will fill your daily requirement. Vitamin D is also present in egg yolks, saltwater fish, liver, and vitamin-fortified milk and cereals. Don't take vitamin D supplements unless your primary health care provider prescribes them — too much of this vitamin can be harmful.

Additional instructions

_____
_____
_____
_____
_____
_____
_____
_____
_____
_____
_____

Taking medications on schedule

Dear Patient,

Taking the right amount of medication at the right time is a crucial part of your treatment. But many people have trouble remembering their medication schedules. Use the tips below to help you recall when to perform this important task.

Premeasure your medication
Your pharmacy sells several devices or "medication planners" to help you remember to take your medication. One type separates your tablets or capsules into individual doses and is helpful if you take your medication more than once a day. These planners usually have compartments with flip-top lids labeled with the time of day — for example, breakfast, lunch, supper, and bedtime.

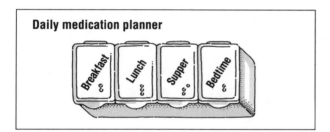

Daily medication planner

Another type of planner compartmentalizes and stores your medications for an entire week.

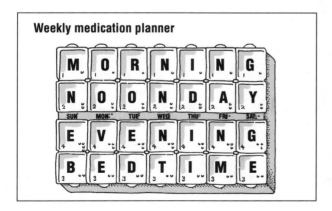

Weekly medication planner

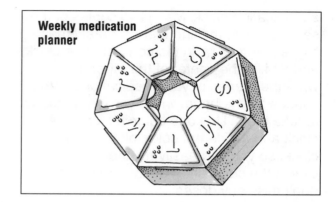

Weekly medication planner

A third type is designed to hold your entire prescription, bottle and all. Computerized numbers on top of the lid show the last time (hour and day) you opened the medication bottle.

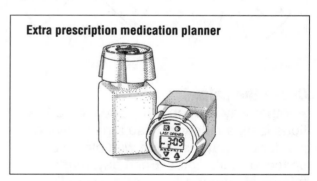

Extra prescription medication planner

If you prefer not to buy a medication planner, you can make one yourself. Here's how: Place a single medication dose in a small envelope and write the time you need to take it on the front. Do this for each dose you need to take that day.

Then put all the small envelopes into a larger one and label the larger one with the day of the week. Do this for each day of the week. Arrange the envelopes in an empty shoe box.

Make a medication clock
To remind you to take your medication at the right time, make a simple device called

(continued)

Taking medications on schedule *(continued)*

a medication clock. Make two copies of the sample clock, making them several times bigger. Write A.M. in the center of one clock, and P.M. in the center of the other. Then write the names of your medications in the spaces for the hours when you're supposed to take them. Use one color ink for the A.M. clock and a different color ink for the P.M. clock, so you can easily tell them apart. Check the clock often during the day, so you don't miss any doses.

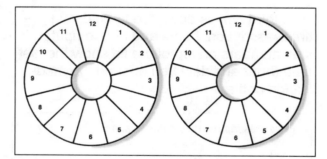

Check the calendar
Another way to keep track of your medications is on a calendar. Use a new calendar just for this purpose, one with plenty of space for daily notes. Each day, mark the names of your medications and the times you're supposed to take them. Do this for a few days at a time or for the whole month. Draw a line through the note after you take each medication. With this method, you can see at a glance if you've taken your medication.

Set an alarm or ask a friend
Last, set your wristwatch or alarm clock to ring at medication time. Or ask a relative, friend, or coworker to remind you to take your medication until you know your schedule.

Additional instructions
_____
_____
_____
_____
_____
_____
_____
_____
_____
_____
_____

Taking another person's temperature

Dear Caregiver,

A fever usually means that your body is fighting an infection or some other illness. To find out if a family member has a fever, you'll probably use a mercury or digital thermometer. You can take a temperature orally, rectally, or under the arm. A normal oral temperature is 97° to 99.5° F (36.1° to 37.5° C). Normal rectal temperature is about 1 degree higher, and normal underarm temperature is 1 to 2 degrees lower.

Follow these same steps to take your own temperature.

Using a mercury thermometer

Before using a mercury thermometer, wipe it with an alcohol-soaked gauze pad and rinse it off.

1 With your thumb and forefinger, grasp the thermometer at the end opposite the bulb. Then quickly snap your wrist to shake down the mercury.

2 Next, hold the thermometer at eye level in good light and rotate it slowly until you see the mercury line clearly. Look for a reading of 95° F (35° C) or lower. Now you're ready to take a temperature.

3 *To take an oral temperature,* place the bulb of the thermometer under the person's tongue, as far back as possible. Remind the person not to bite on the thermometer and not to keep it in place with his teeth. This can affect an accurate reading. Leave the thermometer in place for 4 to 5 minutes — the time needed to register the correct temperature. Then, remove the thermometer and read it at eye level.

To make sure you get an accurate reading, never take the person's oral temperature right after he's smoked a cigarette or sipped a hot or cold beverage. Instead, wait for 20 to 30 minutes.

4 *To take a rectal temperature,* first dip the bulb end of a *rectal* thermometer in petroleum jelly (Vaseline). Then, position the person on his side with his top leg bent. Position an infant on his stomach. Gently insert the thermometer into the rectum — about ½ inch for a baby, 1 inch for a child, and 1½ inches for an adult.

Hold the thermometer in place for 3 minutes. Next, carefully remove it and wipe it with a tissue. Read the thermometer at eye level.

5 *To take an underarm temperature,* put the thermometer's bulb in one armpit, and fold that arm across the chest. (This secures the thermometer.)

Remove the thermometer after 10 minutes, and read it at eye level.

Using a digital thermometer

If you wish, you can use a digital thermometer instead of a mercury one to take an oral temperature reading. Here's how.

1 Remove the thermometer from its protective case.

2 Next, position the thermometer tip under the tongue, as far back as possible. Leave the thermometer in place for at least 45 seconds. (Some thermometers give a series of beeps when the temperature is registered.)

3 Remove the thermometer and read the numbers on display. This is the temperature. Clean the thermometer as the manufacturer instructs, and return it to the protective case.

Additional instructions

_____

_____

_____

_____

Taking your pulse

Dear Patient,

Your primary health care provider wants you to take your pulse — the number of times your heart beats per minute. Take your pulse at rest and during exercise. By comparing these two pulse rates, your primary health care provider can evaluate how well your heart is pumping.

Taking your pulse at rest

Don't check your resting pulse right after exercising or eating a big meal. When you're ready to take you *resting* pulse rate, be sure you have a watch or a clock with a second hand. Sit quietly and relax for 2 minutes. Then place your index and middle fingers on your wrist, as shown here.

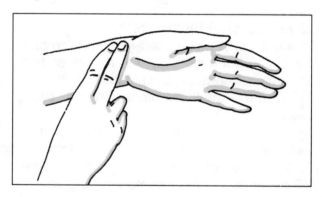

Count the pulse beats for 30 seconds and multiply by 2. (Or count for 60 seconds, but don't multiply, if your primary health care provider has so instructed because of your irregular heart rhythm.) Record this number and the date.

Taking your pulse during exercise

By taking your pulse during exercise, you can help ensure the most benefit from your exercise program.

As soon as you stop exercising, find your neck (carotid) pulse. To do this, place two or three fingers on your windpipe and move them 2 to 3 inches (5 to 8 centimeters) to the left or right. Feel for the pulse point low on your neck and don't press too hard. You can interrupt blood supply to the brain by applying pressure too high on the carotid artery. Pressing too hard may cause an irregular heartbeat.

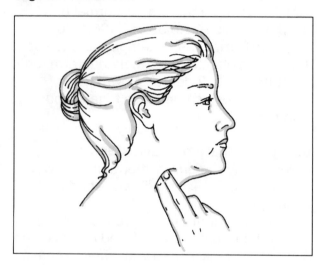

Count the beats for 6 seconds; then add a zero to that figure. This gives you a reliable estimate of your *working* heart rate for 1 minute. (Don't count your pulse for a whole minute. Because your heart rate slows dramatically when you rest, that figure won't be accurate.) Record this number and the date.

If your heart rate during exercise is 10 or more beats above your target rate, don't exercise so hard the next time. But if your working heart rate is lower than your target rate, try to exercise a little harder next time.

Additional instructions

_____

_____

_____

_____

Taking your blood pressure

Dear Patient,

To take your own blood pressure, you can use a digital blood pressure monitor. (You can also use a standard blood pressure cuff and stethoscope, but you'll probably need help from someone else to do so.)

Before you begin, review the instruction booklet that comes with the blood pressure monitor. Operating steps vary with different monitors, so be sure to follow the directions carefully.

Start by taking your blood pressure in both arms. It's common for blood pressure readings to differ by as much as 10 points from arm to arm. If the readings stay consistently similar, the primary health care provider will probably suggest that you use the arm with the higher reading. Here are some guidelines.

1 Sit in a comfortable position and relax for about 2 minutes. Rest your arm on a table so it's level with your heart. (Use the same arm in the same position each time you take your blood pressure.)

2 Wrap the cuff securely around your upper arm just above the elbow. Make sure that you can slide only two fingers between the cuff and your arm. Next, turn on the monitor.

3 Inflate the cuff, as the instruction booklet directs. When the digital scale reads 160, stop inflating. The numbers on the scale will start changing rapidly. When they stop changing, your blood pressure reading will appear on the scale.

4 Record this blood pressure reading, with the date and time. Then deflate and remove the cuff and turn off the machine.

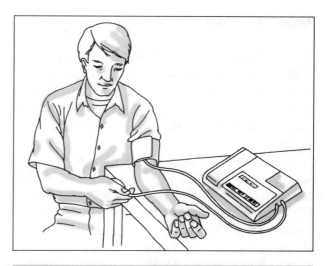

Additional instructions

_____

_____

_____

_____

_____

_____

_____

_____

_____

_____

_____

Taking another person's blood pressure

Dear Caregiver,

You can use a standard blood pressure cuff and stethoscope to take the blood pressure of the person in your care. If you're using an aneroid model, you may need to have it calibrated every 6 months. Just follow these steps.

1 Ask the person to sit comfortably and relax for about 2 minutes. Tell him to rest his arm on a table so it's level with his heart. (Use the same arm in the same position each time you take his blood pressure.) While the person relaxes, hang the stethoscope around your neck.

2 Push up the person's sleeve, and wrap the cuff around his upper arm (just above the elbow) so you can slide only two fingers between cuff and arm.

3 Then, using your middle and index fingers, feel for a pulse in the wrist near the person's thumb.

When you find this pulse, turn the bulb's screw counterclockwise to close it; then squeeze the bulb rapidly to inflate the cuff. Note the reading on the gauge when you can no longer feel his pulse. (This reading, called the *palpatory pressure,* is your guideline for inflating the cuff.) Deflate the cuff by loosening the knob on the bulb.

4 Place the stethoscope's earpieces in your ears. Then place the stethoscope's diaphragm (the disk portion) over the brachial pulse, in the crook of the person's arm.

5 Inflate the cuff 30 points higher than the palpatory pressure (the reading you obtained in step 3). Then loosen the bulb's screw to allow air to escape from the cuff. Listen for the first beating sound. When you hear it, note and record the number on the gauge: This is the *systolic* pressure (the top number of a blood pressure reading).

Slowly continue to deflate the cuff. When you hear the beating stop, note and record the number on the gauge: this is the *diastolic* pressure (the bottom number of a blood pressure reading). Now, deflate and remove the cuff. Record the blood pressure reading, date, and time.

Additional instructions

_____

_____

_____

_____

_____

_____

_____

_____

_____

_____

_____

Checking your PT and INR at home

Dear Patient,

While you're on warfarin (Coumadin) therapy, it's essential to periodically test the thinness of your blood. If your blood is too thin, you may bleed easily. If it's too thick, you may be at risk for blood clots in your legs, lungs, or brain.

To reduce the visits to your primary health care provider, you can use a machine to test your blood at home. This machine measures your prothrombin time (PT) — the speed at which your blood clots — and your international normalized ratio (INR). Together, these measurements show the clotting activity of your blood and help your health care provider evaluate the effectiveness of your drug therapy.

Follow these steps to perform the test.

Getting ready
Follow the instructions included with your machine. First, gather the necessary equipment:
- a mechanical device that makes the incision and collects the blood
- a cuvette
- an alcohol pad
- gauze
- the machine.

1 Turn on the machine, and follow the operating instructions provided with it.

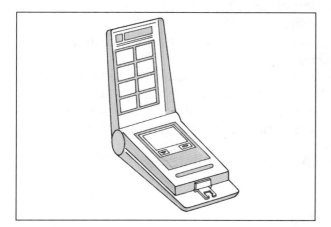

2 While the machine is warming up, wash and dry your hands thoroughly. Choose which fingertip you want to pierce (use your middle or ring finger). To enhance blood flow, hold the finger under warm water for a minute or two. Dry the finger.

3 Hold the finger you plan to pierce below your heart, and use the thumb on the opposite hand to milk the blood toward the fingertip. Then clean the fingertip with an alcohol pad and dry it with gauze.

4 When the machine is ready, place the mechanical device used to make the incision firmly against the side of your finger. Make the incision according to the manufacturer's instructions. Wipe away the first bit of blood that appears.

5 Gently massage from the base of your finger to the tip to form a large drop of blood. Let the drop run into the collection cup. Be sure to add enough blood to reach the fill line.

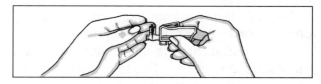

Testing your blood
1 Following the manufacturer's instructions, attach the sample cup or mechanical device to the machine.

2 Press the start button.

3 The machine will display your INR and PT in a few minutes. Call your primary health care provider if the results are higher or lower than those he says are right for you.

Additional instructions
_____
_____
_____

Avoiding infection

Dear Patient,

As your primary health care provider has explained, you have an increased risk of getting an infection. Here are some simple steps you can take to protect yourself.

Follow your primary health care provider's directions

• Take all medications exactly as prescribed. Don't stop taking your medication unless directed by your primary health care provider.
• Keep all medical appointments so that your primary health care provider can monitor your progress and the medication's effects.
• If you're receiving a medication that puts you at risk for infection, be sure to tell your dentist or other doctors.

Minimize your exposure to infection

• Avoid crowds and people who have colds, flu, chickenpox, shingles, or other contagious illnesses.
• Don't receive any immunizations without checking with your primary health care provider, especially live-virus vaccines, such as poliovirus vaccines. These contain weakened but living viruses that can cause illness in anyone who's taking a medication that puts him at risk for infection. Avoid contact with anyone who has recently been vaccinated.
• Practice good personal hygiene, especially hand washing.
• Before preparing food, wash your hands thoroughly. To avoid ingesting harmful organisms, thoroughly wash and cook all food before you eat it.
• Practice good oral hygiene.
• Don't use commercial mouthwashes because their high alcohol and sugar content may irritate your mouth and provide a medium for bacterial growth.
• Don't use unprescribed intravenous drugs — or at least don't share needles.

• If you travel to foreign countries, consider drinking only bottled or boiled water and avoiding raw vegetables and fruits to prevent a possible intestinal infection.
• Wear a mask and gloves to clean bird cages, fish tanks, or cat litter boxes.
• Keep rooms clean and well ventilated. Keep air conditioners and humidifiers cleaned and repaired so they don't harbor infectious organisms.

More prevention tips

• Get adequate sleep at night, and rest often during the day.
• Eat small, frequent meals, even if you've lost your appetite.

Recognize symptoms of infection

Contact your primary health care provider immediately or seek medical treatment for:
• persistent fever or nighttime sweating not related to a cold or the flu
• profound, persistent fatigue unrelieved by rest and not related to increased physical activity, longer work schedules, medication use, or a psychological disorder
• loss of appetite and weight loss
• open sores or ulcerations
• dry, persistent, unproductive cough
• persistent, unexplained diarrhea
• a white coating or spots on your tongue or throat, possibly with soreness, burning, or difficulty swallowing
• blurred vision or persistent, severe headaches
• confusion, depression, uncontrolled excitement, or inappropriate speech
• persistent rash or skin discoloration
• unexplained bleeding or bruising.

Additional instructions

_____

_____

Washing your hands correctly

Dear Patient,

Everyday activities, such as petting your dog or sorting money, leave unwanted germs on your hands. These germs may enter your body and cause an infection. To prevent this, wash your hands several times daily — and always before meals. Here's how.

1 Wet your hands under lots of running water. This carries away contaminants.

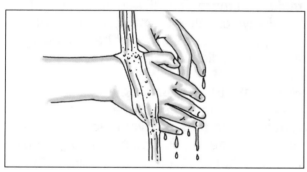

2 Lather your hands and wrists with soap (preferably liquid soap). Although soap and water don't actually kill germs, they do loosen the skin oils and deposits that harbor germs. While you're washing, give your fingernails a good scrub, too.

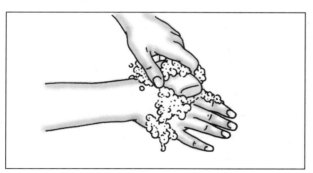

3 Now, thoroughly rinse your hands in running water. Make sure your fingers point downward. That way runoff water won't travel up your arms to bring new germs down to your hands.

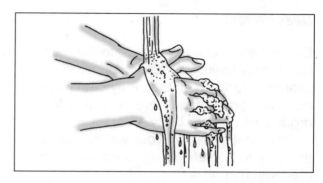

4 If you're at home, dry your hands with a clean cloth or paper towel. Don't dry off with a used towel, which may put germs right back on your hands. If you're in a public place, a hot-air hand dryer is best, but clean paper towels will do.

Help for dry hands

If your hands become dry or scratchy from frequent hand washing, soothe them with a hand lotion. Don't use strong soaps; they aren't needed for good hygiene, and they may cause drying or even allergic reactions.

Additional instructions

_____
_____
_____
_____
_____
_____
_____
_____
_____
_____
_____

Protecting your skin from photosensitivity

Dear Patient,

Exposure to the sun, or even to fluorescent lights, may make your condition worse. Excessive exposure, in fact, may cause rashes, fever, arthritis, and even damage to the organs inside your body.

You needn't spend your waking hours in the dark to be safe though. Just follow the precautions below.

Prepare for going outdoors

Wear a wide-brimmed hat or visor to shield yourself from the sun's rays. Protect your eyes by wearing sunglasses. Put on a dark, densely woven, long-sleeved shirt and trousers to filter out harmful rays.

Buy a sunscreen containing PABA (para-aminobenzoic acid) with a skin protection factor (SPF) of 15 to 45. If you're allergic to PABA, choose a PABA-free product offering equivalent sun protection.

Before you go outside (at least 30 minutes beforehand), rub the sunscreen onto unprotected parts of your body, such as your face and hands. Read the label to determine how often to reapply it. Usually, you'll reapply the sunscreen after swimming or perspiring.

Avoid strong sunlight

Try to stay indoors during the most intense hours of sunlight, from 10 a.m. to 2 p.m. The ideal time to garden, take a walk, play golf, or do any other outdoor activity is just after sunrise or just before sunset.

Remove fluorescent light

At home, replace any fluorescent fixtures or bulbs with incandescent ones. At work, though, avoiding fluorescent light may be difficult. Consider asking your supervisor about moving to a work area closer to a window, so you can use natural light. If you

have a fluorescent light above your desk, turn it off and request a lamp that uses incandescent bulbs.

Be careful with soaps and medications

Certain toiletries, including deodorant soaps, may increase your skin's sensitivity to light.

Try switching to nondeodorant or hypoallergenic soaps. Certain medications, including tetracyclines and phenothiazines, also make you more sensitive to light.

Always check with your primary health care provider or pharmacist before taking any new medication.

Recognize and report rashes

Be alert for the key sign of a photosensitivity reaction: a red rash on your face or other exposed area. If you discover a suspicious rash or other reaction to light, call your primary health care provider. Remember, prompt treatment can prevent damage to the tissues beneath your skin.

Additional instructions

_____

_____

_____

_____

_____

_____

_____

_____

_____

_____

_____

Avoiding allergy triggers

Dear Patient,

To make it easier for you to live with allergies, try to avoid allergy triggers. Here's a list of the most common triggers.

At home

- Such foods as nuts, chocolate, eggs, shellfish, and peanut butter
- Such beverages as orange juice, wine, beer, and milk
- Mold spores, pollens from flowers, trees, grasses, hay, and ragweed. If pollen is the offender, install a bedroom air conditioner with a filter, and avoid long walks when pollen counts are high.
- Dander from rabbits, cats, dogs, hamsters, gerbils, and chickens. Consider finding a new home for the family pet, if necessary.
- Feather or hair-stuffed pillows, down comforters, wool clothing, and stuffed toys. Use smooth (not fuzzy), washable blankets on your bed.
- Insect parts, such as those from dead cockroaches
- Medications such as aspirin
- Vapors from cleaning solvents, paint, paint thinners, and liquid chlorine bleach
- Fluorocarbon spray products, such as furniture polish, starch, cleaners, and room deodorizers
- Scents from spray deodorants, perfumes, hair sprays, talcum powder, and cosmetics
- Cloth-upholstered furniture, carpets, and draperies that collect dust. Hang lightweight, washable cotton or synthetic-fiber curtains, and use washable, cotton throw rugs on bare floors.
- Brooms and dusters that raise dust. Instead, clean your bedroom daily by damp dusting and damp mopping. Keep the door closed.
- Dirty filters on hot-air furnaces and air conditioners that blow dust into the air
- Dust from vacuum cleaner exhaust.

In the workplace

- Dusts, vapors, or fumes from wood products (Western red cedar, some pine and birch woods, mahogany); flour, cereals, and other grains; coffee, tea, or papain; metals (platinum, chromium, nickel sulfate, soldering fumes); and cotton, flax, and hemp
- Mold from decaying hay

Outdoors

- Cold air, hot air, or sudden temperature changes (when you go in and out of air-conditioned stores in the summer)
- Excessive humidity or dryness
- Changes in seasons
- Smog
- Automobile exhaust
- Plants (such as poison ivy and some grasses).

Anyplace

- Overexertion, which may cause wheezing
- Common cold, flu, and other viruses
- Fear, anger, frustration, laughing too hard, crying, or any emotionally upsetting situation
- Smoke from cigarettes, cigars, and pipes. Don't smoke or stay in a smoke-filled room.

Preventive measures

Remember to:
- drink fluids (six to eight glasses daily).
- take all prescribed medications exactly as directed.
- tell your primary health care provider about any and all medications you take— even nonprescription ones.
- schedule only as much activity as you can tolerate. Take frequent rests on busy days.

Additional instructions

_____

_____

_____

INDEX